Scholars from across the globe have been brought together in this thoughtfully prepared anthology to offer us the latest advances in the science and practice of coping, recovery, and healthy lifestyles. The guidance these experts impart is of immense benefit to individuals, instructors, and organizations focused on understanding and enhancing human performance.

David W. Eccles, PhD, Program Director, Graduate Programs in Sport Psychology, Florida State University, USA.

T0386451

Fostering Recovery and Well-being in a Healthy Lifestyle

This insightful book addresses recovery as a comprehensive concept for prevention of health-threats in modern societies through active lifestyles. Several areas of society are addressed, such as sports, work environments, and the military. Internationally renowned experts from different scientific disciplines present results of empirical research as well as applied intervention techniques to effectively manage stress and promote recovery in healthy lifestyles.

Recognising the systemic nature of stress and recovery is critical to designing effective interventions and policies. By promoting a balance between stress and recovery in physiological, psychological, and social terms, individuals and societies can build resilience, promote optimal well-being, and mitigate the negative effects of chronic stress. This book focuses on key research in the area of recovery and healthy living and addresses psychological, somatic, and organisational prevention strategies that foster recovery and healthy lifestyles in society. It offers an expanded understanding of recovery in the health field and applies this to different areas, such as the workplace.

Though written for the scientific community, the book will also benefit applied health scientists, instructors, and students, as well as readers interested in applying effective well-being and recovery techniques in their own lives.

Michael Kellmann is Professor of Sport Psychology at the Faculty of Sport Science at Ruhr University Bochum, Germany. He is also an Honorary Professor in the School of Human Movement and Nutrition Sciences at the University of Queensland, Australia.

Jürgen Beckmann is Professor of Sport Psychology, Emeritus of Excellence at the School of Medicine and Health of Technical University of Munich, Germany. He is currently member of the Psycho-Cardiological Consultation Group at the German Heart Centre Munich. He is also Honorary Professor in the School of Human Movement and Nutrition Sciences at the University of Queensland, Australia.

Advances in Recovery and Stress Research: Multi-Disciplinary Approaches Series

Series Editors

Michael Kellmann, Ruhr University Bochum, Germany, and The University of Queensland, Australia

Jürgen Beckmann, Technical University of Munich, Germany, and The University of Queensland, Australia

Advances in Recovery and Stress Research: Multi-Disciplinary Approaches covers a broad range of areas in which recovery plays a crucial role, providing the current status of research on recovery and stress. In particular, it aims to be unique in addressing fields in which recovery and stress play an important role, but recovery has not received adequate attention, for example, in the areas of health promotion as well as performance promotion in work settings. Another feature of the series is that it contains both up-to-date theoretical and applied perspectives from multi-disciplinary approaches.

Recovery and Well-being in Sport and Exercise
Edited by Michael Kellmann and Jürgen Beckmann

The Importance of Recovery for Physical and Mental Health
Negotiating the Effects of Underrecovery
Edited by Michael Kellmann, Sarah Jakowski and Jürgen Beckmann

Fostering Recovery and Well-being in a Healthy Lifestyle
Psychological, Somatic, and Organizational Prevention Approaches
Edited by Michael Kellmann and Jürgen Beckmann

The Recovery-Stress Questionnaires
A User Manual
Edited by Michael Kellmann and K. Wolfgang Kallus

For more information about this series, please visit: www.routledge.com/ Advances-in-Recovery-and-Stress-Research/book-series/ARSR

Fostering Recovery and Well-being in a Healthy Lifestyle

Psychological, Somatic, and Organizational Prevention Approaches

Edited by Michael Kellmann and Jürgen Beckmann

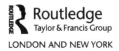

LONDON AND NEW YORK

Designed cover image: Getty Images © Liuzishan

First published 2024
by Routledge
4 Park Square, Milton Park, Abingdon, Oxon OX14 4RN

and by Routledge
605 Third Avenue, New York, NY 10158

Routledge is an imprint of the Taylor & Francis Group, an informa business

British Library Cataloguing-in-Publication Data
A catalogue record for this book is available from the British Library

Library of Congress Cataloging-in-Publication Data
Names: Kellmann, Michael, 1965- editor. | Beckmann, Jürgen, 1955- editor.
Title: Fostering recovery and well-being in a healthy lifestyle :
psychological, somatic, and organizational prevention approaches /
edited by Michael Kellmann and Jürgen Beckmann.
Description: First Edition. | New York, NY : Routledge, 2024. | Series:
Advances in recovery and stress research: multi-disciplinary approaches ;
vol 3 | Includes bibliographical references and index.
Identifiers: LCCN 2023041218 (print) | LCCN 2023041219 (ebook) |
ISBN 9781032168609 (hardback) | ISBN 9781032158648 (paperback) |
ISBN 9781003250654 (ebook)
Subjects: LCSH: Well-being. | Lifestyles. | Health. | Health attitudes.
Classification: LCC HN25 .F67 2024 (print) | LCC HN25 (ebook) |
DDC 613--dc23/eng/20231103
LC record available at https://lccn.loc.gov/2023041218
LC ebook record available at https://lccn.loc.gov/2023041219

ISBN: 978-1-032-16860-9 (hbk)
ISBN: 978-1-032-15864-8 (pbk)
ISBN: 978-1-003-25065-4 (ebk)

DOI: 10.4324/9781003250654

Typeset in Bembo
by SPi Technologies India Pvt Ltd (Straive)

Contents

List of contributors   ix
Series foreword   xi
MICHAEL KELLMANN AND JÜRGEN BECKMANN
Preface   xii
JÜRGEN BECKMANN AND MICHAEL KELLMANN

PART I
Conceptualising the problem   1

1   **Chronic illness and well-being: Promoting quality of
    life with a broadened concept of recovery**   3
    JÜRGEN BECKMANN, MAXIMILIAN HUBER, AND
    CAROLINE S. ANDONIAN-DIERKS

2   **Off-job and on-job recovery as predictors of employee health**   24
    JAN DE JONGE AND TOON W. TARIS

3   **Ambulatory Assessment for recovery and stress
    monitoring in the general population**   38
    SARAH BRÜßLER, BIRTE VON HAAREN-MACK, ANNA VOGELSANG, AND
    MARKUS REICHERT

PART II
Psychological prevention approaches   57

4   **'Switch off when not in use': The benefits of
    detachment from work and sport for recovery**   59
    YANNICK A. BALK

5   **Debriefing sport performance: A strategy to enhance mental
    and emotional recovery and plan for future competition**   73
    JOHN M. HOGG

6 **Engaging in creative behaviours and activities as a well-being and recovery approach** 92
VERONIQUE RICHARD, V. VANESSA WERGIN, AND JOHN CAIRNEY

7 **"Use it right": The relationship between digital media and recovery** 103
JAHAN HEIDARI AND MICHAEL KELLMANN

PART III
Somatic prevention approaches 115

8 **Psychological relaxation techniques to enhance recovery in sports** 117
MICHAEL KELLMANN, MAXIMILIAN PELKA, AND JÜRGEN BECKMANN

9 **Yoga for recovery and well-being in athletes** 131
SELENIA DI FRONSO, MAURIZIO BERTOLLO, AND CLAUDIO ROBAZZA

10 **Sleep well! A key strategy beyond sports** 143
LISA KULLIK AND ASJA KIEL

PART IV
Organisational prevention approaches 163

11 **Optimising fatigue agility and recovery within military settings: Enhancing capability, well-being, and performance** 165
RAYMOND W. MATTHEWS, GERARD J. FOGARTY, EUGENE AIDMAN, AND TOM PATRICK

12 **Building recovery into organisations to foster resilience** 182
JOANA C. KUNTZ

13 **Death due to overwork: Problems and solutions** 199
TOMOHIDE KUBO, XINXIN LIU, AND TOMOAKI MATSUO

14 **Fostering recovery and well-being in a healthy lifestyle: A concluding summary** 218
JÜRGEN BECKMANN AND MICHAEL KELLMANN

Index 223

Contributors

Aidman, Eugene, Defence Science & Technology Group, Australia

Andonian-Dierks, Caroline S., Technical University of Munich, Germany

Balk, Yannick, A., University of Amsterdam and Royal Netherlands Marechaussee, The Netherlands

Beckmann, Jürgen, Technical University of Munich, Germany, and The University of Queensland, Australia

Bertollo, Maurizio, University G. d'Annunzio of Chieti-Pescara, Italy, and University of Suffolk, UK

Brüßler, Sarah, Ruhr University Bochum, Germany

Cairney, John, The University of Queensland, Australia

de Jonge, Jan, Eindhoven University of Technology and Utrecht University, The Netherlands

di Fronso, Selenia, University G. d'Annunzio of Chieti-Pescara, Italy

Fogarty, Gerard, J., University of Southern Queensland, Australia

Heidari, Jahan, Ruhr University Bochum, Germany

Hogg, John, M., Professor Emeritus, University of Alberta, Canada

Huber, Maximilian, Technical University of Munich, Germany

Kellmann, Michael, Ruhr University Bochum, Germany, and The University of Queensland, Australia

Kiel, Asja, Ruhr University Bochum, Germany

Kubo, Tomohide, National Institute of Occupational Safety and Health, Japan

Kullik, Lisa, Ruhr University Bochum, Germany

Kuntz, Joana C., University of Canterbury, New Zealand

Liu, Xinxin, National Institute of Occupational Safety and Health, Japan

Matsuo, Tomoaki, National Institute of Occupational Safety and Health, Japan

Matthews, Raymond, W., Royal Australian Air Force, Australia

Patrick, Tom, Royal Australian Air Force, Australia

Pelka, Maximilian, Ruhr University Bochum, Germany

Reichert, Markus, Ruhr University Bochum, Germany

Richard, Veronique, The University of Queensland, Australia

Robazza, Claudio, University G. d'Annunzio of Chieti-Pescara, Italy

Taris, Toon, W., Utrecht University, The Netherlands

Vogelsang, Anna, Ruhr University Bochum, Germany

von Haaren-Mack, Birte, Karlsruhe Institute of Technology, Germany

Wergin, V. Vanessa, The University of Queensland, Australia

Series foreword

Advances in Recovery and Stress Research: Multi-Disciplinary Approaches covers a broad range of areas in which recovery plays a crucial role, providing the status of research on recovery and stress. In particular, it aims to broaden the understanding of recovery and be unique in addressing fields in which recovery and stress play an important role, but recovery has not received adequate attention. Examples are the areas of health promotion as well as performance promotion in work settings. Another feature of the series is that it contains both up-to-date theoretical and applied perspectives from multi-disciplinary approaches.

It is the idea of the series *Advances in Recovery and Stress Research: Multi-Disciplinary Approaches* to publish a volume each year. We started with *Recovery and well-being in sport and exercise* (Volume 1), followed by *The importance of recovery for physical and mental health: Negotiating the effects of underrecovery* (Volume 2), and now with this Volume 3 *Fostering recovery and well-being in a healthy lifestyle: Psychological, somatic, and organizational prevention approaches*. Volume 4 *The Recovery-Stress Questionnaires: A User* Manual and Volume 5 *Creating urban and workplace environments for recovery and well-being: New perspectives on urban design and mental health* are on the way and Volume 6 is already organised but the title is not finalised. As always, current information on the series can be found at www.routledge.com/Advances-in-Recovery-and-Stress-Research/book-series/ARSR. We thank Routledge for the flexibility and engagement for this adventure to develop the series *Advances in Recovery and Stress Research: Multi-Disciplinary Approaches*.

Michael Kellmann
Jürgen Beckmann

Preface

Stress has been identified as a central cause of impairment of health and well-being in modern societies. A systemic view, in which stress is considered in connection with recovery, was, however, almost not adopted. But for health and well-being, it is crucial to take into consideration that the stress level can be compensated for by suitable recreational measures and resistance resources against negative stress effects are built up. Adequate recovery is an important factor in the prevention of diseases. There is a lack of awareness on the importance of this factor in prevention as well as knowledge on how recovery can be addressed in prevention programmes. Over the last decades, research in the sport context has provided numerous studies that show how to address recovery in order to find a balance between stress and recovery.

This book will address psychological, somatic, and organisational prevention strategies to foster recovery and a healthy lifestyle in society. It will focus on both research and applied counseling aspects to discuss recovery as an underestimated factor in physical and mental health. The contributions expand the possible applicability beyond the area of sport to other fields in which the impact of recovery needs to be addressed, such as the health, well-being, and the workplace.

The editors have approached scientists who are addressing the concept of recovery and highlight prevention approaches to reduce the effects of underrecovery on physical and mental health. The multi-level concept of recovery is pointed out by international experts from general psychology as well as sport, work, and organisational psychology. The approach of the book is interdisciplinary to fully describe prevention approaches to avoid underrecovery. The analysis of effects of underrecovery on health and the individual application of recovery demonstrates the broad range that advancing recovery has for the promotion of physical and mental health.

Jürgen Beckmann
Michael Kellmann

Part I
Conceptualising the problem

1 Chronic illness and well-being

Promoting quality of life with a broadened concept of recovery

Jürgen Beckmann, Maximilian Huber,
and Caroline S. Andonian-Dierks

Introduction

Some illnesses cannot be cured and are therefore called chronic (National Health Council, 2014). Some of those will eventually lead to death over a more or less short period of time like some forms of progressed cancer. There are other illnesses that cannot be healed but because of the progress of modern medicine allow people to have a relatively normal life expectancy. These chronic illnesses, like for example diabetes type 2 nevertheless involve lifelong circumstances. Chronic diseases bear a huge medical as well as a health-economical dimension (Falvo & Holland, 2017).

Research has shown that people who are chronically ill do not necessarily experience reduced well-being. In fact, in several studies those with a more severe chronic illness were found to report higher levels of Quality of Life (QOL) than those with less severe forms of illness (Andonian et al., 2021; Apers et al., 2016, regarding congenital heart defects). This empirical phenomenon that individuals often maintain or even increase their subjective well-being despite (or because of) their chronic illness, is known as the 'paradox of well-being' or in a broader sense 'paradox of satisfaction' (Herschbach, 2002; Swift et al., 2014).

Even though a complete cure may not be possible, a good quality of life can still be achieved for people suffering from a chronic disease. This is to some degree reflected in the broader perspective on recovery advocated by the World Health Organization in 2019 (WHO, 2019). This recovery approach goes beyond 'being cured' or 'being normal again'. In this broader perspective recovery is addressed as a resource that promotes health and well-being. It involves gaining or recapturing meaning and purpose in life as well as self-determination, resulting in personal empowerment and resilience. This chapter will approach several determining factors for achieving well-being and a good QOL despite symptoms of physical and mental illness. It is assumed that the construct of

Beckmann, J., Huber, M., & Andonian-Dierks, C. S. (2024). Chronic illness and well-being: Promoting quality of life with a broadened concept of recovery. In M. Kellmann & J. Beckmann (Eds.), *Fostering Recovery and Well-being in a Healthy Lifestyle: Psychological, Somatic, and Organizational Prevention Approaches* (pp. 3–23). Routledge.

DOI: 10.4324/9781003250654-2

recovery in a broad sense (Beckmann et al., 2023) provides a framework integrating the determinants as a process as well as a resource.

Quality of life

Chronic illnesses are long-lasting illnesses that cannot be completely cured and result in sustained or recurring increased use of healthcare services. Therefore, the goal of promoting recovery in patients with chronic diseases is to increase their well-being and Quality of Life (QOL) although the conditions of the disease can hardly be changed. QOL comprises health, life satisfaction, and well-being of an individual relative to their personal and interpersonal factors, including relationships and culture (Chu et al., 2023; Lundqvist, 2021).

'Good quality of life' might seem like a throwaway phrase in the context of severe chronic illness. Commonly, it is agreed upon that health-related QOL does not equal a lack of symptoms. Rather, it is a subjective measure based on individual health perceptions, goals, and expectations. However, it is difficult to distinguish between health, health-related QOL (HRQOL), and QOL as a more encompassing subjective assessment. HRQOL can be used to address the way health (as measured by health status questionnaires) affects QOL (Karimi & Brazier, 2016).

The concept of QOL dates back to the World Health Organization's definition of health as a "state of complete physical, mental and social well-being, and not merely the absence of disease or infirmity" (World Health Organization, 1946, p. 1). Despite much disagreement, health and medical sciences have adopted this definition and incorporated at least three dimensions in any index measuring QOL: physical health, mental status, and ability to engage in social activities (Post, 2014). Moons et al. (2005, p. 299) expanded the definition of QOL as "the degree of overall life satisfaction that is positively or negatively influenced by an individual's perception of certain aspects of life, including matters both related and unrelated to health". According to this definition, QOL is a holistic umbrella term describing a person's overall sense of well-being, which is influenced by various biopsychosocial factors. Well-being is described as being sensitive to gross and immediate changes in life conditions and does not fully represent the more overarching and stable QOL. In line with the broad conception of recovery advocated by the WHO (2019), recovery appears to be a crucial determinant of both well-being and QOL. The factors that are particularly addressed in this chapter are self-regulation of recovery processes involving the sense of coherence and finding meaning in life.

In a more in-depth consideration, this also gives reason to further reflect on the disease concept itself. Overall, Danzer et al. (2002) point out that there is a gap between being diagnosed with an illness and the individual sense of well-being. Repeatedly, people with chronic somatic diseases such as diabetes mellitus or hepatitis C were found to be entirely satisfied with their health which is one factor determining health-related quality of life (Wilson & Cleary, 1995).

In a study with elderly people, Brinkhof et al. (2021) found that challenges can have considerable social, psychological, and physical consequences that may lead to significant changes in QOL. According to Brinkhof et al. (2021) behavioural coping, positive appraisal, self-management ability, and physical activity are key factors in mastering the challenges. These factors are closely dependent on self-regulation which is a core factor for achieving recovery (Beckmann, 2023a).

Seligman (2012) suggests five key areas for well-being in his PERMA approach: positive emotions (P), engagement (E), positive relationships (R), meaning (M), and achievement (A). Presence of meaning may just be one component of overall well-being (Ryff & Singer, 2008) but appears to be crucial to develop resilience as a study by Krok (2016) suggests. In fact, the other four elements mentioned by Seligman can be seen to contribute to the development of a broad perception of meaningfulness. Meaning appears to be a crucial determinant of well-being and QOL, particularly in the context of illness. It is a central element to Antonovsky's (1987) *Sense of Coherence* (SOC) which is strongly associated with resilience. Thus, the role of meaning in life will be presented in more detail later in this chapter.

Explanatory approaches for the well-being paradox

As pointed out before, research shows that suffering from an illness does not necessarily entail a reduced QOL (Andonian et al., 2021; Apers et al., 2016; Herschbach, 2002; Swift et al., 2014). Some patients with a severe, chronic illness report a poor QOL but others with a comparably bad medical condition report a good QOL. The paradox of well-being has been independently observed in several areas. Social science research has particularly addressed that people with poor income and bad working conditions report higher levels of life satisfaction than better-off people (Olsen & Schober, 1993).

Well-being is a subjective experience or construction which is influenced by a wide range of factors such as culture, social comparison, and personal values. What one person considers satisfying may not be the same for another person. Furthermore, well-being is not an all-or-nothing phenomenon, but rather a complex mix of positive and negative emotions. However, the individual emotional reaction was found to be a strong determinant of well-being (Brown et al., 2020).

According to the *Relative Income and Adaptation Theory*, increases in absolute benefits (e.g., income) do not significantly increase satisfaction (Easterlin, 1995). After reaching the minimal threshold necessary to satisfy basic needs, increases in satisfaction are not based on increases in absolute benefits but on the individual's relative position within the distribution of benefits (Stutzer, 2004). For those suffering from poor health conditions or chronic diseases, not only relative benefits matter but adaptation mechanisms are supposed to emerge (Neff & Olsen, 2007). These mechanisms are assumed to lead to a process of adjusting aspirations leading to a downward revision of aspirations that reflects disadvantaged circumstances. Therefore, people often report being satisfied with their quality of life even if they live in disadvantaged circumstances (Sam et al., 2008) such as a chronic disease because they show a downward revision of aspirations which renders them satisfied with lower levels of aspiration. Of course, this would at least presuppose an acceptance of their situation. In line with *Dissonance Theory* (Festinger, 1957) voluntary acceptance of one's condition should lead to positive changes in the evaluation of this condition (Beckmann & Irle, 1985).

A simple and obvious explanation for the finding that people with a chronically bad medical condition such as a complex congenital heart defect report better QOL than those with less severe illness is that complex impairments are usually recognised earlier in life compared to less complex ones. Therefore, a perceived discrepancy between living with and without the disease is less salient. In addition, those affected have the chance to better adjust to their situation. This finding suggests that the data best fit a 'two factor' model, indicating that overall well-being and illness are two moderately related, yet distinct contributions to our understanding of human health (Iasiello & Van Agteren, 2020; Renshaw & Cohen, 2014).

The *Dual-Continuum Model* of Keyes (2005; Westerhof & Keyes, 2010) reflects these empirical findings. It postulates that illness and well-being are located on two independent continua. This *Dual-Continuum Model* was originally developed for the area of mental health. Therefore, the illness continuum has the endpoints of mental illness and mental health. A second continuum is orthogonal to the first one and expands from low well-being to high well-being. Both continua represent interrelated domains of mental health, each having shared and unique predictors. Low well-being is referred to as 'languishing'. High well-being is denominated as 'flourishing'. Each of the resulting four quadrants depicted in Figure 1.1 are occupied by people. Whereas it is not surprising that people without mental illness and high overall well-being fall into the category of complete mental health and those with severe mental illness and low overall well-being are characterised as struggling, the lower right and the upper left quadrant are less to be expected. Most notable in the present context is the quadrant with high mental illness and well-being, which contradicts classical notions and represents the paradox of well-being addressed at the beginning of the chapter.

Unlike traditional pathogenic-oriented approaches, the *Dual-Continuum Model* represents a more comprehensive concept of psychological well-being (Iasiello & Van Agteren, 2020). This approach allows a person to be considered more or less distressed in some regards, while simultaneously more or less well in others. This leads to several important implications for clinical practice. Patients should be screened for differential levels of mental health and illness to eventually reveal previously 'invisible' groups, especially those considered 'vulnerable' and 'languishing' by Keyes (2005). Furthermore, instead of rigid attempts to fight aversive experiences, successful interventions should include dialectical

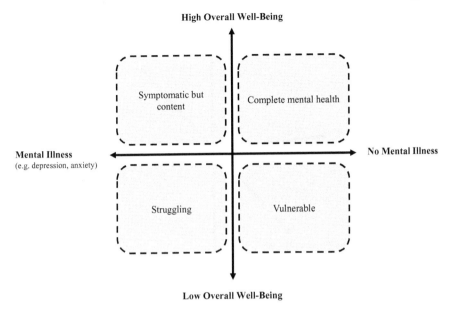

Figure 1.1 Dual-Continuum Model according to Keyes (2005).

elements, bringing positive psychological resources and constructive change together. This consideration is akin to a basic premise of recovery research, that a person can experience a high stress load and at the same time be high in recovery (Kallus, 2016a; Kellmann, 2002; Mierswa & Kellmann, 2015). However, within Kellmann's research approach recovery and stress are functionally linked: recovery functions as a buffer against negative effects of stress. Such a functional connection between the two dimensions is not made in Keyes's (2005) model. Yet empirical findings show overall well-being and mental illness to be associated with shared and unique psychosocial and medical predictors which is a strong indication that the constructs are distinct, but related due to some degree of overlap (Iasiello & Van Agteren, 2020).

Keyes's model addresses only mental illness, but research suggests that it may also apply to somatic illness. According to research by Andonian et al. (2020), the continua do not have to be restricted to mental illness. In their study, the paradox of well-being was replicated with patients who presented a congenital heart defect (CHD) which is a chronic illness condition. In this study patients with higher complexity of CHD causing clinical manifestations like e.g., congestive heart failure, cyanosis, hypoxemia, and neurodevelopmental disabilities, described their overall well-being as significantly superior to those with less complex heart lesions, when considering both psychological and physical health domains in conjunction. This finding suggests an extension to Keyes's *Dual-Continuum Model* by a tri-axial framework. Andonian-Dierks's (2022) novel

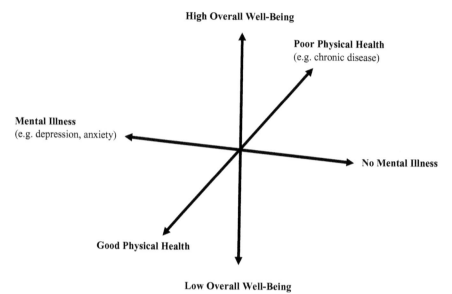

Figure 1.2 *Three-Dimensional Model* of physical health, mental illness, and well-being according to Andonian-Dierks (2022).

Three-Dimensional Model attempts to capture the diversity of subjective health presentations along three different continua: an axis of physical health, an axis of mental illness or emotional distress, and one of overall subjective well-being. Chronic diseases such as congenital heart defects are frequently accompanied by mental health problems (Andonian et al., 2018). As shown in Figure 1.2 according to this model, people with poor physical health (e.g., suffering from chronic diseases) accompanied by mental illness or emotional distress may still experience a decent quality of life. Although this framework does not entirely account for interindividual variability, it allows for a differentiated perspective on contributing factors and appropriate conclusions in the mental health management not only of CHD patients.

Within this context, recovery comes into play as a general resource to foster general well-being. In the following, some impeding and promoting conditions will be addressed.

Recovery as a protective resource

In our understanding recovery means more than simply 'not presenting symptoms anymore'. Kellmann and Kallus (2001) describe recovery as a resource and a buffer. According to Grawe and Grawe-Gerber's (1999) conception of resource-oriented psychotherapy, resources include a client's space of possibilities in which she/he can currently move. The resource orientation in psychotherapy involves activating positive potentials, which are available to people to satisfy their basic needs (Grawe & Grawe-Gerber, 1999). Recovery can be conceptualised as a (goal) state as well as the process of achieving this goal state. Through the recovery process, positive outcomes such as well-being and a high quality of life can be achieved even in the presence of adverse conditions such as a chronic illness. However, it must be noted that most researchers in the medical field still reduce recovery to the process of healing and do not address it as the development of a protective resource.

In line with the WHO (2019) postulation of a broad concept of recovery in the area of mental health, positive psychology has addressed recovery as a resource that enables individuals not only to recover from stress but also to show resilience to health-threatening stress. According to Anthony (1993), this involves a "process of changing one's attitudes, values, feelings, goals, skills and/or roles … a way of living a satisfying, hopeful and contributing life even with the limitations caused by illness" (p. 15). The broader conception of recovery involves a different perception of the human-being. This image is the basis of positive psychology. Positive psychology focuses on strengths instead of weaknesses, and on building a good in life instead of repairing the bad (Peterson et al., 2008). Major components are self-determination, autonomy, and competence (Ryan & Deci, 2017) as well as a growth-orientation (Dweck, 2006; Maslow, 1968). These aspects can be found in the adaptive forms of illness identity which will be described in more detail below. An adaptive illness identity is a favourable precondition for developing well-being and a good quality of life but individuals still need to actively strive for obtaining recovery resources and maintaining them.

It is characteristic of recovery-related resources that they are depleted over time and thus need to be re-established to regain their full functional capacity (Kallus, 2016b). Recovery to re-establish and maintain health can be regarded as a continuous process of acquiring a state of equilibrium (Danzer et al., 2002). In this respect, the replenishment of recovery resources is a process that requires self-regulation (Beckmann, 2023a). Therefore, recovery implies the person to be an active agent who is aware of their individual recovery needs (Beckmann et al., 2023).

Kellmann et al. (2018) distinguish between passive, active, and pro-active approaches to recovery. Passive methods may range from the application of external methods (e.g., massage). However, to even implement a state of rest characterised by inactivity (passive recovery such as sleep) usually necessitates being organised and initiated. Active forms of recovery include, for example, pursuing goals (such as regular physical activity) aimed at compensating for the metabolic responses of physical fatigue. Recovery can be pro-active and involve future goals such as, for example, developing a recovery plan and integrating it into one's weekly schedule. Pro-active recovery (e.g., social activities) implies a high level of self-determination by choosing activities customised to individual needs and preferences.

Recovery is a highly individual-specific process and thus individuals need to find out what kind of recovery is most efficient for them (Kellmann et al., 2018).

In line with this, Danzer et al. (2002) postulate in an even broader sense that health must always be seen in reference to individuals. How people manage to maintain health is based on their individual biographies. In their analysis of the literature on mental health recovery Jacobson and Curtis (2000) identified individual-specific elements of recovery that are in line with this postulation. These individual elements of recovery were related to hope, self-determination, agency, meaning/purpose, and awareness/potentiality.

Recovery constitutes a protective resource that aids in coping with stress and can produce resilience. Rutter (1987) defined resilience as "protective factors which modify, ameliorate, or alter a person's response to some environmental hazard that predisposes to a maladaptive outcome" (p. 316). Resilience is highlighted by Costa et al. (2023) as an important element to ensure physical, social, and psychological health as well as well-being.

In the following, various factors are addressed that influence whether recovery promotes a comprehensive strengthening of resilience and ultimately has a positive effect on well-being and quality of life. The *Three-Dimensional Model* (Andonian-Dierks, 2022) implies that not all patients suffering from mental and/or physical illness manage to experience high well-being or good QOL. The question is what determines whether a person with an illness condition will flourish or languish. What the model describes, and the research supports is that well-being/QOL is not determined by the severity of the mental and/or physical illness. The subjective meaning people with a chronic disease ascribe to their illness is a major influence on how they live (Kleinman, 1988), affecting perception of their well-being and QOL.

The concept of illness identity refers to how chronic illness affects individuals' self-perceptions (Oris et al., 2018). It suggests four different categories of how people perceive and integrate their chronic illness into their sense of self. Two of these categories negatively affect managing the illness whereas two other categories appear to be positive preconditions. The first step in looking at interventions to promote recovery should identify an individual's illness identity and then support them in redefining their values and developing a supportive identity. The therapeutic attitude is therefore alongside the patient by understanding and recognising his or her chronic disease as a real burden while, at the same time, maintaining a solution-oriented supportive approach.

Illness identity

In decades of mind-body dualism the influence of a chronic illness on a person's identity has been largely disregarded. To advance current therapeutic approaches, it is necessary to understand the processes underlying the experience of a chronic illness. Leventhal et al. (1999) introduced a self-regulation model of illness cognition on the interactions between the self and chronic illness. They analyse the processes involved when a person confronts a severe chronic illness that impinges upon self and identity. Particularly, they focus on self-regulation as it applies to the enactment of health and illness behaviours under these conditions. Based on these considerations the concept of *Illness Identity* was developed, which addresses the degree to which a chronic illness is integrated into a person's sense of self (Oris et al., 2018). The concept provides a psychological perspective on the meaning of living with a chronic disease. The illness identity approach assumes that chronic illness threatens central feelings about oneself, presenting a different framework of illness experience than that suggested by pure somatic markers (Leventhal et al., 2003). The framework postulates that individuals form cognitive, affective, and behavioural representations of health threats that affect their conditions of living with the disease (Leventhal et al., 1999). However, a major limitation of Leventhal's model is that it was confined to cognitive illness perceptions and failed to represent the complexity of a patient's illness experience (Breland et al., 2020).

A further development of the illness identity concept postulates that illness identity is not only an expression of the patient's perception of their disease but also how the disease affects the way they think and feel about themselves (Van Bulck et al., 2019). Chronically ill patients need to integrate their illness into their identity to achieve a coherent sense of self (Van Bulck et al., 2019). Illness identity may therefore affect the recovery process, and resulting outcomes in people with a chronic illness. Illness identity comprises four different states, i.e., engulfment, rejection, acceptance, and enrichment (Oris et al., 2018). Each state has been linked to different psychological and behavioural outcomes (Andonian et al., 2020; Oris et al., 2018; Van Bulck et al., 2018). Engulfment and rejection are maladaptive, may interfere with the recovery process, and result in negative psychological and behavioural outcomes whereas acceptance and enrichment support the recovery process leading to better adaptation and positive outcomes.

Engulfment captures the degree to which patients define themselves through their chronic illness. An individual's self-concept becomes reorganised entirely around the experience of the chronic illness (Charmaz, 1995; Leventhal et al., 1999; Oris et al., 2018). In contrast to taking responsibility for one's health, being overtaken by one's condition occurs without choice (Charmaz, 1995). Engulfment leaves no room for an individual self in which one's own needs, orientations, and preferences are considered or are accessible. Hence, the engulfed person can be considered as being highly alienated which is associated with chronic negative affect and impaired self-regulation (Kuhl & Beckmann, 1994). In the long run, this blocking of their very own needs can lead to the experience of an existential vacuum with mental health issues as a consequence (Riethof & Bob, 2019). Not surprisingly engulfment is not found to be linked to flourishing but rather to worsen psychological and physiological outcomes (Andonian et al., 2020; Oris et al., 2018; Van Bulck et al., 2019).

Rejection refers to a state where an individual denies or minimises his or her illness in an attempt to preserve the facade of a normal life (Carver & Vargas, 2011). The illness is regarded as an external threat and individuals refuse to acknowledge it as part of themselves (Leventhal et al., 1999). Even though it was found that rejection is unrelated to emotional distress (Andonian et al., 2020) it implies no active attempts at recovery. Rejection is linked to reduced treatment participation, greater functional impairment, and lower general self-efficacy (Carver & Vargas, 2011; Nahlén Bose et al., 2016; Oris et al., 2018). Hence rejection potentially impairs the recovery process. In the context of clinical psychology, the term denial is used instead of rejection. Research in psycho-cardiology has shown that denial is associated with less help-seeking and the risk of worsening the condition of a cardiac disease (Covino et al., 2011).

While engulfment and rejection represent maladaptive states of illness integration, acceptance and enrichment refer to adaptive ways of illness integration. Engulfment and rejection impair recovery processes and thus affect underrecovery as an imbalance of recovery periods and daily life demands of a person. Acceptance paves the way for recovery. Enrichment already involves recovery in a broader sense.

Acceptance refers to a mode of adaptive illness integration, where individuals adapt to their illness while perceiving the ability to tolerate the unpredictable nature of their condition (Evers et al., 2001; Morea et al., 2008; Oris et al., 2018). Acceptance may have a protective role in the psychological functioning of individuals with chronic diseases as it is associated with beneficial psychological and physiological outcomes (Andonian et al., 2020; Oris et al., 2018). Over the past two decades, research addressing the phenomenon of positive changes as a consequence of illness has expanded (Helgeson et al., 2006; Tedeschi & Calhoun, 2004). Interestingly, acceptance is an important element in mindfulness interventions. By accepting an experience and the thoughts and feelings it provokes, psychological flexibility can be achieved which enables a person to positively manage their contexts and behaviours (Brinkborg et al., 2011).

Enrichment addresses ways in which a chronic illness offers possibilities for positive change and identity transformation, in terms of increased life appreciation, personal resilience, more meaningful relationships, or spiritual growth (Stanton & Revenson, 2007; Tedeschi & Calhoun, 2004). Enrichment, therefore, provides numerous recovery resources and consequently has been associated with QOL after adjusting to several disease-specific and sociodemographic variables (Tomich & Helgeson, 2004). It has also been found to play a moderator role in the relationship between QOL and emotional distress (Morrill et al., 2008). In concrete terms, enrichment appears to be a crucial recovery resource. At first, it may appear counterintuitive that enrichment is linked to experiences of increased symptoms of illness and pain. However, the concept of post-traumatic growth requires that individuals thoroughly explore their illness to form their identities and build valued lives (Oris et al., 2018). Frankl (1959) describes that going through such a process can aid in making the meaning of life more salient which supports coping with hardships. Seery et al. (2010) found that adverse experiences may foster subsequent resilience, with resulting advantages for mental health and well-being.

Some features of enrichment seem to be in parallel with the concept of resilience. In the psychological literature, resilience is consistently linked to the presence of adversities and defined as the capacity or ability "to withstand or recover from significant challenges" (Masten & Narayan, 2012, p. 231). Resilience was initially conceptualised as a process of psychological reintegration, the ability to learn new skills from adverse experiences and develop a new perspective on life, increasing skills in coping with stressful events (Richardson, 2002). According to Rutter (1987, p. 316) resilience provides "protective factors which modify, ameliorate, or alter a person's response to some environmental hazard that predisposes to a maladaptive outcome". Resilience is typically used to understand how the person can reach or maintain positive adaptation despite exposure to stress or adversity (Szedlak et al., 2021).

The research by Andonian et al. (2020) demonstrates that illness identity may provide a valuable tool to detect and predict psychological adaptation to the chronic condition of CHD. Regarding other influential models in the field of health psychology, illness identity could be conceptualised as a dynamic process in which individuals transition through different stages throughout their disease trajectory as proposed in the *Transtheoretical Model of Behaviour Change* (TTM; DiClemente & Prochaska, 1998). The stages postulated by TTM progress through six stages of change: pre-contemplation, contemplation, preparation, action, maintenance, and termination.

Motivational interviewing (MI) is an empirically supported counselling method to evoke intrinsic motivation and achieve personal growth (Tuccero et al., 2016). Supporting individuals with a chronic illness to progress from the two maladaptive illness identities engulfment and rejection to the more adaptive identities of acceptance and enrichment should be the first steps in an MI-based approach to promote well-being and better QOL in people with a chronic disease. Individuals with illness identities of engulfment and rejection are at the pre-contemplation stage of TTM. They are not aware of the consequences of their identities and are typically not considering changing their health-related behaviour. Suggested intervention strategies at this stage involve active listening, expressing empathy, and accepting the client's resistance rather than opposing it. Therapists may ask clients to reconsider their behaviour, become aware of the disadvantages, and identify the benefits of changing. With the illness identity of acceptance, clients have entered the contemplation stage. They acknowledge their problem but may not have the confidence to take a step forward. Clinicians can assist the clients in developing personally adequate recovery strategies that involve building protective resources through changing one's attitudes and aspirations, accepting feelings and roles, and developing skills for a way of living a satisfying life despite the limitations caused by the chronic illness. With the illness identity of enrichment, clients have become aware of opportunities that are available to them and are developing a growth-oriented mindset that guides action and maintenance. They have adopted recovery strategies that prevent relapses due to underrecovery with well-developed coping skills and support systems that result in a strong sense of coherence.

Acceptance and Commitment Therapy (ACT; Hayes et al., 1999) may be particularly effective to increase psychological flexibility and potentially lead to better recovery and self-management within the context of chronic somatic illness. ACT involves acceptance of a disease and the associated impediments such as pain and a restriction of the range of activities through nonjudgmental awareness of related thoughts and feelings. This acceptance should go along with cognitive defusion, i.e., changing how one interacts with thoughts about the experiences to detach oneself from these thoughts. Eventually, a commitment to long-term behaviour change should be reached. Of particular importance within ACT and, in general, for obtaining well-being and good quality of life appears to be having a purpose in life as postulated by logotherapy (Frankl, 2010). Purpose or meaning in life can be seen as the main controller of the well-being continuum. The more people suffering from a chronic illness can focus on something mean-ingful the higher the chances for well-being and good quality of life relatively independent of the illness condition. And because flourishing is associated with resilience it will positively affect the illness itself.

Building resilience: The salutogenic approach

One factor that appears to be associated with positive well-being is the sense of coherence (SOC). Based on a study of Holocaust survivors Antonovsky (1987) addressed in his salutogenic approach factors that support mastering of adverse life conditions. Central to the model is what Antonovsky calls the 'sense of coherence'. SOC is related to resilience and defined as the pervasive, enduring though dynamic, feeling of confidence that one's environment is predictable and that things will work out well. The model postulates generalised resistance resources, which are all the resources that help a person cope with stress and maintain health. The core question is whether stress violates a person's SOC. Antonovsky (1987) defined SOC as:

> a global orientation that expresses the extent to which one has a pervasive, enduring though dynamic feeling of confidence that 1) the stimuli deriving from one's internal and external environments in the course of living are structured, predictable, and explicable; 2) the resources are available to one to meet the demands posed by these stimuli; and 3) these demands are challenges, worthy of investment and engagement.

(p. 19)

The SOC has three components:

- Comprehensibility: A belief that things happen in an orderly and predicta-ble fashion and a sense that you can understand events in your life and reasonably predict what will happen in the future.
- Manageability: A belief that you have the skills or ability, the support, the help, or the resources necessary to take care of things, and that things are manageable and within your control.
- Meaningfulness: A belief that things in life are interesting and a source of satisfaction, that things are really worthwhile, and that there is good reason or purpose to care about what happens.

According to Antonovsky (1987), meaningfulness is the most important of these components. Without the perception of meaning individuals would not have the motivation to comprehend and manage events (DeViva et al., 2016). Experiencing meaning, even in suffering, is a buffer against perceiving life as miserable. It ameliorates negative stress, promotes enrichment, and facilitates a stable recovery-stress balance.

Thus, in a nutshell, Antonovsky (1987) comes to the same proposition as Frankl (1959), namely that maintaining and promoting health involves experiencing meaning in life as an essential component of a strong SOC. Empirical research supports Frankl's and Antonovsky's assumption that meaning is not only associated with resilience but in fact, can increase resilience. For example, Krok (2016) found that meaning in life made individuals more resilient against burnout. People with high levels of meaning report lower levels of perceived stress (Flannery & Flannery, 1990) and fewer symptoms of physical and mental health problems. Building resilience through recovery based on the promotion of a SOC would be another important component of a programme to promote well-being and better QOL in people with a chronic disease. Meaningful activities should constitute a core element.

Meaning in life as a buffer

As stated above, meaning (in life) is a central element in SOC. Perceiving life as meaningful is frequently associated with being resourceful and resilient. It has been considered an indicator of well-being, a facilitator of adaptive coping, and a marker of therapeutic growth. Several studies have supported the link between meaning in life, health, and well-being (Aftab et al., 2019; Mascaro & Rosen, 2005; Steger & Frazier, 2005). Steger et al. (2008) define the presence of meaning as "the degree to which people experience their lives as comprehensible and significant, and feel a sense of purpose or mission in their lives that transcends the mundane concerns of daily life" (p. 661).

However, not all researchers addressing meaning in life consider the transcendence of mundane concerns of daily life a necessary component (Beckmann, 2023b). What appears to be necessary, according to several studies (Church et al., 2014) is the presence of the three basic needs postulated by *Self-Determination Theory* (Deci & Ryan, 2000): autonomy, positive relationships, and competence. Meaning was found to be positively correlated with having a sense of personal control over one's life, or locus of control (Ryff, 1989), as well as positive perceptions of the world itself (Sharpe & Viney, 1973). A meta-analysis by Li et al. (2021) revealed a robust positive association between the presence of meaning in life and subjective well-being.

Imbalances of stress and recovery, particularly because of insufficient recovery, can be related to a perceived void in one's life. Without perceived meaning in life, individuals tend to show apathetic activity, inactivity, and develop psychopathology (Klinger, 2017). In psychotherapy research it was found that improvement of mental health partly depends upon the ability of individuals to find meaning and purpose in their lives (Andresen et al., 2003). People with high levels of meaning report lower levels of perceived stress and fewer symptoms of stress-related disorders (Flannery & Flannery, 1990). Debats et al. (1995) found that individuals who perceive meaning in their lives report more effective coping with stress. In their study, perceived meaningfulness was strongly linked to contact with an individual's self (needs and preferences), whereas meaninglessness was associated with a state of alienation from the self.

Perceived meaning in life appears to be positively related to self-regulation factors that promote adequate recovery in the broad sense postulated in this chapter (Beckmann, 2023b). This relationship is nicely illustrated in the example of a manager with a stressful job who engages in long-distance running. Certainly, running a half-marathon is taxing physical somatic resources. After a run, she says, 'I am exhausted, but it feels good'. Two factors are important to perceive the long-distance running as recovery. First, she voluntarily ran the 21 K. Second, having successfully completed the run is a meaningful accomplishment for her. Thus, self-determination and meaningfulness seem to differentiate a stressful activity from a recovery activity.

Meaning in life can be considered a crucial controlling factor of the well-being continuum (Beckmann, 2023b). The less meaning in life people experience the more likely they will languish. On the contrary, the more meaning in life is experienced the more people will flourish, and that is relatively independent of an illness condition. Therefore, the experience of meaning is an important factor that serves recovery and helps to build a buffer against the negative effects of adversities.

Conclusion and recommendations for practice

Despite even severe, chronic illness people can flourish, experience well-being and a good quality of life. This has been referred to as the paradox of well-being (Herschbach, 2002). In several studies on the *Dual-Continuum Model*, Keyes (2005) and colleagues found well-being to be relatively independent of the objective illness conditions. However, as discussed in this chapter, well-being, and a good quality of life despite illness depends on several factors. So far, no explicit attempt to translate the *Dual-Continuum Model* into intervention approaches is reported in the literature. Attempts to understand the mechanisms underlying the paradox of well-being are crucial for promoting a good quality of life QOL in people with severe chronic diseases. Of course, it must be acknowledged that these mechanisms may vary depending on the type of illness and clients' personality. In psychosomatics and modern psychotherapy, these different aspects have been incorporated (Grawe, et al., 2001).

A broad recovery perspective as advocated by the WHO (2019) appears to provide a good framework for approaching an understanding of the paradox of well-being. Recovery is addressed as providing a resource that functions as a buffer against the stress of illness and the negative experiences associated with it. This broad perspective on recovery involves gaining or recapturing meaning and purpose in life and self-determination, resulting in personal empowerment and resilience despite a chronic illness. The person's capacities for recovery are affected by their perception of the disease, and by the way they think and feel about themselves. This is reflected in the concept of illness identity. If a person is completely engulfed by the illness or denies it their capacities to activate these resources are compromised by underrecovery.

Several steps towards promoting well-being and a good quality of life have been proposed. The first step involves overcoming the maladaptive illness identities of engulfment and rejection and progressing to acceptance and enrichment. Supporting individuals to overcome the maladaptive identities of engulfment and rejection and adopt the adaptive identities of acceptance and enrichment can be fostered by integrative therapeutical approaches such as MI and ACT within the mindfulness approach and Dweck's (2006) growth mind-set approach.

Additionally, to promote well-being and a good QOL despite severely impaired physical and mental health a changed perspective in medicine is needed. This changed perspective must move away from the image of passive patients who are being treated. Instead an orientation needs to be developed that involves a recognition of the individual being actively engaged in recovery. Such an orientation implies even more than granting patients participation. It needs to be oriented toward making chronically ill people active agents of their well-being. An important health care objective enhances all these and contributes to the increase of lifespan years, while maintaining an optimal HRQOL something that is not only a primary concern of patients, their families, and clinicians but is also of global policy interest (Bowling et al., 2003).

References

Aftab, A., Lee, E. E., Klaus, F., Daly, R., Wu, T., Tu, X., Huege, S., & Jeste, D. V. (2019). Meaning in life and its relationship with physical, mental, and cognitive functioning: A study of 1,042 community-dwelling adults across the lifespan. *Journal of Clinical Psychiatry, 81*(1), 19m13064. https://doi.org/10.4088/JCP.19m13064

Andresen, R., Oades, L., & Caputi, P. (2003). The experience of recovery from schizophrenia: Towards an empirically validated stage model. *Australian & New Zealand Journal of Psychiatry, 37*(5), 586–594.

Andonian-Dierks, C. S. (2022). *Quality of life and psychosocial outcomes in adults with congenital heart disease.* [Dissertation, Technical University Munich]. Retrieved May 12, 2023 from https://nbn-resolving.de/urn/resolver.pl?urn:nbn:de:bvb:91-diss-20221017-1639968-1-9

Andonian, C. S., Beckmann, J., Biber, S., Ewert, P., Freilinger, S., Kaemmerer, H., Oberhoffer, R., Pieper, L., & Neidenbach, R. C. (2018). Current research status on the psychological situation of adults with congenital heart disease (ACHD). *Cardiovascular Diagnosis and Therapy, 8*(6), 799–804.

Andonian, C. S., Beckmann, J., Ewert, P., Freilinger, S., Kaemmerer, H., Oberhoffer-Fritz, R., Sack, M., & Neidenbach, R. C. (2020). Assessment of the psychological situation in adults with congenital heart disease. *Journal of Clinical Medicine, 9*(3), 779. https://doi.org/10.3390/jcm9030779

Andonian, C. S., Freilinger, S., Achenbach, S., Ewert, P., Gundlach, U., Hoerer, J., Kaemmerer, H., Pieper, L., Weyand, M., Neidenbach, R. C., & Beckmann, J. (2021). 'Well-being paradox' revisited: A cross-sectional study of quality of life in over 4000 adults with congenital heart disease. *BMJ Open*, *11*(6), e049531. https://doi.org/10.1136/bmjopen-2021-049531

Anthony, W. A. (1993). Recovery from mental illness: The guiding vision of the mental health service system in the 1990s. *Psychosocial Rehabilitation Journal*, *16*(4), 11–23.

Antonovsky, A. (1987). *Unraveling the mystery of health: How people manage stress and stay well*. Jossey-Bass.

Apers, S., Kovacs, A. H., Luyckx, K., Thomet, C., Budts, W., Enomoto, J., Sluman, M. A., Wang, J. K., Jackson, J. L., Khairy, P., Cook, S. C., Chidambarathanu, S., Alday, L., Eriksen, K., Dellborg, M., Berghammer, M., Mattsson, E., Mackie, A. S., Menahem, S., ... Moons, P. (2016). Quality of life of adults with congenital heart disease in 15 countries: Evaluating country-specific characteristics. *Journal of the American College of Cardiology*, *67*, 2237–2245.

Beckmann, J. (2023a). Self-regulation of recovery. In M. Kellmann, S. Jakowsky, & J. Beckmann (Eds.), *The importance of recovery for physical and mental health* (pp. 53–69). Routledge.

Beckmann, J. (2023b). Meaning and meaninglessness in elite sport. In I. Nixdorf, R. Nixdorf, J. Beckmann, T. Loughead, & T. E. MacIntyre (Eds.), *Routledge handbook of mental health in elite sport* (pp. 31–44). Routledge.

Beckmann, J., & Irle, M. (1985). Dissonance and action control. In J. Kuhl & J. Beckmann (Eds.), *Action control: From cognition to behavior* (pp. 129–150). Springer.

Beckmann, J., Kellmann, M., & Jakowski, S. (2023). Recovery is more than just healing. Advocating a broader perspective on recovery in physical and mental health. In M. Kellmann, S. Jakowsky, & J. Beckmann (Eds.), *The importance of recovery for physical and mental health* (pp. 266–270). Routledge.

Bowling, A., Gabriel, Z., Dykes, J., Dowding, L. M., Evans, O., Fleissig, A., Banister, D., & Sutton, S. (2003). Let's ask them: A national survey of definitions of quality of life and its enhancement among people aged 65 and over. *International Journal of Aging and Human Development*, *56*, 269–306.

Breland, J. Y., Wong, J. J., & McAndrew, L. M. (2020). Are common sense model constructs and self-efficacy simultaneously correlated with self-management behaviors and health outcomes: A systematic review. *Health Psychology Open*, *7*(1), 2055102919898846. https://doi.org/10.1177/2055102919898846

Brinkborg, H., Michanek, J., Hesser, H., & Berglund, G. (2011). Acceptance and commitment therapy for the treatment of stress among social workers: A randomized controlled trial. *Behavioral Research and Therapy*, *49*(6), 389–398.

Brinkhof, L. P., Huth, K. S., Murre, J. M. J., de Wit, S., Krugers H. J., & Ridderinkhof, K. R. (2021). The interplay between quality of life and resilience factors in later life: A network analysis. *Frontiers in Psychology*, *12*, 752564. https://doi.org/10.3389/fpsyg.2021.752564

Brown, C. L., Van Doren, N., Ford, B. Q., Mauss, I. B., Sze, J. W., & Levenson, R. W. (2020). Coherence between subjective experience and physiology in emotion: Individual differences and implications for well-being. *Emotion*, *20*(5), 818–829.

Carver, C. S., & Vargas, S. (2011). Stress, coping, and health. In H. S. Friedman (Ed.), *The Oxford handbook of health psychology* (pp. 162–188). Oxford University Press.

Charmaz, K. (1995). The body, identity, and self: Adapting to impairment. *Sociological Quarterly*, *36*(4), 657–680.

Chu, T. L., Harmison, R. J., & Martin, S. B. (2023). Quality of life and recovery. In M. Kellmann, S. Jakowski, & J. Beckmann (Eds.), *The importance of recovery for physical and mental health: Negotiating the effects of underrecovery* (pp. 84–100). Routledge.

Church, A. T., Katigbak, M. S., Ibanez-Reyes, J., de Jesus Vargas-Flores, J., Curtis, G. J., Tanaka-Matsumi, J., Cabrera, H. F., Mastor, K. A., Zhang, H., Shen, J., Locke, K. D., Alvarez, J. M., Ching, C. M., Ortiz, F. A., & Simon, J.-Y. R. (2014). Relating self-concept consistency to hedonic and eudaimonic well-being in eight cultures. *Journal of Cross-Cultural Psychology, 45*(5), 695–712.

Costa, V. T., Noce, F., Bicalho, C. C. F., & de Sousa Pinheiro, G. (2023). Resilience enhances the recovery process. In M. Kellmann, S. Jakowsky, & J. Beckmann (Eds.), *The importance of recovery for physical and mental health* (pp. 101–121). Routledge.

Covino, J. M., Stern, T. W., & Stern, T. A. (2011). Denial of cardiac illness: Consequences and management. *Primary Care Companion CNS Disorders, 13*(5), PCC.11f01166. https://doi.org/10.4088/PCC.11f01166

Danzer, G., Rose, M., Walter, M., & Klapp, B. F. (2002). On the theory of individual health. *Journal of Medical Ethics, 28*(1), 17–19.

Debats, D. L., Drost, J., & Hansen, P. J. (1995). Experiences of meaning in life: A combined qualitative and quantitative approach. *British Journal of Psychology, 86*(3), 359–375.

DeViva, J. C., Sheerin, C. M., Southwick, S. M., Roy, A. M., Pietrzak, R. H., & Harpaz-Rotem, I. (2016). Correlates of VA mental health treatment utilization among OEF/OIF/OND veterans: Resilience, stigma, social support, personality, and beliefs about treatment. *Psychological Trauma: Theory, Research, Practice, and Policy, 8*(3), 310–318.

DiClemente, C. C., & Prochaska, J. O. (1998). Toward a comprehensive, transtheoretical model of change: Stages of change and addictive behaviors. In W. R. Miller & S. Rollnick (Eds.), *Treating addictive behaviors* (pp. 3–24). Plenum Press.

Dweck, C. S. (2006). *Mindset: The new psychology of success.* Random House.

Easterlin, R. A. (1995). Will raising the incomes of all increase the happiness of all? *Journal of Economic Behavior and Organization, 27*, 35–47.

Evers, A. W., Kraaimaat, F. W., van Lankveld, W., Jongen, P. J., Jacobs, J. W., & Bijlsma, J. W. (2001). Beyond unfavorable thinking: The Illness Cognition Questionnaire for chronic diseases. *Journal of Consulting in Clinical Psychology, 69*(6), 1026–1036.

Falvo, D., & Holland, B. E. (2017). *Medical and psychosocial aspects of chronic illness and disability.* Jones & Bartlett Learning.

Festinger, L. (1957). *A theory of cognitive dissonance.* Stanford University Press.

Flannery, R. B., & Flannery, G. J. (1990). Sense of coherence, life stress, and psychological distress: A prospective methodological inquiry. *Journal of Clinical Psychology, 46*(4), 415–420.

Frankl, V. E. (1959). *Man's search for meaning.* Hodder & Stoughton.

Frankl, V. E. (2010). *Logotherapie und Existenzanalyse. Texte aus sechs Jahrzehnten* [Logotherapy and existential analysis. Texts from six decades]. Beltz.

Grawe, K., Donati, R., & Bernauer, F. (2001). *Psychotherapie im Wandel. Von der Konfession zur Profession* [Psychotherapy in transition. From confession to profession] (5th ed.). Hogrefe.

Grawe, K., & Grawe-Gerber, M. (1999). Ressourcenaktivierung. Ein primäres Wirkprinzip der Psychotherapie [Resource activation: A primary change principle in psychotherapy]. *Psychotherapeut, 44*, 63–73.

Hayes, S. C., Strosahl, K. D., & Wilson, K. G. (1999). *Acceptance and commitment therapy: An experiential approach to behavior change.* Guilford Press.

Helgeson, V. S., Reynolds, K. A., & Tomich, P. L. (2006). A meta-analytic review of benefit finding and growth. *Journal of Consulting Clinical Psychology, 74*(5), 797–816.

Herschbach, P. (2002). Das "Zufriedenheitsparadox" in der Lebensqualitätsforschung [The "Well-being Paradox" in quality-of-life research]. *Psychotherapie·Psychosomatik Medizinische Psychologie, 52*(03/04), 141–150.

Iasiello, M., Van Agteren, J., & Muir-Cochrane, E. (2020). Mental health and/or mental illness: A scoping review of the evidence and implications of the dual-continua model of mental health. *Evidence Base, 1*, 1–45. https://doi.org/10.21307/eb-2020-001

Jacobson, N., & Curtis, L. (2000). Recovery as policy in mental health services: Strategies emerging from the states. *Psychiatric Rehabilitation Journal, 23*(4), 333–341.

Kallus, K. W. (2016a). Stress and recovery: An overview. In K. W. Kallus & M. Kellmann (Eds.), *The Recovery-Stress Questionnaires: User manual* (pp. 27–48). Pearson Assessment.

Kallus, K. W. (2016b). RESTQ-Basic: The general version of the RESTQ. In K. W. Kallus & M. Kellmann (Eds.), *The Recovery-Stress Questionnaires: User manual* (pp. 49–85). Pearson Assessment.

Karimi, M., & Brazier, J. (2016). Health, health-related quality of life, and quality of life: What is the difference? *PharmacoEconomics, 34*, 645–649.

Kellmann, M. (2002). Underrecovery and overtraining: Different concepts – Similar impact? In M. Kellmann (Ed.), *Enhancing recovery: Preventing underperformance in athletes* (pp. 3–24). Human Kinetics.

Kellmann, M., Bertollo, M., Bosquet, L., Brink, M., Coutts, A., Duffield, R., Erlacher, D., Halson, S., Hecksteden, A., Heidari, J., Kallus, K. W., Meeusen, R., Mujika, I., Robazza, C., Skorski, S., Venter, R., & Beckmann, J. (2018). Recovery and performance: Consensus statement. *International Journal of Sports Physiology and Performance, 13*, 240–245.

Kellmann, M., & Kallus, K. W. (2001). *The Recovery-Stress Questionnaire for Athletes. User manual.* Human Kinetics.

Keyes, C. L. (2005). Mental illness and/or mental health? Investigating axioms of the complete state model of health. *Journal of Consulting Clinical Psychology, 73*(3), 539–548.

Kleinman, A. (1988). *Rethinking psychiatry: From cultural category to personal experience.* Free Press.

Klinger, E. (2017). The search for meaning in evolutionary goal-theory perspective and its clinical implications. In P. T. P. Wong (Ed.), *The human quest for meaning: Theories, research, and applications* (2nd ed., pp. 23–56). Routledge.

Krok, D. (2016). Can meaning buffer work pressure? An exploratory study on styles of meaning in life and burnout in firefighters. *Archives of Psychiatry and Psychotherapy, 18*, 31–42.

Kuhl, J., & Beckmann, J. (1994). Alienation. Ignoring one's preferences. In J. Kuhl & J. Beckmann (Eds.), *Volition and personality: Action and state orientation* (pp. 375–390). Hogrefe.

Leventhal, H., Idler, E. L., & Leventhal, E. A. (1999). The impact of chronic illness on the self system. In R. J. Contrada & R. D. Ashmore (Eds.), *Self, social identity, and physical health: Interdisciplinary explorations* (pp. 185–208). Oxford University Press.

Leventhal, H., Brissette, I., & Leventhal, E. A. (2003). The common-sense model of self-regulation of health and illness. In L. D. Cameron & H. Leventhal (Eds.), *The self-regulation of health and illness behaviour* (pp. 42–65). Routledge.

Li, J.-B., Dou, K., & Liang, Y. (2021). The relationship between presence of meaning, search for meaning, and subjective well-being: A three-level meta-analysis based on the Meaning in Life Questionnaire. *Journal of Happiness Studies*, *22*(1), 467–489.

Lundquist, C. (2021). Well-being and quality of life. In R. Arnold & D. Fletcher (Eds.), *Stress, well-being, and performance in sport* (pp. 131–147). Routledge.

Mascaro, N., & Rosen, D. H. (2005). Existential meaning's role in the enhancement of hope and prevention of depressive symptoms. *Journal of Personality*, *73*(4), 985–1013.

Maslow, A. H. (1968). *Toward a psychology of being* (2nd ed.). Van Nostrand.

Masten, A. S., & Narayan, A. J. (2012). Child development in the context of disaster, war, and terrorism: Pathways of risk and resilience. *Annual Review of Psychology*, *63*, 227–257.

Mierswa, T., & Kellmann, M. (2015). The influences of recovery for low back pain development: A theoretical model. *International Journal of Occupational Medicine and Environmental Health*, *28*(2), 253–262.

Morea, J. M., Friend, R., & Bennett, R. M. (2008). Conceptualizing and measuring illness self-concept: A comparison with self-esteem and optimism in predicting fibromyalgia adjustment. *Research in Nursing & Health*, *31*(6), 563–575.

Moons, P., Van Deyk, K., Marquet, K., Raes, E., De Bleser, L., Budts, W., & De Geest, S. (2005). Individual quality of life in adults with congenital heart disease: A paradigm shift. *European Heart Journal*, *26*(3), 298–307.

Morrill, E. F., Brewer, N. T., O'Neill, S. C., Lillie, S. E., Dees, E. C., Carey, L. A., & Rimer, B. K. (2008). The interaction of post-traumatic growth and post-traumatic stress symptoms in predicting depressive symptoms and quality of life. *Psychooncology*, *17*(9), 948–953.

Nahlén Bose, C., Elfström, M. L., Björling, G., Persson, H., & Saboonchi, F. (2016). Patterns and the mediating role of avoidant coping style and illness perception on anxiety and depression in patients with chronic heart failure. *Scandinavian Journal of Caring Sciences*, *30*(4), 704–713.

National Health Council. (2014). *About chronic diseases*. Retrieved May 12, 2023 from http://www.nationalhealthcouncil.org/sites/default/files/AboutChronicDisease.pdf

Neff, D. F., & Olsen, W. K. (2007). Measuring subjective well-being from a realist viewpoint. *Methodological Innovations Online*, *2*, 44–66.

Olsen, G. I. & Schober, B. I. (1993). The satisfied poor. Development of an intervention-oriented theoretical framework to explain satisfaction with a life in poverty. *Social Indicators Research*, *28*, 173–193.

Oris, L., Luyckx, K., Rassart, J., Goubert, L., Goossens, E., Apers, S., Arat, S., Vandenberghe, J., Westhovens, R., & Moons, P. (2018). Illness identity in adults with a chronic illness. *Journal of Clinical Psychology in Medical Settings*, *25*(4), 429–440.

Peterson, C., Park, N., & Sweeney, P. J. (2008). Group well-being: Morale from a positive psychology perspective. *Applied Psychology: An International Review*, *57*(Suppl. 1), 19–36.

Post, M. (2014). Definitions of quality of life: What has happened and how to move on. *Topics in Spinal Cord Injury Rehabilitation*, *20*(3), 167–180.

Renshaw, T. L., & Cohen, A. S. (2014). Life satisfaction as a distinguishing indicator of college student functioning: Further validation of the two-continua model of mental health. *Social Indicators Research*, *117*(1), 319–334.

Richardson, G. E. (2002). The metatheory of resilience and resiliency. *Journal of Clinical Psychology*, *58*(3), 307–321.

Riethof, N., & Bob, P. (2019). Burnout syndrome and logotherapy: Logotherapy as useful conceptual framework for explanation and prevention of burnout. *Frontiers in Psychiatry*, 10, 382. https://doi.org/10.3389/fpsyt.2019.00382

Rutter, M. (1987). Psychosocial resilience and protective mechanisms. *American Journal of Orthopsychiatry*, 57, 316–331.

Ryan, R. M., & Deci, E. L. (2017). *Self-determination theory: Basic psychological needs in motivation, development and wellness.* Guilford Press.

Ryff, C. D. (1989). Happiness is everything, or is it? Explorations on the meaning of psychological wellbeing. *Journal of Personality and Social Psychology*, 57(6), 1069–1081.

Ryff, C. D., & Singer, B. H. (2008). Know thyself and become what you are: A eudaimonic approach to psychological wellbeing. *Journal of Happiness Studies*, 9, 13–39.

Sam, D. L., Vedder, P., Liebkind, K., Neto, F., & Virta, E. (2008). Immigration, acculturation and the paradox of adaptation in Europe. *European Journal of Developmental Psychology*, 5, 138–158.

Seery, M. D., Holman, E. A., & Silver, R. C. (2010). Whatever does not kill us: Cumulative lifetime adversity, vulnerability, and resilience. *Journal of Personality and Social Psychology*, 99(6), 1025–1041.

Seligman, M. (2012). *Flourish: A visionary new understanding of happiness and well-being.* Simon & Schuster.

Sharpe, D., & Viney, I. (1973). Weltanschauung and the Purpose-in-life Test. *Journal of Clinical Psychology*, 29(4), 489–491.

Stanton, A. L., & Revenson, T. A. (2007). Adjustment to chronic disease: Progress and promise in research. In H. S. Friedman & R. C. Silver (Eds.), *Foundations of health psychology* (pp. 203–233). Oxford University Press.

Steger, M. F., & Frazier, P. (2005). Meaning in life: One link in the chain from religion to well-being. *Journal of Counseling Psychology*, 52, 574–582.

Steger, M. F., Kashdan, T. B., Sullivan, B. A., & Lorentz, D. (2008). Understanding the search for meaning in life: Personality, cognitive style, and the dynamic between seeking and experiencing meaning. *Journal of Personality*, 76, 199–228.

Stutzer, A. (2004). The role of income aspirations in individual happiness. *Journal of Economic Behavior and Organization*, 54, 89–109.

Swift, H. J., Vauclair, C.-M., Abrams, D., Bratt, C., Marques, S., & Lima, M.-L. (2014). Revisiting the paradox of well-being: The importance of national context. *Journals of Gerontology Series B: Psychological Sciences and Social Sciences*, 69(6), 920–929.

Szedlak, C., Smith, M. J., & Callary, B. (2021). Developing a 'letter to my younger self' to learn from the experiences of expert coaches. *Qualitative Research in Sport, Exercise, and Health*, 13(4), 569–585.

Tedeschi, R. G., & Calhoun, L. G. (2004). Posttraumatic growth: Conceptual foundations and empirical evidence. *Psychological Inquiry*, 15(1), 1–18.

Tomich, P. L., & Helgeson, V. S. (2004). Is finding something good in the bad always good? Benefit finding among women with breast cancer. *Health Psychology*, 23(1), 16–23.

Tuccero, D., Railey, K., Briggs, M., & Hull, S. K. (2016). Behavioral health in prevention and chronic illness management: Motivational interviewing. *Primary Care: Clinics in Office Practice*, 43(2), 191–202.

Van Bulck, L., Goossens, E., Luyckx, K., Oris, L., Apers, S., & Moons, P. (2018). Illness identity: A novel predictor for healthcare use in adults with congenital heart disease.

Journal of the American Heart Association, 7(11), e008723. https://doi.org/10.1161/JAHA.118.008723

Van Bulck, L., Luyckx, K., Goossens, E., Oris, L., & Moons, P. (2019). Illness identity: Capturing the influence of illness on the person's sense of self. *European Journal of Cardiovascular Nursing*, *18*(1), 4–6.

Westerhof, G., & Keyes, C. L. (2010). Mental illness and mental health: The two continua model across the lifespan. *Journal of Adult Development*, *17*, 110–119.

Wilson, I. B., & Cleary, P. D. (1995). Linking clinical variables with health-related quality of life. A conceptual model of patient outcomes. *Journal of the American Medical Association*, *273*, 59–65.

World Health Organization. (1946). *Constitution of the World Health Organization*. Retrieved February 16, 2023 from https://apps.who.int/gb/bd/PDF/bd47/EN/constitution-en.pdf?ua=1

World Health Organization. (2019). *Recovery practices for mental health and well-being: WHO Quality rights core training: Mental health and social services: Course guide*. Retrieved June 21, 2022 from https://apps.who.int/iris/handle/10665/329602

2 Off-job and on-job recovery as predictors of employee health

Jan de Jonge and Toon W. Taris

Introduction

The world of work is constantly changing. More and more employees are experiencing escalating demands at work. Digitisation (Hu et al., 2021), flexibilisation of work schedules and work places (Shifrin & Michel, 2022), and changes in values and attitudes toward work and life (Smith et al., 2022) have implications for how employees will, can and should recover from work. Moreover, information and communication technology (ICT) allows people to work anytime and anywhere, which makes them available for work 24 hours, seven days a week. As a result, work demands such as extended working days, work pressure and blurred work-private boundaries are accelerating. Work stress research has shown that this kind of work demands are becoming increasingly problematic (van Veldhoven, 2024). A negative consequence of high work demands and overtime work is that employees' off-work time is shortened as well as its recovery potential. The toll employees pay for this is expressed in increased health-related risks such as burnout, depression, poor performance, intention to leave, and sickness absenteeism (for an overview, see Peeters et al., 2024).

While there is mounting evidence on the health-related consequences of high work demands, less attention has been paid to the role of recovery from work demands and work-related stress (Sonnentag et al., 2022). Moreover, when employees experience high work demands, they tend to detach less from their work during off-job time, they engage less in physical activity, which is associated with more health problems. Understanding how employees recover from work is therefore commensurately important. Several research omissions can be mentioned here. First, while there is ample research on recovery from work such as recovery activities after work, weekends, vacations and sabbaticals in relation to employee health, less research has investigated recovery *during* the work day

de Jonge, J., & Taris, T. W. (2024). Off-job and on-job recovery as predictors of employee health. In M. Kellmann & J. Beckmann (Eds.), *Fostering Recovery and Wellbeing in a Healthy Lifestyle: Psychological, Somatic, and Organizational Prevention Approaches* (pp. 24–37). Routledge.

DOI: 10.4324/9781003250654-3

(Chan et al., 2022). This is remarkable, considering that people spend anywhere from a third to a half of their day working (Lyubykh et al., 2022). During this time, they are likely to have formally scheduled breaks such as coffee or lunch breaks, as well as various types of informal (mini-)breaks such as a toilet visit or a chat with a colleague to socialise. Second, even fewer studies have been conducted that investigated off-job recovery and on-job recovery simultaneously. Last but not least, the type of recovery seems to be important for effective recovery as well, such as cognitive, emotional, and physical detachment from work (de Jonge et al., 2012). For this reason, the present chapter aims to understand how different dimensions of both off-job recovery and on-job recovery can benefit employees and organisations through improved employee health. Employee health refers here to the overall health status of employees in the workplace, encompassing physical, emotional, and cognitive health (de Jonge & Dormann, 2003).

This chapter starts by explaining the recovery from work concept and presenting three prominent theoretical frameworks used in recovery research. We introduce the distinction between off-job and on-job recovery, and then focus on the recovery concept of detachment from work. Moreover, we review the research evidence of their impact on health outcomes. Next, we present findings of an empirical study that combined both types of recovery in the prediction of employee health. The chapter ends with an overall summary of findings and their implications for today's practice.

Theoretical perspectives on recovery from work

Recovery from work can generally be defined as a dynamic process of unwinding and restoration during which an employee's functioning and stressful experiences return to their pre-stress levels (i.e., how far one's 'battery' is charged at the end of the recovery process; Sonnentag et al., 2022). Generally, recovery can take two functions (Heidari et al., 2022). First, recovery can be considered the reverse of the stress process, in which detrimental effects of demanding and stressful situations are at least alleviated or eliminated (i.e., this involves a more passive process). Second, recovery can also be (pro-)active, in that it involves the use of coping strategies to compensate (i.e., buffer) stressful experiences. In this stage, recovery can act as a self-regulatory mechanism.

To understand how and when recovery occurs as well as what makes a complete recovery, we will look through the lenses of three theoretical frameworks; that is, the *Conservation of Resources (COR) Theory* (Hobfoll, 1998, 2002), the *Effort-Recovery (E-R) Model* (Meijman & Mulder, 1998), and the *Stressor-Detachment (S-D) Model* (Sonnentag & Fritz, 2015). These frameworks generally assume that an employee's reservoir of resources may be depleted during and after a work day, which makes recovery necessary. According to Hobfoll's (1998, 2002) *COR Theory*, resources generally refer to external entities such as objects (e.g., housing situation) or conditions (e.g., job autonomy), to personal characteristics (e.g., self-esteem), and to energies (e.g., vigour). In this context, Hunter and Wu (2016) mentioned *human energy* as the cornerstone resource for recovery. Human energy entails physical energy (i.e., the physical capacity to do the job) and energetic activation (i.e., the degree to which people feel energised to do the job). In addition to energy, Quinn and associates (2012) have also identified motivation and concentration as key to the process of resource production and depletion.

Unfortunately, energy, motivation, and concentration resources are not unlimited but rather function like batteries that periodically need recharging (Hunter & Wu, 2016). The *E-R Model* proposes that these resources are expended and recharged by the opposite stress processes of reactivity and recovery. Reactivity refers to the immediate physiological and psychological reactions to work demands. In the case physiological and psychological systems are sustained activated, mental and physical effort drains resources and may lead to negative health outcomes such as concentration problems, depressive feelings and fatigue. For that very reason, energy management during and after a working day is a constant challenge for employees (Steidle et al., 2017). If recovery through effective energy management is successful, employee health and performance will return to their baseline. If not, health and performance will be affected and the employee starts the next working day in a suboptimal state. The three theoretical frameworks further propose that successful recovery can be reached in the following ways. First, according to the *E-R Model* and *S-D Model*, work imposes certain demands on employees. To meet them, resources will be expended. Recovery usually occurs when these demands are interrupted (e.g., during a work break) or end (after work). Employees are then able to replenish their resources and successfully recover from work. Second, according to *COR Theory*, recovery can be obtained by investing in new resources during leisure time such as learning new skills or engaging in leisure activities that positively contribute to an employee's self-esteem. Consequently, employees are better able to deal with future work demands. To summarise, the *E-R Model* describes the recovery process as a reduction of strain built up in the stress process because of effort invested to deal with demands at work. Next to strain reduction, building new personal resources is a central facet of successful work-stress recovery as explained by *COR Theory*.

Finally, the effectiveness of recovery during or after work also depends on the type of recovery activities people perform during this time, and how they perceive these activities (Trougakos & Hideg, 2009). Sonnentag and Fritz (2015) proposed the *Stressor-Detachment (S-D) Model* that emphasises the important role of *psychological detachment* in the work stress process. This model emphasises that it is not primarily the acute stress–reaction that is detrimental for an employee but rather the sustained activation (Ursin & Olff, 1993; see also Brosschot et al., 2006). Essential to this phenomenon is that the activation of psycho-physiological systems in response to exertion does not cease immediately upon completion of exposure. Increased psycho-physiological activation persists because the regulatory mechanisms responsible for de-activation are put out of action by higher mechanisms in the central nervous system. For instance, people continue to ruminate about their work demands during the night which impairs sleep. In general, the *S-D Model* proposes that work stressors impair psychological detachment and, in turn, poor psychological detachment influences employee health and well-being. Thus, low psychological detachment from work during off-job time is seen as a mechanism that can explain why work stressors such as work demands that are experienced as being too high lead to elevated levels of work-related strain.

Off-job and on-job recovery

De Bloom et al. (2015) argued that off-job and on-job recovery are distinctive yet complementary to each other, as each takes place in different contexts and at different times and might have differing impacts on employee health. Off-job recovery usually takes place outside the workplace setting and/or after set work hours, whereas on-job recovery usually occurs at a physical workplace or during dedicated work hours (Chan et al., 2022). However, distinguishing both types of recovery in this particular way is accompanied with two remarks (Chan et al., 2022). First, what actually is the 'workplace' is becoming more difficult to define, as the boundary between work and home is becoming more and more blurred. Nowadays, and particularly during and after the COVID-19 pandemic, more employees work outside traditional workspaces. Moreover, the mental distinction between work and home life has become more diffuse and flexible (Kelliher et al., 2019). Second, both off-job and on-job recovery seem to share identical psychological mechanisms for recovery, whether recovery is studied within a workplace context or else (such as home or sports). It seems highly unlikely that employees develop separate recovery mechanisms with regard to off-job and on-job contexts. So, the psychological and physiological experience of energy loss and recovery function is viewed as a single system, regardless of where the straining forces come from. For that very reason, Chan et al. (2022) concluded that the psychological and physiological mechanisms of the recovery process are functionally equivalent regardless of context. Their conclusion has implications for recovery research as it might indicate that much of our understanding of off-job and on-job recovery is directly transferable between these contexts.

Detachment from work and its effects on employee health

The present chapter focuses on the recovery concept of *detachment from work*. Detachment can be seen as the most central diversionary strategy as far as job-related recovery is concerned (Balk, this volume, Chapter 4; Sonnentag & Geurts, 2009). Etzion et al. (1998) defined detachment from work as an "individual's sense of being away from the work situation" (p. 579). It is an experience of leaving one's work behind during work breaks or after work has been done (i.e., 'switching completely off'). Low detachment from work implies that the functional psycho-physiological systems) remain in a state of sustained activation.

To recover from high work demands, Geurts and Sonnentag (2006) suggested that it is important that employees engage in recovery activities that appeal to other bodily systems than those used at work, or do not engage at all in effort-related activities. In a similar vein, Kallus and Kellmann (2000) pointed out that a change of systems is crucial for efficient recovery. For instance, an employee whose job requires high emotional effort would be better off avoiding engagement in recovery activities that put high demands on the same (i.e., emotional) systems. Similarly, a construction worker with a highly demanding physical job would be better off avoiding engagement in recovery activities that put high demands on the same (i.e., physical) systems. In this context, several authors assume that detachment from work should encompass cognitive, emotional, and physical absence from work (de Jonge et al., 2012; Geurts & Sonnentag, 2006). Further, they propose that a full degree of off-job and on-job recovery is attained when the employee feels that both cognitive and emotional as well as physical systems called upon during work have returned to their baseline levels during work breaks and after work. This implies that a completely detached employee is able to stop thinking about work-related issues ('cognitive detachment'), is no longer bothered by work-related negative emotions ('emotional detachment') and is able to shake off physical exertion from work ('physical detachment').

Generally, detachment from work can be further split into detachment *after* and *during* work. Empirical evidence for the beneficial effects of detachment *after* work on employee health have been extensively reported in the literature (Sonnentag et al., 2022; Wendsche & Lohmann-Haislah, 2017). For instance, a meta-analytical study by Wendsche and Lohmann-Haislah (2017) indicated positive associations between detachment after work and employee health. More specifically, empirical research studies on detachment after work showed that employees who fully detach after work report less psychological and physical health problems (Shimazu et al., 2012), less emotional exhaustion (Fritz et al., 2010), and better subjective health (de Bloom et al., 2015).

With respect to detachment *during* work, a systematic review and meta-analysis by Albulescu et al. (2022) revealed that micro-breaks are efficient in boosting high levels of vigour and alleviating fatigue. Another systematic review on work breaks by Lyubykh et al. (2022) indicated that a lack of, or incomplete, work breaks are related to higher levels of stress, increased emotional exhaustion, cognitive irritation, and sleeping problems. In addition, a small number of research studies on detachment during work breaks demonstrated that relaxing lunch breaks were related to less somatic health symptoms (Hunter & Wu, 2016), less fatigue (Trougakos et al., 2014), and less emotional exhaustion (Bosch et al., 2018; Sianoja et al., 2018). Last but not least, several studies on detachment from work have included the role of sleep. Sleep seems to be essential to complete the recovery process to a large extent (Kullik & Kiel, this volume, Chapter 10). For example, Clinton et al. (2017) detected a positive association between detachment from work and sleep quality. A study by Cropley and his team (2006) showed that the inability to stop thinking about work issues during off-job time was related with more sleep problems. In a quasi-experimental study with a recovery experience training program, Hahn et al. (2011) revealed that training participants showed higher psychological detachment one to three weeks after the training. In addition, training participants showed also a better sleep quality several weeks after the training. Thus, it may be concluded that sleep problems can be considered key outcomes of insufficient recovery, too (Kullik & Kiel, this volume, Chapter 10).

Empirical study

To illustrate the theoretical part of this chapter, we highlight a pre-pandemic empirical study that combined both on-job and off-job recovery as predictors of employee health (de Jonge, 2020). Specifically, this study tried to disentangle the particular role of different detachment dimensions (i.e., cognitive, emotional, physical) both after work and during work on employee health. Based on the theoretical arguments and empirical findings discussed earlier, it was hypothesised that detachment after work as well as detachment during work are both positively associated with employee health. Relations between the two contexts in terms of their mutual prediction of employee health are often neither specified nor adequately studied (Chan et al., 2022; Sonnentag et al., 2017). Furthermore, we are not aware of any research study that *simultaneously* investigated detachment after work and detachment during work in relation to the three detachment dimensions expressed earlier (i.e., cognitive, emotional, and physical). To further develop off-job and on-job recovery research, it is necessary to investigate the two contexts simultaneously to outline their commonalities and distinctions. So, this study explored the following research question: What kind of detachment (i.e., after work or during work) and which detachment dimensions (i.e., cognitive, emotional, physical) are associated with employee health?

An online cross-sectional survey study was performed in a general hospital in the Netherlands. In total, 541 health care employees of nine different departments received a questionnaire, and 368 people returned it (68.0% response rate). Most of them were nurses or nurses' aides (37.4%), laboratory staff (28.6%), and operating room assistants (22.8%). The remaining people were administration staff (3.8%), managers (3.6%), 'else' (2.7%), and doctors (1.1%). Demographics showed that 81.9% of the participants were female, and 18.1% were male. Mean age was 44.5 years (SD = 11.4) with an empirical range of 20 to 63 years. Most of the employees had finished higher vocational education (55.1%). Finally, 54.5% of them worked at least 32 hours (i.e., four days) per week. Mean working time was 29.7 hours per week (SD = 7.5), and 69.6% of them worked irregular shifts.

The measures used in this study were derived from earlier, well-validated, scales that are presented in Table 2.1. Internal consistencies (Cronbach's Alpha) ranged from α = .61 to α = .95. Example items of detachment after work were "After work, I put all thoughts of work aside" (cognitive), "After work, I put all emotions from work aside" (emotional), and "After work, I shake off the physical exertion from work" (physical).

Table 2.1 Measures of the cross-sectional survey study (N = 368).

Measure	# Items	Scale range	Cronbach's α / Pearson's r/p
Off-job recovery (de Jonge et al., 2012)			
- Cognitive detachment after work	3	1 – 5	α = .79
- Emotional detachment after work	3	1 – 5	α = .77
- Physical detachment after work	4	1 – 5	α = .75
On-job recovery (de Jonge et al., 2012)			
- Cognitive detachment during work	1	1 – 5	
- Emotional detachment during work	1	1 – 5	
- Physical detachment during work	1	1 – 5	
Concentration problems (Meijman, 1991)	4	1 – 5	α = .95
Emotional exhaustion (Schaufeli & van Dierendonck, 2000)	5	1 – 7	α = .87
Depressive feelings (Spitzer et al., 1994)	2	1 – 3	r = .63, p < .001
Sleep problems (Appels et al., 1987)	3	1 – 3	α = .61
Physical health problems (Hildebrandt & Douwes, 1991)	4	1 – 3	α = .73

Off-job and on-job recovery as predictors of health

Hierarchical multiple regression analyses (controlled for demographics) were used to examine the associations between 1) detachment after and during work, and 2) employee health outcomes (Table 2.2). The six detachment variables were stepwise entered in the regression model to detect those accounting for the most variance in the respective health outcome. This procedure continued until adding predictors did not contribute anything to the regression model anymore. Standardised beta-weights (β) and their significance for respective predictor variables were presented.

As far as *off-job recovery* is concerned, stepwise entering detachment after work in the second step of the regression analysis revealed that both cognitive and physical detachment after work contributed to the explanation of concentration problems. Furthermore, emotional and physical detachment after work contributed to the explanation of emotional exhaustion, while only emotional detachment contributed to the explanation of depressive feelings. With regard to sleep problems, both emotional and physical detachment after work contributed to their explanation. Finally, only physical detachment after work contributed to the explanation of physical health problems. All these findings indicated that the higher the detachment after work was, the less health problems were reported by employees.

As far as *on-job recovery* is concerned, stepwise entering detachment during work in the second step of the analysis showed that *none* of the 'detachment during work' predictors contributed to the explanation of the five health outcomes. In other words, employee health was not affected by detachment during work in this study.

Table 2.2 Stepwise regression analyses of employee health with detachment after and during work as predictor variables.

	Concentration problems	Emotional exhaustion	Depressive feelings	Sleep problems	Physical health problems
	β	β	β	β	β
Detachment from work					
Cognitive detachment after work	-0.12*				
Emotional detachment after work		-0.22***	-0.16**	-0.16**	
Physical detachment after work	-0.15**	-0.25***		-0.14*	-0.30***
Cognitive detachment during work					
Emotional detachment during work					
Physical detachment during work					
Model F test	$F_{(7,360)} =$ 4.33***	$F_{(7,360)} =$ 9.79***	$F_{(6,361)} =$ 3.93***	$F_{(7,360)} =$ 7.31***	$F_{(6,361)} =$ 6.72***

Note: $N = 368$; adapted from de Jonge (2020); * $p < .05$; ** $p < .01$; *** $p < .001$ (two-tailed).

Conclusions and recommendations for practice

This chapter highlight the concept of recovery from work and discussed associations between off-job and on-job recovery and employee health. We focused on the central recovery concept of *detachment from work* that can be split into 1) detachment after and during work, and 2) cognitive, emotional, and physical detachment. Detachment after work and detachment during work are distinctive yet complementary to each other, as each take place in different contexts (i.e., outside or at the workplace), at different times, and might have separate impacts on employee health. However, what actually is the 'workplace' is becoming more difficult to define nowadays, as the boundary between work and home is more and more blurred. In addition, the mental distinction between work and home life has become more diffuse and flexible. Finally, both types of detachment seem to share identical psychological mechanisms for recovery, whether recovery is studied within a workplace context or else (e.g., home or sports).

Systematic reviews, meta-analyses and distinctive empirical research studies indicated beneficial effects of detachment after and during work on employee health. However, relations between the two contexts in terms of their mutual prediction of employee health are often neither specified nor adequately studied (Chan et al., 2022; Sonnentag et al., 2017). Furthermore, there exists no research study that simultaneously investigated detachment after and during work in relation to different detachment dimensions (i.e., cognitive, emotional, physical). To further develop off-job and on-job recovery research, it is necessary to investigate the two contexts to outline the commonalities and distinctions between them. For that very reason, we highlighted a pre-pandemic empirical study that combined both on-job and off-job recovery as predictors of employee health, as well as three different dimensions of detachment from work. The goal was to understand how different dimensions of both detachment after work and detachment during work breaks (i.e., cognitive, emotional, physical) can benefit employees and organisations through improved individual health. Results demonstrate that when employees experienced more cognitive detachment after work, they reported less concentration problems. Second, when employees experienced more emotional detachment after work, they reported less feelings of emotional exhaustion, less depressive feelings, and less sleep problems. Finally, in the case employees experienced more physical detachment after work, they reported less concentration problems, less feelings of emotional exhaustion, less sleep problems and less physical health problems. Overall, results demonstrated empirical support for the positive associations between detachment *after* work and employee health. However, no support was found for additional significant associations between detachment *during* work and employee health.

The findings of the example study advance recovery research in several ways. First, this study shows that the *E-R Model* (Meijman & Mulder, 1998), *COR Theory* (Hobfoll, 1998, 2002), and the *S-D Model* (Sonnentag & Fritz, 2015) are helpful and beneficial for understanding detachment after work and detachment during work breaks. In sum, the entire recovery process includes both strain recovery and resource recovery. Whereas strain recovery (i.e., the unwinding of psycho-physiological systems as depicted in the *E-R Model*) is thought to occur automatically (more like a passive process), for resource recovery (i.e., the restoration and building of personal resources according to *COR Theory*), the active investment of other resources is required (Venz et al., 2024). Whereas this process of work-stress recovery implies that recovery is more important in the case of higher job demands and higher job strain, the *S-D Model* suggests that recovery is most difficult when demands and strain are highest. In other words, low psychological detachment from work implies that strain will not be sufficiently reduced because the psycho-physiological systems remain activated. In the worst case, job-related strain may even increase (i.e., one's 'battery' is not recharged but emptied even further). Altogether, the three frameworks complement each other in describing the work-rest cycle of recovery. At the end of a successful recovery process, job-related strain is reduced, psycho-physiological systems are back to baseline, and depleted resources are restored. On top of that, possibly additional resources are built, such that people reach a state of being recovered as well as full of new resources. Furthermore, the current study extends these frameworks by focusing on three different detachment dimensions: cognitive, emotional, and physical detachment from work. Introducing and exploring these three dimensions demonstrated a promising avenue for examining off-job and on-job recovery. Study findings show an interesting pattern: cognitive detachment after work was associated with cognitive health (i.e., concentration problems), emotional detachment after work with emotional health (i.e., emotional exhaustion), and physical detachment after work with physical health (i.e., physical health problems). Several researchers have argued that the associations between detachment and outcomes largely depend on the respective types of detachment and corresponding outcomes (Balk et al., 2019; de Jonge et al., 2012). So, it might be that specific detachment dimensions correspond to, or match, specific health outcomes to show a particular health effect. This line of thinking is referred to as the *matching hypothesis* (de Jonge & Dormann, 2006). Cognitive types of detachment from work are proposed to cause particularly cognitive types of health, whereas other areas of health (e.g., emotional health symptoms) are not likely to be affected. In other words, using the same bodily systems during work and non-work could lead to system overload and may affect an identical health outcome. Furthermore, study findings also show that physical detachment after work acted as some sort of panacea for nearly all health outcomes. Apparently, shaking off the physical exertion from work and/ or physically distancing oneself from work is in general important for employee health (de Jonge et al., 2012).

This chapter contributes to a better understanding of the simultaneous health effects of off-job and on-job recovery. Although employees in the example study reported detaching from their work during work breaks (that initially showed zero-order relations with health as well), it was *not* a significant predictor for individual health *in combination with* detachment after work. This goes against previous research demonstrating how important detachment during work breaks is for employee health (Albulescu et al., 2022). So, it seems that fully detaching from work after work has been done is more effective than detachment during work breaks in the case both types were studied simultaneously. Bosch et al. (2018) argued that complete detachment during work might be very difficult in work break settings. Formal work breaks are embedded in the work context and are mostly taken at the workplace or within the company area, and quite often still encompass contact with colleagues. In addition, formal and informal work breaks provide significantly less time for complete detachment than off-job recovery activities. Employees still have to put effort in those breaks due to, e.g., informal (work-related) talks with bosses and colleagues. These work breaks are also directly followed by new work activities, thus closer to new work demands and associated work stress.

To summarise, all these findings add to recovery research, and suggests that cognitive, emotional, and physical detachment from work after regular working hours are powerful off-job recovery experiences (i.e., rebuilding energy resources) in case of employee health.

Practical recommendations

The current findings have implications for practice as well. Modern technologies such as smartphones and social media imply that employees can and often will stay tuned to their work while having leisure time. This could create a 24/7 availability for work demands, could make boundaries between work and home obscure, and may hamper detachment from work. Given the chapter's findings that recovery from work seems to be crucial for employee health, we should uncover ways how to facilitate and improve adequate recovery from work (Kuntz, this volume, Chapter 12). First, results suggest that physical detachment after work is important for all kinds of employee health. So, physically distancing oneself from work and/or being able to shake off physical exertion from work seem to be beneficial for employees' health. Next, as regards cognitive and emotional health, findings suggest not a 'one-size-fits-all' approach, but a more nuanced view. Employees who are able to stop thinking about work-related issues may report less concentration problems. In addition, employees who are no longer bothered by work-related negative emotions may report less emotional exhaustion, less depressive feelings, and less sleep problems. The practical question is how to facilitate and improve detachment from work after work has been done? Managers and organisations play an important role here and should create a work climate in which working beyond regular work hours is not 'business as usual', as this kind of activity impedes necessary recovery processes. Managers should also act as role models by not being available during non-work time and should not contact their employees during this time as well. Further, it is important to identify not only the work-related risk factors that accompany an employee's poor recovery, but also to explore recovery opportunities during and after working hours. Employees are then able to replenish their energy resources and fully detach from work. Finally, employees should spend recovery time on activities that they like most (Hunter & Wu, 2016). For instance, ten Brummelhuis and Trougakos (2014) showed that the recovery potential is highest in case recovery activities are intrinsically motivated, and employees have fun doing them.

Taken together, research on off-job and on-job recovery has shown beneficial health effects. It has also provided insights for employees how to detach during and after work. To achieve this, managers and organisations are important to facilitate off-job and on-job recovery. Ultimately, it should encourage employees to actively engage in recovery activities, and to include this in their working lives.

References

Albulescu, P., Macsinga, I., Rusu, A., Sulea, C., Bodnaru, A., & Tulbure, B. T. (2022). "Give me a break!": A systematic review and meta-analysis on the efficacy of micro-breaks for increasing well-being and performance. *PloS One, 17*(8), e0272460. https://doi.org/10.1371/journal.pone.0272460

Appels, A., Höppener, P., & Mulder, P. (1987). A questionnaire to assess premonitory symptoms of myocardial infarction. *International Journal of Cardiology*, *17*, 15–24.

Balk, Y. A., de Jonge, J., Geurts, S. A. E., & Oerlemans, W. G. M. (2019). Antecedents and consequences of perceived autonomy support in elite sport: A diary study linking coaches' recovery and athletes' performance satisfaction. *Psychology of Sport and Exercise*, *44*, 26–34.

Bosch, C., Sonnentag, S., & Pinck, A. S. (2018). What makes for a good break? A diary study on recovery experiences during lunch break. *Journal of Occupational and Organizational Psychology*, *91*, 134–157.

Brosschot, J. F., Gerin, W., & Thayer, J. F. (2006). The perseverative cognition hypothesis: A review of worry, prolonged stress-related physiological activation, and health. *Journal of Psychosomatic Research*, *60*, 113–124.

Chan, P. H., Howard, J., Eva, N., & Herman, H. M. (2022). A systematic review of at-work recovery and a framework for future research. *Journal of Vocational Behavior*, *137*, 103747. https://doi.org/10.1016/j.jvb.2022.103747

Clinton, M. E., Conway, N., & Sturges, J. (2017). "It's tough hanging-up a call": The relationships between calling and work hours, psychological detachment, sleep quality, and morning vigor. *Journal of Occupational Health Psychology*, *22*, 28–39.

Cropley, M., Dijk, D. J., & Stanley, N. (2006). Job strain, work rumination, and sleep in school teachers. *European Journal of Work and Organizational Psychology*, *15*, 181–196.

de Bloom, J., Kinnunen, U., & Korpela, K. (2015). Recovery processes during and after work: Associations with health, work engagement, and job performance. *Journal of Occupational and Environmental Medicine*, *57*, 732–742.

de Jonge, J. (2020). What makes a good work break? Off-job and on-job recovery as predictors of employee health. *Industrial Health*, *58*(2), 142–152.

de Jonge, J., & Dormann, C. (2003). The DISC Model: Demand Induced Strain Compensation mechanisms in job stress. In M. F. Dollard, A. H. Winefield, & H. R. Winefield (Eds.), *Occupational stress in the service professions* (pp. 43–74). Taylor & Francis.

de Jonge, J., & Dormann, C. (2006). Stressors, resources, and strain at work: A longitudinal test of the triple match principle. *Journal of Applied Psychology*, *91*(6), 1359–1374.

de Jonge, J., Spoor, E., Sonnentag, S., Dormann, C., & van den Tooren, M. (2012). "Take a break?!": Off-job recovery, job demands and job resources as predictors of health, active learning, and creativity. *European Journal of Work and Organizational Psychology*, *21*(3), 321–348.

Etzion, D., Eden, D., & Lapidot, Y. (1998). Relief from job stressors and burnout: Reserve service as a respite. *Journal of Applied Psychology*, *83*, 577–585.

Fritz, C., Yankelevich, M., Zarubin, A., & Barger, P. (2010). Happy, healthy and productive: The role of detachment from work during nonwork time. *Journal of Applied Psychology*, *95*, 977–983.

Geurts, S. A. E., & Sonnentag, S. (2006). Recovery as an explanatory mechanism in the relation between acute stress reactions and chronic health impairment. *Scandinavian Journal of Work and Environmental Health*, *32*, 482–492.

Hahn, V. C., Binnewies, C., Sonnentag, S., & Mojza, E. J. (2011). Learning how to recover from job stress: Effects of a recovery training program on recovery, recovery-related self-efficacy, and well-being. *Journal of Occupational Health Psychology*, *16*, 202–216.

Heidari, J., Jakowski, S., & Kellmann, M. (2022). The value of recovery-stress monitoring for athletes' well-being. In M. Kellmann & J. Beckmann (Eds.), *Recovery and well-being in sport and exercise* (pp. 3–16). Routledge.

Hildebrandt, V. H., & Douwes, M. (1991). *Lichamelijke Belasting en Arbeid: Vragenlijst Bewegingsapparaat* [Physical demands and work: Motion questionnaire]. Dictoraat-Generaal van de Arbeid.

Hobfoll, S. E. (1998). *Stress, culture and community: The psychology and philosophy of stress.* Plenum.

Hobfoll, S. E. (2002). Social and psychological resources and adaptation. *Review of General Psychology, 6,* 307–324.

Hu, X. J., Barber, L. K., Park, Y., & Day, A. (2021). Defrag and reboot? Consolidating information and communication technology research in IO psychology. *Industrial and Organizational Psychology, 14*(3), 371–396.

Hunter, E. M., & Wu, C. (2016). Give me a better break: Choosing workday break activities to maximize resource recovery. *Journal of Applied Psychology, 101,* 302–311.

Kallus, K. W., & Kellmann, M. (2000). Burnout in athletes and coaches. In Y. Hanin (Ed.), *Emotions in sport* (pp. 209–230). Human Kinetics.

Kelliher, C., Richardson, J., & Boiarintseva, G. (2019). All of work? All of life? Reconceptualising work-life balance for the 21st century. *Human Resource Management Journal, 29*(2), 97–112.

Lyubykh, Z., Gulseren, D., Premji, Z., Wingate, T. G., Deng, C., Bélanger, L. J., & Turner, N. (2022). Role of work breaks in well-being and performance: A systematic review and future research agenda. *Journal of Occupational Health Psychology, 27*(5), 470–487.

Meijman, T. F. (1991). *Over Vermoeidheid* [About fatigue; Doctoral thesis, University of Groningen, The Netherlands]. University of Groningen research portal. Retrieved February 13, 2023 from https://hdl.handle.net/11370/7b5b160b-904b-4b08-9811-d79ad859a8fb

Meijman, T. F., & Mulder, G. (1998). Psychological aspects of workload. In P. J. D. Drenth, H. Thierry, & C. J. de Wolff (Eds.), *Handbook of work and organizational psychology* (Vol. 2, pp. 5–33). Psychology Press.

Peeters, M. C. W., de Jonge, J., & Taris, T. W. (Eds.). (2024). *An introduction to contemporary work psychology* (2nd ed.). Wiley-Blackwell.

Quinn, R. W., Spreitzer, G. M., & Lam, C. F. (2012). Building a sustainable model of human energy in organizations: Exploring the critical role of resources. *Academy of Management Annals, 6*(1), 337–396.

Schaufeli, W. B., & van Dierendonck, D. (2000). *Utrechtse Burnout Schaal (UBOS): Handleiding* [Manual Utrecht Burnout Scale: UBOS]. Swets & Zeitlinger.

Shifrin, N. V., & Michel, J. S. (2022). Flexible work arrangements and employee health: A meta-analytic review. *Work & Stress, 36*(1), 60–85.

Shimazu, A., Sonnentag, S., Kubota, K., & Kawakami, N. (2012). Validation of the Japanese version of the Recovery Experience Questionnaire. *Journal of Occupational Health, 54,* 196–205.

Sianoja, M., Syrek, C. J., de Bloom, J., Korpela, K., & Kinnunen, U. (2018). Enhancing daily well-being at work through lunchtime park walks and relaxation exercises: Recovery experiences as mediators. *Journal of Occupational Health Psychology, 23*(3), 428–442.

Smith, T. A., Butts, M. M., Courtright, S. H., Duerden, M. D., & Widmer, M. A. (2022). Work-leisure blending: An integrative conceptual review and framework to guide future research. *Journal of Applied Psychology, 107*(4), 560–580.

Sonnentag, S., Cheng, B. H., & Parker, S. L. (2022). Recovery from work: Advancing the field toward the future. *Annual Review of Organizational Psychology and Organizational Behavior, 9,* 33–60.

Sonnentag, S., & Fritz, C. (2015). Recovery from job stress: The stressor-detachment model as an integrative framework. *Journal of Organizational Behavior, 36*(S1), S72–S103.

Sonnentag, S., & Geurts, S. A. E. (2009). Methodological issues in recovery research. In S. Sonnentag, P. L. Perrewé, & D. C. Ganster (Eds.), *Current perspectives on job-stress recovery* (Vol. 7, pp. 1–36). Emerald Group Publishing Limited.

Sonnentag, S., Venz, L., & Casper, A. (2017). Advances in recovery research: What have we learned? What should be done next? *Journal of Occupational Health Psychology, 22,* 365–380.

Spitzer, R. L., Williams, J. B., Kroenke, K., Linzer, M., deGruy, F. V., Hahn, S. R., Brody, D., & Johnson, J. G. (1994). Utility of a new procedure for diagnosing mental disorders in primary care. The PRIME-MD 1000 study. *Journal of the American Medical Association, 272*(22), 1749–1756.

Steidle, A., Gonzalez-Morales, M. G., Hoppe, A., Michel, A., & O'Shea, D. (2017). Energizing respites from work: A randomized controlled study on respite interventions. *European Journal of Work and Organizational Psychology, 26*(5), 650–662.

ten Brummelhuis, L. L., & Trougakos, J. P. (2014). The recovery potential of intrinsically versus extrinsically motivated off-job activities. *Journal of Occupational and Organizational Psychology, 87,* 177–199.

Trougakos, J. P., & Hideg, I. (2009). Momentary work recovery: The role of within-day work breaks. In S. Sonnentag, P. L. Perrewé, & D. C. Ganster (Eds.), *Current perspectives on job-stress recovery* (Vol. 7, pp. 37–84). Emerald Group Publishing Limited.

Trougakos, J. P., Hideg, I., Cheng, B. H., & Beal, D. J. (2014). Lunch breaks unpacked: The role of autonomy as a moderator of recovery during lunch. *Academy of Management Journal, 57,* 405–421.

Ursin, H., & Olff, M. (1993). Psychobiology of coping and defence strategies. *Neuropsychobiology, 28*(1–2), 66–71.

van Veldhoven, M. (2024). Job demands. In M. C. W. Peeters, J. de Jonge, & T. W. Taris (Eds.), *An introduction to contemporary work psychology* (2nd ed., pp. 147–169). Wiley-Blackwell.

Venz, L., Wöhrmann, A., Vieten, L., & Michel, A. (2024). Recovery from work stress. In M. C. W. Peeters, J. de Jonge, & T. W. Taris (Eds.), *An introduction to contemporary work psychology* (2nd ed., pp. 321–344). Wiley-Blackwell.

Wendsche, J., & Lohmann-Haislah, A. (2017). A meta-analysis on antecedents and outcomes of detachment from work. *Frontiers in Psychology, 7,* 2072. https://doi.org/10.3389/fpsyg.2016.02072

3 Ambulatory Assessment for recovery and stress monitoring in the general population

Sarah Brüßler, Birte von Haaren-Mack, Anna Vogelsang, and Markus Reichert

Introduction

High-performance sport comes with enormous demands for human physical and mental capacity. Findings gained from studying elite athletes can therefore serve as a blueprint which may well translate to expedient interventions in the general population. Given that athletes, just like everybody else, have only limited resources to compensate for mismatches between stress and recovery, Kellmann (2002a) developed a model (*Scissors-Model*), which is used to describe the relationship between stress states and recovery demands. This is based on the idea of a comprehensive development of athletes where many factors must be considered to optimally coordinate training processes, to succeed in competitions, and to promote mental health. Here, not only proximal performance determinates such as training load are important, but also distal factors such as lifestyle and environmental conditions (Heidari et al., 2022). To develop strategies in using Ambulatory Assessment for research and practice while accounting for the interrelations between recovery and stress, the following chapter is based on theoretical foundations not only from the field of sport psychology, but also from occupational psychology.

The *Scissors-Model* (Kellmann, 2002a), which constitutes a state-of-the-art model in elite sports and sport psychology research, proposes that an increase in stress must be met by a simultaneous increase in recovery to keep the recovery-stress state stable. If the growing need for recovery demands is not met (e.g., because of limited resources such as time), a vicious cycle may result in an individually increasing stress experience. Conversely, optimal performance and mental health is related to a balanced recovery-stress state. According to this model, high stress levels do not necessarily negatively affect individual's mental health and performance. Instead, the higher the stressstate of a person, the more

Brüßler, S., von Haaren-Mack, B., Vogelsang, A., & Reichert, M. (2024). Ambulatory Assessment for recovery and stress monitoring in the general population. In M. Kellmann & J. Beckmann (Eds.), *Fostering Recovery and Well-being in a Healthy Lifestyle: Psychological, Somatic, and Organizational Prevention Approaches* (pp. 38–55). Routledge.

DOI: 10.4324/9781003250654-4

recovery efforts are necessary to reach the individual's optimal recovery-stress state (Kellmann, 2002a, 2010).

Besides this theory, models on the relationship between recovery and stress have been developed targeting the general population. For example, the *Effort-Recovery Model* (Meijman & Mulder, 1998) suggests that recovery or reduced recovery and the demands and stressors associated with it occur repeatedly in recovery-stress cycles that differ in length. Cycles are longer, when, for example, the recovery effect of prolonged holidays is considered, and shorter, when breaks throughout the workday are undertaken and their influence on recovery and well-being is added up at the end of the day (Sonnentag et al., 2017). Additionally, there are various other short- (i.e., daily) and long-term intraindividual varia-tions that can negatively or positively influence a person's recovery, such as (work-) family conflicts, fluctuating job demands and resources, physical or emotional pain, recovery related self-efficacy as a relatively time-stable assump-tion about the recovery possibility during certain activities or the ability of self-regulation in general (Beckmann & Kellmann, 2004; Sonnentag & Kruel, 2006; Sonnentag et al., 2022).

Based on the theoretical assumptions described above, two main approaches have emerged in occupational and organisational psychology research: The first approach, *recovery activities*, that promote recovery from work-related stress, such as physical activity, hobby or social activities with family and friends (Sonnentag et al., 2017, 2022). The second approach focuses on *recovery experiences* underly-ing these recovery activities. Here, four recovery experiences that can occur during different recovery activities are shown to be particularly influential: detachment from work, mastery, relaxation, and control (Balk, this volume, Chapter 4; Sonnentag & Fritz, 2007).

Taken together, theoretical assumptions used in elite sports and occupational approaches all underline the importance of maintaining a balance between recovery and stress, the need to conduct recovery activities, and the processual character of the interaction between recovery and stress. By additionally investi-gating recovery experiences, Sonnentag and Fritz (2007) suggest gaining more insight in underlying psychological mechanisms of these processes. Recovery has long been known in elite sport as a key factor for optimal performance and monitoring recovery and stress of athletes can be very helpful to optimally con-trol daily training load, to maintain performance capacity and health, and to prevent injury or burnout (Jakowski, 2022; Kellmann et al., 2018). Therefore, possible variables and their interrelatedness influencing recovery and stress of top athletes have been intensively researched for a long time (Kellmann, 2002b; Kellmann & Beckmann, 2022; Kellmann et al., 2018). Nowadays, new insights are gained, for example, due to the continuing improvement in data collection and evaluation methods and thus the understanding of recovery and stress pro-cesses continues to grow (Sonnentag et al., 2022).

From a holistic perspective, the overall goal is to achieve a balance between effective training stimuli and adequate rest and recovery periods (Kellmann et al., 2018). To achieve this optimal balance, it is crucial to measure the athletes' stress, recovery processes and its consequences on an individual level as accurately as possible (Coutts et al., 2022; Heidari et al., 2018). Although recovery is central to elite sport performance, athletes and coaches still face challenges in its assessment. For example, while the stress elicited from training can be objectively quantified through the given weight, the training duration, the performance or the calculated load intensity, and load volume (Bourdon et al., 2017; Heidari et al., 2019), some athletes might still report greater fatigue than others, possibly because of different mental load (Coutts et al., 2022). In addition to the objective (training) parameters, there are psychometric methods necessary to measure the recovery-stress state. A widely used questionnaire is the Recovery-Stress Questionnaire (RESTQ; Kallus, 2016) which, in addition to being used in the general population, was developed specifically for athletes (RESTQ-Sport; Kellmann & Kallus, 2016), as well as coaches, work and clinical settings, children and adolescents (Kallus & Kellmann, 2016). Seven sub-facets capture the general stress level, five facets capture general recovery in addition to specific measures, such as sport specific stress and recovery. These facets can be summarised in a profile that shows the recovery-stress balance which covers a time frame of the last three days and nights (Heidari et al., 2018; Kallus & Kellmann, 2016).

Thus far, stress, recovery, and their influencing variables as well as individual changes are not fully understood, and it remains unclear how it is possible for an athlete to attempt the next training session as refreshed as possible based on physical load only. While one athlete might perceive the demands of studying next to training as a positive challenge, another one might feel overwhelmed. To identify an optimal relationship between recovery and stress, it seems thus insufficient to measure the training load intensity and volume solely (Bourdon et al., 2017; Heidari et al., 2018; Saw et al., 2016). Every person's training and recovery attitudes are individual. Thus, the monitoring of a person's recovery and stress should therefore allow to account for dynamic changes and situation-specific intraindividual variations (e.g., contextual influences) across different temporal cycles (e.g., hours, days, weeks) and address additional complex individual influences (de Jonge & Taris, this volume, Chapter 2; Sonnentag et al., 2022).

To better understand the complex multifactorial relationship between stress, resources, recovery, and well-being in research and practice while addressing processual dynamic changes and situation-specific variations, Ambulatory Assessment has key strengths that will be introduced in the following. Two prime research examples will be exemplified, and it is discussed how already available monitoring approaches can benefit humans in their everyday life recovery processes.

Ambulatory Assessment for recovery and stress monitoring

Ambulatory Assessment (AA), also known as Ecological Momentary Assessment (EMA), is an umbrella term for a battery of assessment methods, including self-report, observational, physiological, biological, and behaviour monitoring used to study people in their everyday life (Reichert, Braun, Lautenbach, et al., 2020; Reichert, Giurgiu, et al., 2020) and has expanded rapidly over time (for an overview see Trull & Ebner-Priemer, 2020). The development and distribution of smartphones has been a game-changer for AA methods (Wilhelm et al., 2012), allowing not only to collect self-report data, but also 'passive' data through built-in sensors (e.g., video clips, audio and pictures, and geolocations through Global Positioning; Reichert, Braun, Gan, et al., 2020; Reichert, Braun, Lautenbach, et al., 2020; Reichert, Giurgiu, et al., 2020). Data collection through these methods has advantages that are particularly important for understanding the rapidly changing states of recovery and stress.

Everyday life/real life perspective

Amongst the most obvious advantages of AA methods is the ability to collect intrapersonal and environmental parameters in people's everyday life, thus AA studies are more ecologically valid compared to laboratory studies (Trull & Ebner-Priemer, 2013). In particular, given that recovery and stress represent constructs that vary constantly, the continuous monitoring is especially important and is therefore difficult to capture or replicate in the laboratory. Furthermore, to explain variations in the phenomena of interest, it is important to not only assess the phenomena itself (e.g., mood, relaxation, well-being), but also contextual characteristics such as environment, time of day, or interpersonal conflicts. AA can also be used to measure a wide range of physical stress signals, such as changes in heart rate, speech or brain activity (Can et al., 2019) while people follow their daily routine. As such, AA data provide not only intensive longitudinal but also ecologically valid data (Trull & Ebner-Priemer, 2013).

Retrospective bias

Although the argument of obtaining data in real-time or near-real-time speaks for itself, the improved measurement accuracy through AA methods over retrospective queries of events, behaviours or experiences has been scientifically demonstrated (Solhan et al., 2009; Trull & Ebner-Priemer, 2013). Researchers have often tried to illustrate dynamic processes through collecting data by means of retrospective self-reports. Retrospective questionnaires often lead to biased responses, potentially attributable to the recency effect, the mood-congruent memory effect, and the affective valence effect, all of which describe that information is more easily reproduced when it is personally relevant, occurs frequently, is particularly significant or unusual, or coincides with the current mood of the query (Mehl & Conner, 2014; Trull & Ebner-Priemer, 2013). Compared to retrospective reports, AA approaches are significantly less affected by these methodological problems (Trull & Ebner-Priemer, 2013).

Between- vs. within-person perspective

While precious cross-sectional studies in recovery and stress mainly focus on differences between persons, AA enables to assess within-subject processes.

Between-person findings and within-person processes differ conceptually, methodologically, and statistically and can therefore also differ in their direction of effect (Reichert et al., 2022). For example, psychological stress can predict both, decreased and increased physical activity (Stults-Kolehmainen & Sinha, 2014). While this ambiguous observation has been challenging researchers for decades, the ecological fallacy may account for the contradictory findings as shown by our original research (Reichert et al., 2022). In particular, the physical activity-stress association in a sample of children aged seven to eleven years reversed as a function of the analyses level. On the between-person level, children who experienced higher stress on average were the ones that were less active. However, on the within-person level and analysed within the same data, children were more active on days where they experienced more stress (Figure 3.1; Reichert et al., 2022).

By studying within-subject processes as described here, time-dynamic processes as such can be understood and studied to generate scientific findings of psychological determinants and consequences of recovery and stress in everyday life, which may serve the evidence-based development of specific recovery interventions (Zawadzki et al., 2017).

Context perspective

The relationship between context, experience, and behaviour of individuals is a relatively new field of research, since traditional survey methods, such as questionnaires, only partially allow the investigation of contextual influences. AA, on the other hand, offers the opportunity to collect context-sensitive information and to understand both behaviour and state of mind as context-dependent. Examples of captured contexts are time of day, social interactions, and the current location (e.g., via geolocation tracking), thus behaviour and experiences can be considered in the context of several environmental parameters such as population density, noise, or traffic (Reichert et al., 2018; Tost et al., 2019). In particular, it may be interesting to investigate which recovery strategies under which contextual conditions work best to recover from stress (e.g., in terms of affective states) at work, after competitions or training sessions.

When using AA methods for monitoring recovery and stress, the implementation in sport can serve as a role model for the general population. Compared to the RESTQ, which covers a period of three days (Kallus & Kellmann, 2016), the Short Recovery and Stress Scale (SRSS) is increasingly used for monitoring recovery and stress in sport (Kellmann & Kölling, 2019). The SRSS is a short version form of the Acute Recovery and Stress Scale (Kellmann & Kölling, 2019) and suitable for multiple measurements per day, a huge advantage when capturing constructs such as recovery or stress characterised by high within-subject variance and short-term variations. As an example, for monitoring recovery experiences in the general population, the Recovery Experience Questionnaire (Sonnentag & Fritz, 2007) proved to be a suitable monitoring tool in various research settings.

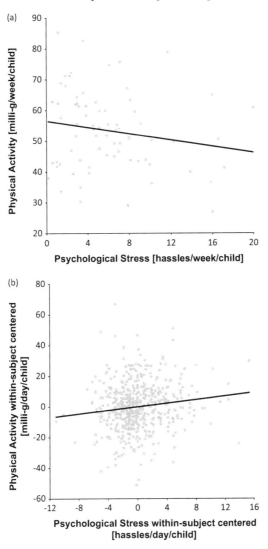

Figure 3.1 Within-person and between-person association of psychological stress and physical activity.

Note: The negative between-person (a) and positive within-person (b) association of psychological stress (PS) and physical activity (PA) in 74 children. (a) Scatterplot with regression line (black line), (b) estimated mean effect of PS on PA within the typical subject (black line). For better visualisation of the within-subject association, values on the PS (x-axis) and PA (y-axis) were centred on each subject's mean (b).

Reprinted with permission from Reichert, M., Brüßler, S., Reinhard, I., Braun, U., Giurgiu, M., Hoell, A., Zipf, A., Meyer-Lindenberg, A., Tost, H., & Ebner-Priemer, U. W. (2022). The association of stress and physical activity: Mind the ecological fallacy. *German Journal of Exercise and Sport Research, 52*(2), 282–289.

Taken together, the advantages of AA methods suggest a great potential to advance the progress of knowledge in terms of recovery and stress processes in elite sports as well as the general population. Therefore, in the following section, current research in monitoring recovery and stress in everyday life is presented.

Two prime research examples for monitoring recovery and stress in everyday life

While AA has been applied for decades in psychological studies (Trull & Ebner-Priemer, 2013), it only recently gained attention in exercise, sport, and movement sciences (Reichert, Braun, Gan, et al., 2020; Reichert, Braun, Lautenbach, et al., 2020; Reichert, Giurgiu, et al., 2020). In this field, the two most prominent lines of AA-based research looked at the association between physical activity and affective well-being (Liao et al., 2015) and the association between physical activity and stress reactivity (von Haaren et al., 2015, 2016), both of which provide valuable insights into how AA approaches can benefit the monitoring of recovery and stress.

Physical activity and affective well-being

Physical activity is well-evidenced to benefit affective well-being in cross-sectional and laboratory studies (Buecker et al., 2020). Across the last decade, AA studies were used to research the association between physical activity and affective well-being in everyday life and within persons, acknowledging the time-dynamic nature of this real-life process (Reichert et al., 2016). In essence, these studies showed that physical activity is positively related to affective well-being on a momentary level and within persons in their everyday life (Liao et al., 2015). However, and interestingly to the issue of monitoring recovery and stress, studies showed that these effects are moderated by a host of influences, for example, the intensity and duration of physical activity, contextual factors, and neurobiological underpinnings (Liao et al., 2015; Reichert et al., 2017; Reichert, Giurgiu, et al., 2020).

For example, Reichert et al. (2017) could show that exercise such as jogging, playing tennis, or soccer and non-exercise activity (NEA) such as climbing stairs, gardening, or dishwashing influenced the three basic dimensions of mood, i.e., affective valence, energetic arousal, and calmness within persons in distinct ways. While exercise was related to an increase in affective valence and calmness, NEA enhanced energetic arousal but decreased calmness. The study had been conducted in a sample of 106 adults that wore an accelerometer for continuously measuring NEA across seven days as they went about their daily routines and repeatedly reported their mood states in real time on GPS-triggered smartphone e-diaries. Translated to the recovery and stress field, Reichert et al. (2017) emphasised the need to tailor physical activity types to the momentary needs of participants to foster recovery processes.

Tost et al. (2019) investigated contextual influences on affective well-being, and they analysed how inner-city green spaces relate to affective well-being. First, AA data of 33 citizens were collected, including repeated ratings of affective valence via e-diaries on smartphones, time-stamped geolocation-tracking, and physical activity data via accelerometry. Second, geoinformatics were applied to quantify the citizens' relative green space exposure prior to AA ratings. Multilevel statistics revealed that momentary inner-city greenspace exposure was related to affective valence within citizens. The same association could be replicated in an independent sample consisting of 52 participants. Given that fMRI data had been collected within the replication study, neural correlates could be examined, revealing that participants who showed larger affective benefits from greenspace exposure reflected less activation in the dorso-lateral prefrontal cortex during the processing of negative emotion in an established fMRI-paradigm shown to robustly activate neural emotion circuitry. Interestingly, and in contrast to low-responsive individuals, these participants additionally reflected enhanced levels of trait anxiety, and they reported to spend more time at green-deprived neighbourhoods, characterised by an increased incidence of psychiatric disorders. In sum, momentary green space exposure within cities functions as resilience factor that can make up for constrained prefrontal resources (Tost et al., 2019), which in turn offers direct implications for recovery and stress in the general population.

Reichert, Braun, Gan et al. (2020) provided insights into how NEA is involved in the regulation of affective well-being. In a representative community-based sample, NEA was related to gray matter volume (GMV) of the subgenual anterior cingulate cortex (sgACC), a core region both implicated in the regulation of affect, as well as in risk for and recovery from affective disorders, which constitute a highly comorbid condition in eating disorder (Godart et al., 2007). Low ACC volumes have been repeatedly associated with affective disorders (Drevets et al., 1997; Meyer-Lindenberg & Tost, 2012). On a between-person level, in Reichert, Braun, Gan et al's. (2020) study, high NEA-levels were related to high GMV in this region, which in turn moderated the momentary energetic within-in-person benefit from NEA in humans' everyday life: Low sgACC volume predicted a stronger NEA-susceptibility, which resulted in a stronger adverse within-person influence of NEA on energy. However, it concurrently resulted in an increased energy-benefit when being active. Importantly, perceived energy was in turn positively and robustly related to affective well-being and mental health metrics. The validity of this particular and related mechanisms remains to be tested in patient groups and especially in persons with affective disorders. Translated to the field of recovery and stress, this innovative methodological approach combining AA with structural neuroimaging appears highly promising to gain neurobiological, yet ecological valid insights into neurobiological underpinnings that mediate individual recovery processes in everyday life. In sum and in the long run, the AA studies exemplified can pave the way towards evidenced-based and tailored real-life interventions informed by intensity and duration of physical activity, contextual factors, and neurobiological underpinnings.

Physical activity and stress reactivity

While the AA approach has been used in numerous studies to assess changes in affective states during the day and week as responses to daily life stressors, studies on the potential of acute, recent, and regular physical activity during daily life are still in their infancy. Thus, for example, the role of physical activity as a stress buffer and a recovery driver has yet to be proven in the real-life setting. There are very few studies that address research questions such as how physical activity during daily life moderates changes in affect as response to daily stressors. In one such approach von Haaren et al. (2016) addressed stress reactivity and recovery to stress in students. To test the cross-stressor adaptation hypothesis in a real-life setting, von Haaren et al. (2016) conducted a randomised controlled trial in 61 inactive students and used an exam period as real-life stressor. The results confirmed insights from the laboratory indicating that exercise appears to be a useful preventive strategy to buffer the effects of stress on the autonomic nervous system (Klaperski et al., 2014). Particularly, 61 inactive students were assigned into an aerobic exercise intervention and a wait list control group. Two real-life assessment periods were used for the AA approach: The pre-intervention baseline assessment was set to the beginning of the semester representing a regular academic period where students experience low stress. The post-intervention assessment was set to a real-life stressor, i.e., an academic examination period with two assessment periods (post 1 and post 2). Ambulatory ECG (36h including one night) to determine heart rate variability (HRV), physical activity and perceived stress were assessed pre- and post-intervention for a two-day period. Separate models for the night and the day were calculated to test whether the exercise intervention led to reduced physiological responses in HRV during the day and the night (recovery) during the exam period. Students of the intervention group showed reduced physiological responses during the day and night, confirming the cross-stressor hypothesis in a real-life setting (von Haaren et al., 2016).

To determine whether the same exercise intervention leads to reduced emotional stress reactivity during daily life, perceived stress and mood was assessed with an AA approach during the pre-intervention (pre) and during the exam period (post 1 and post 2). Participants rated their mood and their perceived stress during all three assessment periods over two days throughout their daily routine. Multilevel models were calculated for the pre (baseline) and both post (exam) assessment periods separately. The results showed that during the exam period, especially in moments of higher perceived stress, participants of the exercise intervention group reported lower negative affect compared to their inactive counterparts. Thus, the stress–buffer hypothesis for physical activity was confirmed in a real-life setting (von Haaren et al., 2015). While these real-life studies provide important preliminary insights into the effects of regular exercise on stress reactivity (Kallus, 2023) and recovery during daily life, many open questions remain unanswered: In particular, how regular, and daily physical activity buffers affective responses to accumulated stressors, prolonged stress periods and insufficient recovery has yet to be determined. In addition, whether physical activity, and if yes, in what form and under which circumstances, can accelerate recovery of affective responses to stress is an important future subject worth to consider.

Available monitoring approaches to potentially benefit humans in their recovery process

Although the aforementioned studies are insightful showing that the adaptation and reaction to training stimuli as well as other stressors and strains on a daily basis are highly individual, the question that remains pertains to how to transfer this science-based knowledge to the individual recovery process. To gain an optimal understanding of the intraindividual variations and its influences within the recovery-stress continuum, continuous monitoring of recovery is necessary alongside stress, its appraisal, and reactions, as well as other influencing factors such as sleep, nutrition, and social life. By systematically manipulating these factors, our understanding of intraindividual variations in recovery and stress can be expanded and potential moderators may be detected. Ultimately, each and every one of us can become the ever-learning manager of his/her own recovery process. As such, using smartphones for continuous data collection and evaluation, as already used in numerous dairy studies (Sonnentag et al., 2022), is certainly of value. Many companies have embraced the opportunity and offer apps and devices to monitor recovery and stress for the general population.

There are various, often fitness-related wearables available that offer recovery monitoring via heart rate variability (HRV) or heart rate (HR) (for example Oura[1], Garmin[2], Polar[3]). WHOOP[4] is one out of many examples for a commercial company selling its customers a combination of app and wearable, representative for many providers in the recovery and stress monitoring segment. WHOOP4.0 is a wearable wrist-based biosensor using photoplethysmography to measure HR and HRV over 24 hours a day. The generated data can be read out from the sensor and interpreted via a smartphone app. HRV describes the fluctuation of the amount of time between single heart beats and represents the ability of the heart to respond to a variety of environmental und physiological stimuli. HRV is also often used as a noninvasive physiological measure of stress because it is linked to the autonomic nervous system and allows to reflect imbalances between sympathetic and parasympathetic activity (Ernst, 2017; Kim et al., 2018; Malik et al., 1996; Thayer et al., 2012). WHOOP4.0 uses these data, in addition to the sleep duration, to predict a personal recovery score, based on a constantly learning algorithm (WHOOP, 2023). This score varies within an individual. For example, alcohol consumption negatively and physical exercise positively impacts sleep and recovery. The visualisation of the fluctuating recovery score in the app facilitates behaviour change and helps to detect parameters that have detrimental effects on recovery. WHOOP4.0 also seems to be able to assess sleep sufficiently well, provided that accurate bedtimes are entered manually in the app (Bellenger et al., 2021; Miller et al., 2020). Pre-processed individual data can be downloaded in 24-hour sections and the recovery score can, if desired, be recalculated by researchers (Khazeni, 2022). Of note, researchers should be aware that the raw data of commercial devices such as WHOOP is not accessible and therefore, it remains challenging to assess the validity of the measurements.

Besides its many advantages, systematic measurement errors have been reported that however, do not constrain the assessment of daily variations for the use in the general population. While these fitness-related wearables are reliable and insightful for personal use, provided data must be interpreted with caution, especially regarding scientific guidelines of good research due to a lack of scientific validation (Burchartz et al., 2020; Reichert, Giurgiu, et al., 2020).

In sum, to achieve accurate assessments of stress and recovery, it should be kept in mind that the interplay between recovery and stress is complex and various influencing factors (and resources) co-exist. Acknowledging a multitude of variables (e.g., mood, subjective stress, physiological markers like heart rate or hormone levels) may greatly improve prediction of recovery related outcomes (Carpenter et al., 2016). To date, commercial providers have solely focused on the measurement of physiological parameters.

Limitations and open issues

Digitisation comes with promising possibilities for monitoring recovery and stress, not only in elite sport, but also in the general population. However, there are also limitations and open issues that merit discussion.

Subjective vs. objective data on recovery and stress: An open issue

In general, whether the monitoring of recovery and stress in everyday life should rely on subjective vs. objective data or a combination of both is up to debate (Campbell & Ehlert, 2012; Can et al., 2019; Kölling & Kellmann, 2020). Here, again, professional sport may serve as an example. Daily life stressors, such as training, and increasing internal and external performance pressure may impose stress on athletes (Eccles & Kazmier, 2019; Eklund & Defreese, 2015). Besides subjective measures, objective methods such as performance, biochemical, and physiological measures are all options for monitoring athletes' recovery and well-being. While performance represents the ultimate test of readiness for competition, a daily maximum performance test is practically impossible to implement (Currell & Jeukendrup, 2008). However, with many physiological markers, such as hormone concentrations or inflammation levels, it is difficult to distinguish abnormal changes or signs of overtraining from normal reactions to intense training stimuli (Meeusen et al., 2013; Meyer et al., 2020).

A systematic review by Saw et al. (2016) comparing well-being monitoring options in relation to athletes' responses to acute and chronic training load did not find a correlation between subjective and objective measures of well-being and recovery in athletes. The authors concluded that subjective measures using questionnaires (mood, perceived stress) reflected both acute and chronic training loads more sensitively and consistently compared to objective measures such as heart rate variability, blood markers or oxygen consumption during exercise (Saw et al., 2016).

If subjective measures of changes in recovery prove to be more sensitive compared to physiological parameters in the context of professional sports, this is welcome news for monitoring one's recovery in everyday life. In research on the relationship between stress, recovery, well-being, and health from the field of occupational and organisational psychology, but also from health psychology, mainly subjective psychometric scales are used to capture the predictors and outcome variables (Bennett et al., 2018; Sonnentag et al., 2022). This type of assessment, combined with the advantages of AA methods, provides an opportunity to map one's own recovery and stress processes in a time-critical manner and thus to better understand and influence them, as well as uncover potential recovery resources.

It is important to keep in mind that subjective measurements via questionnaires as well as more objective measurements via multiple sensors worn on the body can be burdensome and may influence a person's behaviour. Using smartphones for assessments might bypass some of the burden, given that many people constantly carry around their smartphones without perceiving it as 'foreign' sensor (Gimpel et al., 2015; Smets et al., 2018).

In sum, future research will show whether technological developments resulting in more fine-grained and high-resolution, device-based, and objective measurements may be able to enrich subjective information on recovery and stress over and above subjective self-reports (e.g., approaches that passively measure internal stressors via voice recording, audio feature detection, geolocation tracking, and environmental feature classification).

Data security

With the technological development and opportunities of new technologies, large amounts of personal data can be collected and stored. This is accompanied by an increased need for attention to the security and privacy of such data that are, for example collected via AA methods. Especially health related data (e.g., on recovery and stress), as well as geolocation data can reveal the most private and personal information. For example, smartphones or other devices may be lost, misplaced, or stolen, and the transmission of data to servers may be read out (Carpenter et al., 2016; Reichert, Braun, Lautenbach, et al., 2020). Therefore, in the research-context, very strict rules apply when using personal data. In addition to the consent of the participants, the encryption of the data on the AA devices, the encrypted transmission of the data and the encrypted storage are indispensable, just to name a few necessary data security measures (Reichert, Giurgiu, et al., 2020; Reichert et al., 2021).

Besides the research setting, several precautions can be taken to maintain data security in a private recovery monitoring setting. All devices and apps used should be password-protected. Collected data must be encrypted at the time of collection such that information from a lost smartphone or any other mobile device cannot be read and identified. One should keep in mind that data leaks can always happen. Considering which kind of personal data should have which level of security can help to decide on how to store this data. For this reason, recovery monitoring data should be stored locally on a secure server. Servers in Europe are subject to the General Data Protection Regulation and therefore have a certain security standard, which can nevertheless vary between countries (Carpenter et al., 2016). In summary, to secure recorded AA data, password-protection of apps and devices used for recovery monitoring, as well as several layers of data encryption must be considered.

Conclusion and recommendations for practice

Taken together, AA methods encompassing psychological, behavioural, physio-logical, and biological data assessment strategies allowing to consider context and to account for dynamic changes bear huge potential to move the field of recovery and stress forward. This may be promising if the key methodological strengths of AA are combined with existing knowledge and approaches from organisational and occupational psychology as well as from professional sports. Insights from existing studies may be transferred and further developed for example by implementing advanced data analysis such as artificial intelligence approaches (e.g., machine learning based on constant learning algorithms) to improve predictions (Flach, 2012; McClernon & Choudhury, 2013).

This will not only help individuals in the general population to track their recovery and stress processes in depth, it will also set the basis for evidence-based and tailored interventions which build upon individual time and context-de-pendent needs to achieve an optimal recovery-stress homeostasis.

Notes

1 Oura: https://ouraring.com/de
2 Garmin: https://www.garmin.com/en-US/garmin-technology/running-science/physio
   logical-measurements/recovery-time/
3 Polar: https://support.polar.com/en/recovery-pro
4 WHOOP: https://www.whoop.com

References

Beckmann, J., & Kellmann, M. (2004). Self-regulation and recovery: Approaching and understanding of the process of recovery from stress. *Psychological Reports, 95,* 1135–1136.
Bellenger, C. R., Miller, D. J., Halson, S. L., Roach, G. D., & Sargent, C. (2021). Wrist-based photoplethysmography assessment of heart rate and heart rate variability: Validation of WHOOP. *Sensors, 21*(10), 3571. https://doi.org/10.3390/S21103571
Bennett, A. A., Bakker, A. B., & Field, J. G. (2018). Recovery from work-related effort: A meta-analysis. *Journal of Organizational Behavior, 39*(3), 262–275.

Bourdon, P. C., Cardinale, M., Murray, A., Gastin, P., Kellmann, M., Varley, M. C., Gabbett, T. J., Coutts, A. J., Burgess, D. J., Gregson, W., & Cable, N. T. (2017). Monitoring athlete training loads: Consensus statement. *International Journal of Sports Physiology and Performance, 12*(Suppl. 2), S2-161–S2-170.

Buecker, S., Simacek, T., Ingwersen, B., Terwiel, S., & Simonsmeier, B. A. (2020). Physical activity and subjective well-being in healthy individuals: A meta-analytic review. *Health Psychology Review, 15*(4), 574–592.

Burchartz, A., Anedda, B., Auerswald, T., Giurgiu, M., Hill, H., Ketelhut, S., Kolb, S., Mall, C., Manz, K., Nigg, C. R., Reichert, M., Sprengeler, O., Wunsch, K., & Matthews, C. E. (2020). Assessing physical behavior through accelerometry – State of the science, best practices and future directions. *Psychology of Sport and Exercise, 49,* 101703. https://doi.org/10.1016/J.PSYCHSPORT.2020.101703

Campbell, J., & Ehlert, U. (2012). Acute psychosocial stress: Does the emotional stress response correspond with physiological responses? *Psychoneuroendocrinology, 37*(8), 1111–1134.

Can, Y. S., Arnrich, B., & Ersoy, C. (2019). Stress detection in daily life scenarios using smart phones and wearable sensors: A survey. *Journal of Biomedical Informatics, 92,* 103139. https://doi.org/10.1016/J.JBI.2019.103139

Carpenter, R. W., Wycoff, A. M., & Trull, T. J. (2016). Ambulatory assessment. *Assessment, 23*(4), 414–424.

Coutts, A. J., Crowcroft, S., & Kempton, T. (2022). Developing athlete monitoring systems: Theoretical basis and practical applications. In M. Kellmann & J. Beckmann (Eds.), *Recovery and well-being in sport and exercise* (pp. 17–31). Routledge.

Currell, K., & Jeukendrup, A. E. (2008). Validity, reliability and sensitivity of measures of sporting performance. *Sports Medicine, 38*(4), 297–316.

Drevets, W. C., Price, J. L., Simpson, J. R., Todd, R. D., Reich, T., Vannier, M., & Raichle, M. E. (1997). Subgenual prefrontal cortex abnormalities in mood disorders. *Nature, 386,* 824–827.

Eccles, D. W., & Kazmier, A. W. (2019). The psychology of rest in athletes: An empirical study and initial model. *Psychology of Sport and Exercise, 44,* 90–98.

Eklund, R., & Defreese, J. D. (2015). Athlete burnout: What we know, what we could know, and how we can find out more. *International Journal of Applied Sports Sciences, 27*(2), 63–75.

Ernst, G. (2017). Heart-rate variability – More than heart beats? *Frontiers in Public Health, 5,* 240. https://doi.org/10.3389/FPUBH.2017.00240

Flach, P. (2012). *Machine learning: The art and science of algorithms that make sense of data.* Cambridge University Press.

Gimpel, H., Regal, C., & Schmidt, M. (2015). myStress: Unobtrusive smartphone-based stress detection. *ECIS 2015 Research-in-Progress Papers* (Paper 16). Retrieved May 16, 2023 from https://aisel.aisnet.org/ecis2015_rip/16

Godart, N. T., Perdereau, F., Rein, Z., Berthoz, S., Wallier, J., Jeammet, P., & Flament, M. F. (2007). Comorbidity studies of eating disorders and mood disorders. Critical review of the literature. *Journal of Affective Disorders, 97*(1–3), 37–49.

Heidari, J., Beckmann, J., Bertollo, M., Brink, M., Kallus, K. W., Robazza, C., & Kellmann, M. (2019). Multidimensional monitoring of recovery status and implications for performance. *International Journal of Sports Physiology and Performance, 14*(1), 2–8.

Heidari, J., Jakowski, S., & Kellmann, M. (2022). The value of recovery-stress monitoring for athletes' well-being. In M. Kellmann & J. Beckmann (Eds.), *Recovery and well-being in sport and exercise* (pp. 3–16). Routledge.

Heidari, J., Kölling, S., Pelka, M., & Kellmann, M. (2018). Monitoring the recovery-stress state in athletes. In M. Kellmann & J. Beckmann (Eds.), *Sport, recovery, and performance: Interdisciplinary insights* (pp. 3–18). Routledge.

Jakowski, S. (2022). Self-tracking via smartphone app: Potential tool for athletes' recovery self-management?: A survey on technology usage and sleep behaviour. *German Journal of Exercise and Sport Research*, *52*(2), 253–261.

Kallus, K. W. (2016). RESTQ-Basic: The general version of the RESTQ. In K. W. Kallus & M. Kellmann (Eds.), *The Recovery-Stress Questionnaires: User manual* (pp. 49–85). Pearson Assessment.

Kallus, K. W. (2023). Recovery and stress reactivity. In M. Kellmann, S. Jakowski, & J. Beckmann (Eds.), *The importance of recovery for physical and mental health: Negotiating the effects of underrecovery* (pp. 33–50). Routledge.

Kallus, K. W., & Kellmann, M. (Eds.). (2016). *The Recovery-Stress Questionnaires: User manual*. Pearson Assessment.

Kellmann, M. (2002a). Underrecovery and overtraining: Different concepts – Similar impact? In M. Kellmann (Ed.), *Enhancing recovery: Preventing underperformance in athletes* (pp. 3–24). Human Kinetics.

Kellmann, M. (Ed.). (2002b). *Enhancing recovery: Preventing underperformance in athletes*. Human Kinetics.

Kellmann, M. (2010). Preventing overtraining in athletes in high-intensity sports and stress/recovery monitoring. *Scandinavian Journal of Medicine and Science in Sports*, *20*(2), 95–102.

Kellmann, M., & Beckmann, J. (Eds.). (2022). *Recovery and well-being in sport and exercise*. Routledge.

Kellmann, M., Bertollo, M., Bosquet, L., Brink, M., Coutts, A. J., Duffield, R., Erlacher, D., Halson, S. L., Hecksteden, A., Heidari, J., Kallus, K. W., Meeusen, R., Mujika, I., Robazza, C., Skorski, S., Venter, R., & Beckmann, J. (2018). Recovery and performance in sport: Consensus statement. *International Journal of Sports Physiology and Performance*, *13*(2), 240–245.

Kellmann, M., & Kallus, K. W. (2016). Recovery-Stress Questionnaire for Athletes. In K. W. Kallus & M. Kellmann (Eds.), *The Recovery-Stress Questionnaires: User manual* (pp. 86–131). Pearson Assessment.

Kellmann, M., & Kölling, S. (2019). *Recovery and stress in sport: A manual for testing and assessment*. Routledge.

Kellmann, M., Kölling, S., & Hitzschke, B. (2016). *Das Akutmaß und die Kurzskala zur Erfassung von Erholung und Beanspruchung im Sport – Manual* [The Acute and the Short Recovery and Stress Scale for Sports – manual]. Sportverlag Strauß.

Khazeni, K. (2022, April 30). *Analyzing Whoop health data*. RPubs. Retrieved May 16, 2023 from https://rpubs.com/kkhazeni/WhoopAnalysis

Kim, H. G., Cheon, E. J., Bai, D. S., Lee, Y. H., & Koo, B. H. (2018). Stress and heart rate variability: A meta-analysis and review of the literature. *Psychiatry Investigation*, *15*(3), 235. https://doi.org/10.30773/PI.2017.08.17

Klaperski, S., von Dawans, B., Heinrichs, M., & Fuchs, R. (2014). Effects of a 12-week endurance training program on the physiological response to psychosocial stress in men: A randomized controlled trial. *Journal of Behavioral Medicine*, *37*(6), 1118–1133.

Kölling, S., & Kellmann, M. (2020). Current considerations and future directions of psychometric training monitoring of recovery-stress states. *Deutsche Zeitschrift für Sportmedizin*, *71*(2), 29–34.

Liao, Y., Shonkoff, E. T., & Dunton, G. F. (2015). The acute relationships between affect, physical feeling states, and physical activity in daily life: A review of current evidence. *Frontiers in Psychology, 6*, 1975. https://doi.org/10.3389/fpsyg.2015.01975

Malik, M., Camm, A. J., Bigger, J. T., Breithardt, G., Cerutti, S., Cohen, R. J., Coumel, P., Fallen, E. L., Kennedy, H. L., Kleiger, R. E., Lombardi, F., Malliani, A., Moss, A. J., Rottman, J. N., Schmidt, G., Schwartz, P. J., & Singer, D. H. (1996). Heart rate variability. Standards of measurement, physiological interpretation, and clinical use. *European Heart Journal, 17*(3), 354–381.

McClernon, F. J., & Choudhury, R. R. (2013). I am your smartphone, and I know you are about to smoke: The application of mobile sensing and computing approaches to smoking research and treatment. *Nicotine & Tobacco Research, 15*(10), 1651–1654.

Meeusen, R., Duclos, M., Foster, C., Fry, A., Gleeson, M., Nieman, D., Raglin, J., Rietjens, G., Steinacker, J., Urhausen, A., European College of Sport Science, & American College of Sports Medicine. (2013). Prevention, diagnosis, and treatment of the overtraining syndrome: Joint consensus statement of the European College of Sport Science (ECSS) and the American College of Sports Medicine (ACSM). *European Journal of Sport Science, 13*(1), 1–24.

Mehl, M., & Conner, T. (Eds.). (2014). *Handbook of research methods for studying daily life.* The Guilford Press.

Meijman, T. F., & Mulder, G. (1998). Psychological aspects of workload. In P. J. D. Drenth, H. Thierry, & C. J. de Wolff (Eds.), *Handbook of work and organizational: Work psychology* (pp. 5–33). Psychology Press/Erlbaum (UK) Taylor & Francis.

Meyer, T., Ferrauti, A., Kellmann, M., & Pfeiffer, M. (Eds.). (2020). *Regenerationsmanagement im Spitzensport (Tiel 2)* [Regeneration management in elite sports (Part 2)]. Bundesinstitut für Sportwissenschaft.

Meyer-Lindenberg, A., & Tost, H. (2012). Neural mechanisms of social risk for psychiatric disorders. *Nature Neuroscience, 15*(5), 663–668.

Miller, D. J., Lastella, M., Scanlan, A. T., Bellenger, C., Halson, S. L., Roach, G. D., & Sargent, C. (2020). A validation study of the WHOOP strap against polysomnography to assess sleep. *Journal of Sport Science, 38*(22), 2631–2636.

Reichert, M., Braun, U., Gan, G., Reinhard, I., Giurgiu, M., Ma, R., Zang, Z., Hennig, O., Koch, E. D., Wieland, L., Schweiger, J., Inta, D., Hoell, A., Akdeniz, C., Zipf, A., Ebner-Priemer, U. W., Tost, H., & Meyer-Lindenberg, A. (2020). A neural mechanism for affective well-being: Subgenual cingulate cortex mediates real-life effects of nonexercise activity on energy. *Science Advances, 6*(45), eaaz8934. https://doi.org/10. 1126/SCIADV.AAZ8934

Reichert, M., Braun, U., Lautenbach, S., Zipf, A., Ebner-Priemer, U., Tost, H., & Meyer-Lindenberg, A. (2020). Studying the impact of built environments on human mental health in everyday life: Methodological developments, state-of-the-art and technological frontiers. *Current Opinion in Psychology, 32*, 158–164.

Reichert, M., Brüßler, S., Reinhard, I., Braun, U., Giurgiu, M., Hoell, A., Zipf, A., Meyer-Lindenberg, A., Tost, H., & Ebner-Priemer, U. W. (2022). The association of stress and physical activity: Mind the ecological fallacy. *German Journal of Exercise and Sport Research, 52*(2), 282–289.

Reichert, M., Gan, G., Renz, M., Braun, U., Brüßler, S., Timm, I., Ma, R., Berhe, O., Benedyk, A., Moldavski, A., Schweiger, J. I., Hennig, O., Zidda, F., Heim, C., Banaschewski, T., Tost, H., Ebner-Priemer, U. W., & Meyer-Lindenberg, A. (2021). Ambulatory assessment for precision psychiatry: Foundations, current developments and future avenues. *Experimental Neurology, 345*, 113807. https://doi.org/10.1016/J.EXPNEUROL.2021.113807

Reichert, M., Giurgiu, M., Koch, E., Wieland, L. M., Lautenbach, S., Neubauer, A. B., von Haaren-Mack, B., Schilling, R., Timm, I., Notthoff, N., Marzi, I., Hill, H., Brüßler, S., Eckert, T., Fiedler, J., Burchartz, A., Anedda, B., Wunsch, K., Gerber, M., … Liao, Y. (2020). Ambulatory assessment for physical activity research: State of the science, best practices and future directions. *Psychology of Sport and Exercise, 50*, 101742. https://doi.org/10.1016/j.psychsport.2020.101742

Reichert, M., Tost, H., Braun, U., Zipf, A., Meyer-Lindenberg, A., & Ebner-Priemer, U. W. (2018). GPS-triggered electronic diaries and neuroscience to unravel risk and resilience factors of city dwellers mental health in everyday life. *European Neuropsychopharmacology, 28*, S86. https://doi.org/10.1016/j.euroneuro.2017.12.120

Reichert, M., Tost, H., Reinhard, I., Schlotz, W., Zipf, A., Salize, H. J., Meyer-Lindenberg, A., & Ebner-Priemer, U. W. (2017). Exercise versus nonexercise activity: E-diaries unravel distinct effects on mood. *Medicine and Science in Sports and Exercise, 49*(4), 763–773.

Reichert, M., Tost, H., Reinhard, I., Zipf, A., Salize, H. J., Meyer-Lindenberg, A., & Ebner-Priemer, U. W. (2016). Within-subject associations between mood dimensions and non-exercise activity: An ambulatory assessment approach using repeated real-time and objective data. *Frontiers in Psychology, 7*, 918. https://doi.org/10.3389/FPSYG.2016.00918

Saw, A. E., Main, L. C., & Gastin, P. B. (2016). Monitoring the athlete training response: Subjective self-reported measures trump commonly used objective measures: A systematic review. *British Journal of Sports Medicine, 50*(5), 281–291.

Smets, E., De Raedt, W., & Van Hoof, C. (2018). Into the wild: The challenges of physiological stress detection in laboratory and ambulatory settings. *IEEE Journal of Biomedical and Health Informatics, 23*(2), 463–473.

Solhan, M. B., Trull, T. J., Jahng, S., & Wood, P. K. (2009). Clinical assessment of affective instability: Comparing EMA indices, questionnaire reports, and retrospective recall. *Psychological Assessment, 21*(3), 425–436.

Sonnentag, S., Cheng, B. H., & Parker, S. L. (2022). Recovery from work: Advancing the field toward the future. *Annual Review of Organizational Psychology and Organizational Behavior, 9*, 33–60.

Sonnentag, S., & Fritz, C. (2007). The Recovery Experience Questionnaire: Development and validation of a measure for assessing recuperation and unwinding from work. *Journal of Occupational Health Psychology, 12*(3), 204–221.

Sonnentag, S., & Kruel, U. (2006). Psychological detachment from work during off-job time: The role of job stressors, job involvement, and recovery-related self-efficacy. *European Journal of Work and Organizational Psychology, 15*(2), 197–217.

Sonnentag, S., Venz, L., & Casper, A. (2017). Advances in recovery research: What have we learned? What should be done next? *Journal of Occupational Health Psychology, 22*(3), 365–380.

Stults-Kolehmainen, M. A., & Sinha, R. (2014). The effects of stress on physical activity and exercise. *Sports Medicine, 44*(1), 81–121.

Thayer, J. F., Åhs, F., Fredrikson, M., Sollers, J. J., & Wager, T. D. (2012). A meta-analysis of heart rate variability and neuroimaging studies: Implications for heart rate variability as a marker of stress and health. *Neuroscience & Biobehavioral Reviews, 36*(2), 747–756.

Tost, H., Reichert, M., Braun, U., Reinhard, I., Peters, R., Lautenbach, S., Hoell, A., Schwarz, E., Ebner-Priemer, U., Zipf, A., & Meyer-Lindenberg, A. (2019). Neural correlates of individual differences in affective benefit of real-life urban green space exposure. *Nature Neuroscience*, *22*(9), 1389–1393.

Trull, T. J., & Ebner-Priemer, U. (2013). Ambulatory assessment. *Annual Review of Clinical Psychology*, *9*(1), 151–176.

Trull, T. J., & Ebner-Priemer, U. (2020). Ambulatory assessment in psychopathology research: A review of recommended reporting guidelines and current practices. *Journal of Abnormal Psychology*, *129*(1), 56–63.

von Haaren, B., Haertel, S., Stumpp, J., Hey, S., & Ebner-Priemer, U. (2015). Reduced emotional stress reactivity to a real-life academic examination stressor in students participating in a 20-week aerobic exercise training: A randomised controlled trial using Ambulatory Assessment. *Psychology of Sport and Exercise*, *20*, 67–75.

von Haaren, B., Ottenbacher, J., Muenz, J., Neumann, R., Boes, K., & Ebner-Priemer, U. (2016). Does a 20-week aerobic exercise training programme increase our capabilities to buffer real-life stressors? A randomized, controlled trial using ambulatory assessment. *European Journal of Applied Physiology*, *116*, 383–394.

WHOOP. (2023). *Strain*. Retrieved April 25, 2023, from https://support.whoop.com/s/article/WHOOP-Strain

Wilhelm, P., Perez, M., & Pawlik, K. (2012). Conducting research in daily life: A historical review. In M. R. Mehl & T. S. Conner (Eds.), *Handbook of research methods for studying daily life* (pp. 62–86). The Guilford Press.

Zawadzki, M. J., Smyth, J. M., Sliwinski, M. J., Ruiz, J. M., & Gerin, W. (2017). Revisiting the lack of association between affect and physiology: Contrasting between-person and within-person analyses. *Health Psychology*, *36*(8), 811–818.

Part II

Psychological prevention approaches

4 'Switch off when not in use'

The benefits of detachment from work and sport for recovery

Yannick A. Balk

Introduction

Work stress has increased significantly over the past two decades, a development mostly driven by an intensification of psychological job demands (Rigó et al., 2021). In a comparable trend, the psychological demands surrounding training and competition in sport have increased and these demands will likely only increase further (Soligard et al., 2016). Maintaining the delicate balance between stress and recovery is essential for individuals to achieve optimal health, well-being, and performance (Kellmann et al., 2018). In contrast, insufficient recovery from the demands of work or sport can lead to prolonged stress reactions and chronic strain, which can ultimately lead to diverse negative outcomes (Kellmann, 2002; McEwen, 1998). For example, employees are at risk of occupational burnout (Ahola et al., 2006), lower productivity (Halkos & Bousinakis, 2010), a higher rate of sickness absence (Götz et al., 2018), and an earlier exit from the labour force (Kubo et al., this volume, Chapter 13; Mäcken, 2019). Likewise, potential consequences of prolonged stress and chronic strain for athletes are underrecovery, overtraining syndrome, decreased performance, and ill-health (Kellmann et al., 2018).

The concept of recovery essentially centres around the notion that balance is regained by restoring the invested physiological and psychological resources after engaging in a demanding or stressful activity (Kellmann et al., 2018; McEwen, 1998). Examples of demands that require physiological and psychological effort are high workload, perceived pressure, physical and mental exertion, and having to deal with conflict. Such demands may all play a role when working in teams, giving a presentation to your superiors, playing a tennis match, coaching a football team, acting in a play, or singing on stage. As such, the principles underlying the balance between recovery and stress appear to be largely universal, operating similarly in various work domains, sport, and the performing arts. Hence, the

Balk, Y. A. (2024). 'Switch of when not in use': The benefits of detachment from work and sport for recovery. In M. Kellmann & J. Beckmann (Eds.), *Fostering Recovery and Well-being in a Healthy Lifestyle: Psychological, Somatic, and Organizational Prevention Approaches* (pp. 59–72). Routledge.

DOI: 10.4324/9781003250654-6

insights regarding recovery discussed in the current chapter are relevant to all individuals who invest precious physiological and psychological resources in their pursuit of certain goals such as a surgeon, a tennis player, or an opera singer.

Psychological recovery

What is clear in the light of increasing demands in both work and sport as well as compromised time for rest, is that recovery has become increasingly important. Recovery is generally defined as a physiological and psychological restorative process relative to time (Kellmann et al., 2018). So, both physiological and psychological recovery are needed to achieve *complete* recovery.

Box 4.1

Imagine start-up owner Gerald, who has to give a presentation to a group of investors who can make or break the immediate future of his start-up company. The presentation went well, but Gerald feels he was struggling with some of the questions they asked him. The day after the meeting he finds himself still thinking back to the meeting over and over again. He wonders: What could I have said differently? Could I have prepared myself better? As a result, 24 hours after the meeting Gerald still feels tense while the physiological and psychological reaction to that stressful activity should have diminished by now. Stress reactions can develop into more adverse reactions when there is continued exposure to stress, thereby limiting the replenishment of important physiological and psychological resources. For instance, according to the perseverative cognition hypothesis, psychophysiological activity will be extended after a stressful or demanding situation due to "repeated or chronic activation of the cognitive representation of one or more psychological stressors" (Brosschot et al., 2006, p. 114). Likewise, the *Cognitive Activation Theory of Stress* (Ursin & Eriksen, 2010) proposes that it is not primarily the acute reaction to stressful stimuli that is detrimental to individuals' health and well-being, but rather the sustained activation, even when stressors are no longer present. So, when an individual is unable to regulate negative thoughts and emotions about a prior demanding or stressful situation (e.g., high pressure to perform, a disappointing performance), the stress response is not 'switched off' and psychophysiological activation remains high. This compromises the recovery process and can cause chronic stress and health problems. This is a real threat for athletes as well, as research by Allen et al. (2009) showed that golfers' anger persisted for two days after a game depending on their attributions (i.e., whether they perceived the cause to be stable rather than unstable). Fortunately, Gerald realises that the outcome of the meeting is now beyond his control and decides to meet with a friend for a walk outside to clear his mind.

Furthermore, recovery can be considered a *process* as well as an *outcome* (Sonnentag & Geurts, 2009). Recovery as an outcome refers to one's physiological and psychological state after a certain recovery period, which can be, for instance at the end of the day, after engaging in a certain activity, or after waking up. Physiological recovery outcomes involve the restoration of physiological resources such as muscle strength, heart rate, and the absence of physical fatigue (e.g., muscle soreness, heavy arms and legs). Psychological recovery outcomes pertain to the restoration of mental resources such as attention, motivation, mental energy, and mood. As such, one's physiological and psychological states act as a resource that functions as a stress-buffer for upcoming activities as well (Kellmann & Kallus, 2001). Recovery as a process refers to those activities and experiences that result in a change in one's physiological and psychological state. Accordingly, recovery processes precede recovery outcomes and, consequently, determine whether adequate recovery is obtained. Regarding recovery processes, physical inactivity is generally considered the most effective way to restore physiological resources. However, ceasing physical activity does not guarantee a cessation of mental activity (Eccles & Kazmier, 2019). It turns out that the psychological recovery process is somewhat more complex than the physiological recovery process.

Detachment: A key recovery experience

Since adverse effects on health and well-being may arise from prolonged continued exposure to stress, a fundamental aspect of the psychological recovery process is experiencing a mental break from the demands of a previous stressful activity (Kellmann, 2002; Kellmann et al., 2018). A mental break means that (negative) cognitions and emotions are halted, which allows the physiological and psychological stress response to be 'switched off' and, as a result, regain homeostatic balance.

According to the *Stressor-Detachment Model* of Sonnentag and Fritz (2015), a central recovery experience that provides such a mental break is detachment. Detachment originally referred to "the individual's sense of being away from the work situation" (Etzion et al., 1998, p. 579). Sonnentag and Bayer (2005) introduced the concept of psychological detachment as they argued that detachment goes beyond being just physically detached from work. Psychological detachment involves ceasing work-related activities and cognitively disengaging from work during non-work time (Sonnentag & Fritz, 2015), which is reflected in the items of the often-used Recovery Experience Questionnaire ("I forget about work", "I get a break from the demands of work"; Sonnentag & Fritz, 2007). In an attempt to further refine the recovery experience of detachment, more recent work showed that detachment can be considered a multidimensional construct consisting of a physical, cognitive, and emotional element (Balk & de Jonge, 2021; Balk et al., 2017; de Jonge et al., 2012). Physical detachment refers to shaking off the physical exertion from training or competition. Physical relaxation can be considered the primary way of achieving physical detachment, and physical inactivity is often the typical way in which athletes spend their leisure time (Franssen et al., 2022; Weiler et al., 2015). Yet, physical detachment also involves distancing oneself from the physical environment of a previous demanding or stressful activity, for instance when an athlete leaves the sports arena. Cognitive detachment means putting all thoughts about a stressful activity aside. Think of a civil engineer focuses on his family and forgets about work when at home. Cognitive detachment enables an individual to recover as there are no intrusive thoughts related to the past or future (Beckmann, 2002; Sonnentag & Fritz, 2007). Finally, emotional detachment refers to taking distance from negative emotions resulting from a previous stressful activity. Imagine a firefighter who is not upset anymore by emotional events that took place earlier at work. Lasting negative emotions potentially interfere with recovery as a result of heightened arousal and energy depletion (Lundqvist & Kenttä, 2010). In contrast, positive emotions will likely benefit the recovery process through replenishing both physiological and psychological resources (Fredrickson et al., 2000; Meier et al., 2016). The cognitive and emotional elements of detachment together are sometimes referred to as mental detachment (Balk et al., 2018; Loch et al., 2019). To avoid confusion, in this chapter the general term *detachment* is used unless otherwise specified. Detachment is considered an active, self-regulatory process of ceasing thoughts and emotions related to a previous activity (Balk & Englert, 2020; Beckmann, 2023; Beckmann & Kellmann, 2004; Sonnentag & Bayer, 2005). While physical detachment by means of physical rest can be considered the primary way of dealing with physical fatigue, cognitive and emotional detachment can be considered the primary way of dealing with mental fatigue (Eccles & Kazmier, 2019; Russell et al., 2019).

Consequences of detachment

The importance of detachment for employees is relatively well-researched in the context of work and organisational psychology. More recently, the role of detachment for individuals in performance domains such as sport and dance has been investigated as well. In general, the benefits of detachment for various recovery outcomes are clear.

Work

Within the context of work there has been a plethora of studies on the role of detachment from work for employees' health, well-being, and performance. In their seminal study introducing the concept of psychological detachment, Sonnentag and Fritz (2007) showed that detachment was negatively related to health complaints, burnout, and depressive symptoms, and positively related to life satisfaction. Similarly, a study among 291 employees found that detachment from work was related to fewer health complaints and that it attenuated the positive association between interpersonal conflicts at work and health complaints (Sonnentag et al., 2013). However, other studies showed conflicting results for the health-promoting effects of detachment. For instance, de Bloom et al. (2012) found that detachment from work during vacation predicted an increase in health and well-being after vacation, whereas another study by the same authors found that detachment from work during vacation did not predict a change in health and well-being after vacation (de Bloom et al., 2013). Nonetheless, a meta-analysis conducted by Wendsche and Lohmann-Haislah (2017) concluded that detachment from work is positively associated with both physical health (e.g., lower physical discomfort) and psychological health (e.g., increased life satisfaction, improved sleep quality).

In addition to health-related outcomes, studies among employees have shown that detachment from work is also important for employee well-being (Sonnentag & Fritz, 2015). For instance, research showed that a lack of detachment from work during the evening was related to a low level of positive emotions in the evening (Rodríguez-Muñoz et al., 2017), high evening strain (Debrot et al., 2018), evening energetic depletion (Germeys & de Gieter, 2018) and other negative states at bedtime (Garrosa-Hernández et al., 2013; Sonnentag & Lischetzke, 2018). Furthermore, detachment moderated the negative association between job stressors and employee well-being. That is, job stressors were generally more strongly related to indicators of poor well-being when detachment was low (Sonnentag & Fritz, 2015). These findings suggest that distancing oneself from work and ceasing work-related thoughts can provide a mental break from job stressors and thereby lower their negative impact (Sonnentag & Fritz, 2015). Interestingly, meta-analyses (Bennett et al., 2018; Wendsche & Lohmann-Haislah, 2017) reported stronger correlations between detachment from work and negative indicators of well-being, such as exhaustion, physical discomfort, and fatigue, compared to positive indicators of well-being, such as vigour. This suggests that detachment from work might be more effective in preventing negative states instead of promoting positive states (Sonnentag, 2018).

In contrast to health and well-being outcomes, associations between detachment from work and job performance are relatively weak. More specifically, detachment is positively associated with employees' task performance but negatively associated with contextual performance indicators, such as personal initiative and organisational citizenship behaviour, as well as creativity (Wendsche & Lohmann-Haislah, 2017). Work motivation appears to not be affected by employees' detachment from work (Wendsche & Lohmann-Haislah, 2017). One notable study linking detachment from work and performance was conducted among 31 elite-level sport coaches (Balk, de Jonge, Geurts, & Oerlemans, 2019). Coaches' daily off-job emotional detachment predicted higher levels of positive affect the next morning, which in turn predicted higher levels of work engagement during the day. More interestingly, coaches experiencing higher work engagement were rated as being more autonomy-supportive by their athletes. Autonomy-supportive behaviour is a key determinant of well-being and satisfaction with performance among athletes (Balk, de Jonge, Geurts, & Oerlemans, 2019; Mageau & Vallerand, 2003). Thus, coaches' emotional detachment from work is not only important for their own well-being and work engagement but also benefits the quality of their interactions with their athletes, thereby positively affecting their daily sport experiences.

Taken together, detachment from work is an important recovery experience for employees, particularly through mitigating the negative effects of job stressors on health and well-being. However, associations between detachment form work and performance are less unequivocal.

Sport and dance

The role of detachment in the context of sport has only recently gained traction in the field of sport and performance psychology. Without referring to detachment directly, Beckmann and Kellmann (2004) described how the process of distancing (i.e., the mental deactivation of a stressful activity) is important for recovery. More recent empirical studies provided evidence for the beneficial role of detachment from sport for athletes' recovery outcomes as well. For instance, detachment was found to be positively related to mental energy and sleep, and negatively related to injury in a sample of recreational athletes (Balk, de Jonge, Oerlemans, & Geurts, 2019). Differentiating between cognitive and emotional detachment, a diary study by Balk et al. (2017) found that elite athletes' daily emotional detachment was positively associated with daily cognitive and emotional recovery at the end of the day. Moreover, emotional detachment weakened the negative relation between daily emotional sport demands and emotional recovery. More specifically, on days where athletes reported higher emotional sport demands, they felt less emotionally recovered when emotional detachment was low, while athletes did not experience such a decline in emotional recovery when emotional detachment was high. A study among full-time dance students reported similar findings, showing that higher emotional detachment was related to increased positive affect and negatively related to health problems (Balk et al., 2018). Again, emotional detachment weakened the negative relation between emotional demands and positive affect. In a study by Eccles and Kazmier (2019), athletes reported that rest for them meant getting a break from thinking about one's sport. In other words, continuously thinking about one's sport was considered detrimental to feeling recovered. However, due to their constant involvement in sport-related activities and social activities, which typically involve teammates and conversations about their sport, athletes feel they are always thinking about their sport (Eccles & Kazmier, 2019). As a result, not being able to 'switch off' is mentally fatiguing and can develop into reduced motivation to engage in one's sport (Eccles & Kazmier, 2019; Russell et al., 2019).

Taken together, detachment seems to provide performers with an important mental break from previous demands. A tentative conclusion based on the aforementioned studies, is that regulating post-performance negative emotions (i.e., emotional detachment) might be of particular importance for adequate recovery. This is in line with the idea that mood repair is one of the core functions of recovery (Sonnentag & Fritz, 2007). Yet, there is still a strong need for a better understanding of the role of detachment in relation to performance in domains such as sport and dance.

Antecedents of detachment from work and sport

Detachment provides a mental break from a previous demanding or stressful activity, which allows important resources to be replenished. Paradoxically, however, it appears that individuals tend to experience lower levels of detachment when one has been confronted with high demands or stress (Sonnentag, 2018). There appear to be several factors that may either impede or benefit the extent to which employees and athletes experience detachment.

Wendsche and Lohmann-Haislah (2017) concluded in their meta-analysis that detachment from work is influenced by both work-related and personal characteristics. In general, high job demands are generally associated with lower levels of detachment from work (Bennett et al., 2018). For instance, Kinnunen and Feldt (2013) found that time pressure, decision-making demands, and long work hours predicted a decrease in detachment over the course of one year. With regard to short-term effects, Sonnentag and Bayer (2005) found that time pressure and daily work hours were negatively related to detachment during the evening. Other stressors such as negative events at work (Bono et al., 2013), high self-control demands (Germeys & de Gieter, 2018), and interpersonal stressors such as bullying and conflicts (Rodríguez-Muñoz et al., 2017; Volmer et al., 2012) were also negatively related to detachment from work during non-work time.

Similar to job demands, personal characteristics can impede detachment. Both neuroticism and heavy work investment have shown a negative association with detachment from work (Wendsche & Lohmann-Haislah, 2017). A study among academics found that more perfectionistic academics reported significantly higher levels of fatigue, emotional exhaustion, and anxiety after an Easter respite which was explained by a greater tendency to worry and ruminate about work (Flaxman et al., 2012). Increased worry and rumination about work also explained the negative association between perfectionistic concerns on the one hand, and were sleep quality and workday functioning on the other hand among government agency employees (Flaxman et al., 2018).

Fortunately, there are also factors that promote detachment from work. A study among German teachers found that support from colleagues was associated with a reduced risk of experiencing difficulties detaching from work (Varol et al., 2021). A meta-analysis by Bennett et al. (2018) reported no association between general job resources and detachment from work. However, Wendsche and Lohmann-Haislah (2017) found support for the positive association between two specific job resources, namely social support and job control, with detachment from work.

Studies among athletes also signify a paradoxical relation between sport-related demands and detachment from sport. Specifically, athletes reporting higher levels of cognitive and emotional sport demands tend to report lower levels of cognitive and emotional detachment (Balk & de Jonge, 2021). Similarly, dance students' self-reported emotional demands are negatively correlated with emotional detachment (Balk et al., 2018). To better understand how sport-related demands and subsequent detachment from sport are connected, Balk and de Jonge (2021) conducted a daily diary study among 85 elite athletes to investigate associations between daily physical, cognitive, and emotional sport demands and daily physical, cognitive, and emotional detachment. The authors found that high daily physical and emotional sport demands were associated with increased physical fatigue after training and competition. In turn, high physical fatigue was associated with lower physical and cognitive detachment after training/competition. Physical fatigue mediated the association between physical and emotional sport demands and physical and cognitive detachment. These findings point toward an 'underrecovery trap', in which high levels of physical fatigue can interfere with athletes' physical and mental recovery (Balk & de Jonge, 2021). That is, when the need for recovery is high, as indicated by increased levels of fatigue, athletes seem to experience suboptimal mental recovery as they do not mentally disconnect from their sport. This is in line with the view that excessive strain is not necessarily caused by high demands but rather a lack of recovery that leads to a state of underrecovery (Kellmann, 2002).

In a follow-up study, Balk et al. (2021) followed 39 Dutch elite athletes to investigate the role of daily sport-related rumination and worry as the underlying mechanism linking daily post-training physical fatigue and vigour on the one hand, and subsequent cognitive and emotional detachment on the other hand. Results showed that daily physical fatigue was positively associated with sport-related rumination and worry during recovery time, whereas daily vigour was negatively associated with sport-related worry during recovery. In turn, worry was negatively associated with both cognitive detachment and emotional detachment. Worry mediated the relation between physical fatigue and cognitive detachment. So, athletes' high physical fatigue and vigour seem to induce worrisome thoughts about upcoming demands (Figure 4.1). Taken together, it

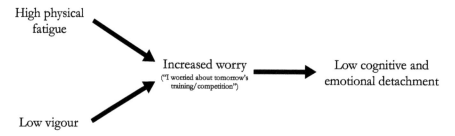

Figure 4.1 Process in which post-performance energetic states (high fatigue, low vigour) impair cognitive and emotional detachment via increased worry. Adapted from Balk et al. (2021).

is important for athletes to employ strategies aimed at regulating both post-performance energetic states as well as sport-related worry to optimise the mental recovery process.

There are behavioural approaches to promoting detachment from sport as well. For instance, athletes indicated that a break from constantly thinking about is generally facilitated through avoiding teammates, engaging in an activity unrelated to one's sport, and going to a space not synonymous with one's sport (Eccles & Kazmier, 2019).

Conclusion and recommendations for practice

Adequate recovery restores one's invested physiological and psychological resources after engaging in a demanding or stressful activity. However, cognitive and emotional processes may extend the duration of stress responses, thereby impeding recovery. In both work and sport, detachment protects against the negative effect of stressors on health and well-being by providing a mental break from a previous demanding or stressful activity.

Evidently, educating individuals about the importance of detachment for sustainable health, well-being, and performance remains important. In addition, I would like to recommend one specific approach aimed at enhancing detachment, regardless of the performance domain. Specifically, after a demanding or stressful activity individuals are encouraged to engage in a two-step *mental cool-down* consisting of a relaxation exercise and promoting the transition to rest and recovery. This mental cool-down can be implemented after a workday, after training or competition, or after any other demanding performance.

First, engaging in relaxation techniques can improve one's ability to self-regulate physical and psychological states (Kellmann et al., this volume, Chapter 8). Examples of relaxation strategies are deep breathing, imagery, progressive muscle relaxation, biofeedback, and listening to music (Kellmann et al., this volume, Chapter 8; Loch et al., 2019). An additional benefit of using these strategies is that they provide a certain level of distraction, thereby kickstarting the process of switching off as well. Deploying other strategies and behaviours that guide one's attention away from a previous stressful activity or that can reduce worry should be encouraged. For instance, effective strategies to regulate cognitions and emotions include expressive writing and worry postponement (Brosschot & van der Doef, 2006; Hudson & Day, 2012), as well as debriefing (Hogg, this volume, Chapter 5). In support of this, a meta-analysis by Karabinski et al. (2021) found that interventions focusing on mindfulness, emotion regulation are effective in promoting detachment. Similarly, a recent study by Nien et al. (2023) among athletes showed that both a 30-minute mindfulness and relaxation protocol were effective in reducing state anxiety and negative affect. The mindfulness protocol used a combination of three mindfulness exercises, whereas the relaxation protocol combined progressive muscle relaxation and diaphragmatic breathing. Brain activity measures suggested that decreased levels of state anxiety and negative affect might be the result of greater attentional control (Nien et al., 2023).

Second, improving the transition to the recovery phase can benefit subsequent detachment. Boundary management routines such as making a to-do list for the next day, creating plans to resolve incomplete goals, or changing one's professional outfit for a casual outfit can have a positive effect on such a transition and, as a result, detachment (Ashforth et al., 2000; Karabinski et al., 2021; Smit, 2016). Eccles et al. (2021) describe several strategies to help athletes switch off from thinking about their sport. These strategies centre around two principles: 1) achieving a focus different from sport and 2) avoiding cues that remind of sport. Strategies to switch focus include engaging in activities unrelated to one's sport that are intrinsically interesting, such as a hobby, which makes it more difficult to think about sport. To avoid cues that remind of sport it is recommended to avoid seeing physical items and being in places that remind of one's sport, as well as to avoid people who will talk about one's sport.

Ideally, a mental cool-down is accompanied by situational or organisational adjustments. For instance, leaders and supervisors should encourage employees to mentally switch off from work as well (Sonnentag & Schiffner, 2019). Similarly, clear organisational policies concerning IT and off-job communication are likely important to support employees in detaching from work. In contrast, organisational norms and expectations about taking work home are negatively linked to employees' ability to detach and recover during non-work time (Foucreault et al., 2018). Detachment from sport is hindered when an organisation or its staff members are involved with an athletes' personal life. For instance, monitoring resting behaviours and sleep as well as communicating during leisure time increases the chance that athletes stay mentally connected to their sport. A specific recommendation to sport coaches and other staff members is to limit communication between the last training session and the next day (e.g., no contact after 8 p.m.), which helps to establish sport-home boundaries for athletes. Rest and recovery in sport is often undervalued at both cultural and societal levels (Eccles et al., 2020), which can impact on the extent to which athletes push themselves and allow themselves to detach from sport. As recovery is a fundamental aspect underlying athletic health and well-being, there is a responsibility for coaches, management, media, and policymakers to encourage a healthy balance between stress and rest.

References

Ahola, K., Honkonen, T., Isometsä, E., Kalimo, R., Nykyri, E., Koskinen, S., Aromaa, A., & Lönnqvist, J. (2006). Burnout in the general population. *Social Psychiatry and Psychiatric Epidemiology, 41*, 11–17.

Allen, M. S., Jones, M. V., & Sheffield, D. (2009). Causal attribution and emotion in the days following competition. *Journal of Sports Sciences, 27*(5), 461–468.

Ashforth, B. E., Kreiner, G. E., & Fugate, M. (2000). All in a day's work: Boundaries and micro role transitions. *Academy of Management Review, 25*, 472–491.

Balk, Y. A., & de Jonge, J. (2021). The "underrecovery trap": When physical fatigue impairs the physical and mental recovery process. *Sport, Exercise, and Performance Psychology, 10*, 88–101.

Balk, Y. A., de Jonge, J., Geurts, S. A. E., & Oerlemans, W. G. (2019). Antecedents and consequences of perceived autonomy support in elite sport: A diary study linking coaches' off-job recovery and athletes' performance satisfaction. *Psychology of Sport and Exercise, 44*, 26–34.

Balk, Y. A., de Jonge, J., Oerlemans, W. G. M., & Geurts, S. A. E. (2017). Testing the triple-match principle among Dutch elite athletes: A day-level study on demands, detachment and recovery. *Psychology of Sport and Exercise, 33*, 7–17.

Balk, Y. A., de Jonge, J., Oerlemans, W. G. M., & Geurts, S. A. E. (2019). Physical recovery, mental detachment and sleep as predictors of injury and mental energy. *Journal of Health Psychology, 24*, 1828–1838.

Balk, Y. A., de Jonge, J., van Rijn, R., & Stubbe, J. (2018). "Leave it all behind": The role of mental demands and mental detachment in relation to dance students' health and well-being. *Medical Problems of Performing Artists, 33*, 258–264.

Balk, Y. A., & Englert, C. (2020). Recovery self-regulation in sport: Theory, research, and practice. *International Journal of Sports Science and Coaching, 15*, 273–281.

Balk, Y. A., Tamminen, K. A., & Eccles, D. W. (2021). Too tired to switch off? How post-training physical fatigue impairs mental recovery through increased worry. *Sport, Exercise, and Performance Psychology, 10*, 489–503.

Beckmann, J. (2002). Interaction of volition and recovery. In M. Kellmann (Ed.), *Enhancing recovery: Preventing underperformance in athletes* (pp. 269–282). Human Kinetics.

Beckmann, J. (2023). Self-regulation of recovery. In M. Kellmann, S. Jakowski, & J. Beckmann (Eds.), *The importance of recovery for physical and mental health: Negotiating the effects of underrecovery* (pp. 53–69). Routledge.

Beckmann, J., & Kellmann, M. (2004). Self-regulation and recovery: Approaching an understanding of the process of recovery from stress. *Psychological Reports, 95*, 1135–1153.

Bennett, A. A., Bakker, A. B., & Field, J. G. (2018). Recovery from work-related effort: A meta-analysis. *Journal of Organizational Behavior, 39*, 262–275.

Bono, J. E., Glomb, T. M., Shen, W., Kim, E., & Koch, A. J. (2013). Building positive resources: Effects of positive events and positive reflection on work stress and health. *Academy of Management Journal, 56*, 1601–1627.

Brosschot, J. F., Gerin, W., & Thayer, J. F. (2006). The perseverative cognition hypothesis: A review of worry, prolonged stress-related physiological activation, and health. *Journal of Psychosomatic Research, 60*, 113–124.

Brosschot, J. F., & van der Doef, M. (2006). Daily worrying and somatic health complaints: Testing the effectiveness of a simple worry reduction intervention. *Psychology & Health, 21*, 19–31.

de Bloom, J., Geurts, S. A. E., & Kompier, M. A. (2012). Effects of short vacations, vacation activities and experiences on employee health and well-being. *Stress and Health, 28*, 305–318.

de Bloom, J., Geurts, S. A. E., & Kompier, M. A. (2013). Vacation (after-) effects on employee health and well-being, and the role of vacation activities, experiences and sleep. *Journal of Happiness Studies, 14*, 613–633.

Debrot, A., Siegler, S., Klumb, P. L., & Schoebi, D. (2018). Daily work stress and relationship satisfaction: Detachment affects romantic couples' interactions quality. *Journal of Happiness Studies, 88*, 2283–2301.

de Jonge, J., Spoor, E., Sonnentag, S., Dormann, C., & van den Tooren, M. (2012). "Take a break?!" Off-job recovery, job demands, and job resources as predictors of health, active learning, and creativity. *European Journal of Work and Organizational Psychology, 21*(3), 321–348.

Eccles, D. W., Balk, Y., Gretton, T. W., & Harris, N. (2020). "The forgotten session": Advancing research and practice concerning the psychology of rest in athletes. *Journal of Applied Sport Psychology, 34*, 3–24.

Eccles, D. W., Caviedes, G., Balk, Y. A., Harris, N., & Gretton, T. W. (2021). How to help athletes get the mental rest needed to perform well and stay healthy. *Journal of Sport Psychology in Action, 12*, 259–270.

Eccles, D. W., & Kazmier, A. W. (2019). The psychology of rest in athletes: An empirical study and initial model. *Psychology of Sport and Exercise, 44*, 90–98.

Etzion, D., Eden, D., & Lapidot, Y. (1998). Relief from job stressors and burnout: Reserve service as a respite. *Journal of Applied Psychology, 83*, 577–585.

Flaxman, P. E., Ménard, J., Bond, F. W., & Kinman, G. (2012). Academics' experiences of a respite from work: Effects of self-critical perfectionism and perseverative cognition on postrespite well-being. *Journal of Applied Psychology, 97*, 854–865.

Flaxman, P. E., Stride, C. B., Söderberg, M., Lloyd, J., Guenole, N., & Bond, F. W. (2018). Relationships between two dimensions of employee perfectionism, postwork cognitive processing, and work day functioning. *European Journal of Work and Organizational Psychology, 27*, 56–69.

Franssen, W. M., Vanbrabant, E., Cuveele, E., Ivanova, A., Franssen, G. H., & Eijnde, B. O. (2022). Sedentary behaviour, physical activity and cardiometabolic health in highly trained athletes: A systematic review and meta-analysis. *European Journal of Sport Science, 22*(10), 1605–1617.

Fredrickson, B. L., Mancuso, R. A., Branigan, C., & Tugade, M. M. (2000). The undoing effects of positive emotions. *Motivation and Emotion, 24*, 237–258.

Foucreault, A., Ollier-Malaterre, A., & Ménard, J. (2018). Organizational culture and work–life integration: A barrier to employees' respite? *The International Journal of Human Resource Management, 29*, 2378–2398.

Garrosa-Hernández, E., Carmona-Cobo, I., Ladstätter, F., Blanco, L. M., & Cooper-Thomas, H. D. (2013). The relationships between family-work interaction, job-related exhaustion, detachment, and meaning in life: A day-level study of emotional well-being. *Journal of Work and Organizational Psychology, 29*, 169–177.

Germeys, L., & de Gieter, S. (2018). A diary study on the role of psychological detachment in the spillover of self-control demands to employees' ego depletion and the crossover to their partner. *European Journal of Work and Organizational Psychology, 27*, 140–152.

Götz, S., Hoven, H., Müller, A., Dragano, N., & Wahrendorf, M. (2018). Age differences in the association between stressful work and sickness absence among full-time employed workers: Evidence from the German socio-economic panel. *International Archives of Occupational and Environmental Health, 91*, 479–496.

Halkos, G., & Bousinakis, D. (2010). The effect of stress and satisfaction on productivity. *International Journal of Productivity and Performance Management, 59*, 415–431.

Hudson, J., & Day, M. C. (2012). Athletes' experiences of expressive writing about sports stressors. *Psychology of Sport and Exercise, 13*, 798–806.

Karabinski, T., Haun, V. C., Nübold, A., Wendsche, J., & Wegge, J. (2021). Interventions for improving psychological detachment from work: A meta-analysis. *Journal of Occupational Health Psychology, 26*, 224–242.

Kellmann, M. (2002). Underrecovery and overtraining: Different concepts – Similar impact? In M. Kellmann (Ed.), *Enhancing recovery: Preventing underperformance in athletes* (pp. 3–24). Human Kinetics.

Kellmann, M., Bertollo, M., Bosquet, L., Brink, M., Coutts, A. J., Duffield, R., Erlacher, D., Halson, S. L., Hecksteden, A., Heidari, J., Kallus, K. W., Meeusen, R., Mujika, I., Robazza, C., Skorski, S., Venter, R., & Beckmann, J. (2018). Recovery and performance in sport: Consensus statement. *International Journal of Sports Physiology and Performance*, *13*, 240–245.

Kellmann, M., & Kallus, K.W. (2001). *The Recovery-Stress Questionnaire for Athletes: User manual*. Human Kinetics.

Kinnunen, U., & Feldt, T. (2013). Job characteristics, recovery experiences and occupational well-being: Testing cross-lagged relationships across 1 year. *Stress and Health*, *29*, 369–382.

Loch, F., Ferrauti, A., Meyer, T., Pfeiffer, M., & Kellmann, M. (2019). Resting the mind – A novel topic with scarce insights. Considering potential mental recovery strategies for short rest periods in sports. *Performance Enhancement & Health*, *6*, 148–155.

Lundqvist, C., & Kenttä, G. (2010). Positive emotions are not simply the absence of the negative ones: Development and validation of the Emotional Recovery Questionnaire (EmRecQ). *The Sport Psychologist*, *24*, 468–488.

Mäcken, J. (2019). Work stress among older employees in Germany: Effects on health and retirement age. *PLoS One*, *14*, e0211487. https://doi.org/10.1371/journal.pone.0211487

Mageau, G. A., & Vallerand, R. J. (2003). The coach-athlete relationship: A motivational model. *Journal of Sports Sciences*, *21*, 883–904.

McEwen, B. S. (1998). Stress, adaptation, and disease. Allostasis and allostatic load. *Annals of the New York Academy of Sciences*, *840*, 33–44.

Meier, L. L., Cho, E., & Dumani, S. (2016). The effect of positive work reflection during leisure time on affective well-being: Results from three diary studies. *Journal of Organizational Behavior*, *37*, 255–278.

Nien, J. T., Gill, D. L., Chou, T. Y., Liu, C. S., Geng, X., Hung, T. M., & Chang, Y. K. (2023). Effect of brief mindfulness and relaxation inductions on anxiety, affect and brain activation in athletes. *Psychology of Sport and Exercise*, *67*, 102422. https://doi.org/10.1016/j.psychsport.2023.102422

Rigó, M., Dragano, N., Wahrendorf, M., Siegrist, J., & Lunau, T. (2021). Work stress on rise? Comparative analysis of trends in work stressors using the European working conditions survey. *International Archives of Occupational and Environmental Health*, *94*, 459–474.

Rodríguez-Muñoz, A., Antino, M., & Sanz-Vergel, A. I. (2017). Cross-domain consequences of workplace bullying: A multi-source daily diary study. *Work & Stress*, *31*, 297–314.

Russell, S., Jenkins, D., Rynne, S., Halson, S. L., & Kelly, V. (2019). What is mental fatigue in elite sport? Perceptions from athletes and staff. *European Journal of Sport Science*, *19*, 1367–1376.

Smit, B. W. (2016). Successfully leaving work at work: The self-regulatory underpinnings of psychological detachment. *Journal of Occupational and Organizational Psychology*, *89*, 493–514.

Soligard, T., Schwellnus, M., Alonso, J. M., Bahr, R., Clarsen, B., Dijkstra, H. P., Gabbett, T., Gleeson, M., Hägglund, M., Hutchinson, M. R., Janse van Rensburg, C., Khan, K. M., Meeusen, R., Orchard, J. W., Pluim, B. M., Raftery, M., Budgett, R., & Engebretsen, L. (2016). How much is too much? (Part 1) International Olympic Committee consensus statement on load in sport and risk of injury. *British Journal of Sports Medicine*, *50*, 1030–1041.

Sonnentag, S. (2018). The recovery paradox: Portraying the complex interplay between job stressors, lack of recovery, and poor well-being. *Research in Organizational Behavior*, *38*, 169–185.

Sonnentag, S., & Bayer, U. V. (2005). Switching off mentally: Predictors and consequences of psychological detachment from work during off-job time. *Journal of Occupational Health Psychology*, *10*, 393–414.

Sonnentag, S., & Fritz, C. (2007). The recovery experience questionnaire: Development and validation of a measure assessing recuperation and unwinding from work. *Journal of Occupational Health Psychology*, *12*, 204–221.

Sonnentag, S., & Fritz, C. (2015). Recovery from job stress: The stressor-detachment model as an integrative framework. *Journal of Organizational Behavior*, *36*, S72–S103.

Sonnentag, S., & Geurts, S. A. E. (2009). Methodological issues in recovery research. In S. Sonnentag, P. L. Perrewé, & D. C. Ganster (Eds.), *Current perspectives on job-stress recovery* (Vol. 7, pp. 1–36). Emerald Group Publishing Limited.

Sonnentag, S., & Lischetzke, T. (2018). Illegitimate tasks reach into after-work hours: A multi-level study. *Journal of Occupational Health Psychology*, *23*, 248–261.

Sonnentag, S., Unger, D., & Nägel, I. J. (2013). Workplace conflict and employee well-being: The moderating role of detachment from work during off-job time. *International Journal of Conflict Management*, *24*, 166–183.

Sonnentag, S., & Schiffner, C. (2019). Psychological detachment from work during nonwork time and employee well-being: The role of leader's detachment. *The Spanish Journal of Psychology*, *22*, E3. https://doi.org/10.1017/sjp.2019.2

Ursin, H., & Eriksen, H. R. (2010). Cognitive activation theory of stress (CATS). *Neuroscience & Biobehavioral Reviews*, *34*, 877–881.

Varol, Y. Z., Weiher, G. M., Wendsche, J., & Lohmann-Haislah, A. (2021). Difficulties detaching psychologically from work among German teachers: Prevalence, risk factors and health outcomes within a cross-sectional and national representative employee survey. *BMC Public Health*, *21*, 2046. https://doi.org/10.1186/s12889-021-12118-4

Volmer, J., Binnewies, C., Sonnentag, S., & Niessen, C. (2012). Do social conflicts with customers at work encroach upon our private lives? A diary study. *Journal of Occupational Health Psychology*, *17*, 304–315.

Weiler, R., Aggio, D., Hamer, M., Taylor, T., & Kumar, B. (2015). Sedentary behaviour among elite professional footballers: Health and performance implications. *BMJ Open Sport & Exercise Medicine*, *1*, e000023. http://dx.doi.org/10.1136/bmjsem-2015-000023

Wendsche, J., & Lohmann-Haislah, A. (2017). A meta-analysis on antecedents and outcomes of detachment from work. *Frontiers in Psychology*, *7*, 2072. https://doi.org/10.3389/fpsyg.2016.02072

5 Debriefing sport performance

A strategy to enhance mental and emotional recovery and plan for future competition

John M. Hogg

Introduction

In the post-performance sport setting, there is a need for athletes and coaches to deliberately and exactly evaluate, assimilate, and share, all detailed performance information, and to be totally accountable for the outcomes whether these are successful or not. For optimum mental and emotional recovery, the performance needs to be mentally recalled, relived, and fully disclosed to establish whether or not objectives were met, and to determine if new lessons have to be learned and acted upon.

This chapter considers the essential elements of an effective performance debriefing procedure, its connections to psychological theory, the significance of accurate reflection, feedback, and evaluation, working models to assist with the mental recovery and well-being of the participants, and the roles and responsibilities of coaches and athletes to ensure purposeful training and successful competitive experiences. Although performance appraisal has received adequate consideration in the sport psychology literature (Holder, 1997), it has recently enjoyed increased attention in other professional fields from which there is much to learn cross-culturally.

This chapter is written from a pragmatic perspective. For over 30 years the author was a head swim coach at the club, university and international levels of competition. The author has also been associated with several team and individual sports as a performance psychologist and has worked with athletes from various sports to help them mentally excel in sport and life.

Debriefing: Definitions, conceptual development and understanding

Performance evaluation is a vital ritual in the service of understanding, learning, processing, and improving personal strengths and coping with challenges.

Hogg, J. M. (2024). Debriefing sport performance: A strategy to enhance mental and emotional recovery and plan for future competition. In M. Kellmann & J. Beckmann (Eds.), *Fostering Recovery and Well-being in a Healthy Lifestyle: Psychological, Somatic, and Organizational Prevention Approaches* (pp. 73–91). Routledge.

DOI: 10.4324/9781003250654-7

Debriefing is a performance enhancement technique, a carefully structured learning process, and an effective intervention procedure providing significant post-performance information over an extended period of time for both developmental and elite athletes. It is a powerful tool enabling performers to mentally recall what happened, to assess their responses, and to explore possibilities for any improvement learned from the experience (Boud et al., 1985). Debriefing has many meanings and uses in different disciplines. It is succinctly defined in the healthcare literature as "facilitated or guided reflection in the cycle of experiential learning" (Fanning & Gaba, 2007, p. 117). It is a structural process that identifies the root causes of behaviour. It gives order and meaning to the performance, yields important actionable lessons, and evaluates the contribution of everyone involved in the determination of whether or not the performance was deemed a success or failure. It should follow a precise protocol in terms of its delivery.

Debriefing, both as a construct and as a procedure, is of surprisingly recent origin. It has received attention in several professional areas, and readers interested in its development within a social psychology framework are referred to its historical evolvement (Harris, 1988).

Debriefing procedures were initially used in military settings. The debriefing of bomber pilots during World War II, referred to as AAR (after action review), continues to be practiced the world over today, and is considered a contributing factor to the remarkable safety record of modern-day aviation (Murphy & Duke, 2011). Protocols are documented in emergency service organisations (Eppich et al., 2021), in surgical procedures, and simulated healthcare (Garden et al., 2015), in business administration (Reyes et al., 2018), in organisational development, and leadership (Sundheim, 2013), in education and curriculum development (Rudolph et al., 2008), and in crisis intervention (Meyer, 2001). These areas of application refined debriefing, sharing information about ideal conditions (timing, place, delivery, age, culture, developmental stage), the need for competent facilitators, and the individual and collective benefits to be gained.

Debriefing found importance in individual sports (Hogg, 2002), and in team sports (Macquet et al., 2015; Middlemas et al., 2018). The process of debriefing as a formative performance assessment tool occurs when athletes and coaches are engaged in an evaluative activity either in an intense or deliberate training practice or following a major competitive event, with the intended purpose of analysing and assessing performance outcomes, addressing athletes' mental and emotional recovery, and determining what might be improved upon to ensure future performance success and fulfillment (Hogg, 1998).

Following a debriefing session, athletes should be: 1) fully aware of any progress, 2) know exactly where they stand relative to their performance goals, 3) released of negative emotional states, and 4) physically and mentally recovered and re-energised. Mental recovery is aided by relaxation and tension releasing exercises, by mental toughness skills (resilience and unshakeable self-belief), by emotionally coping with any body-mind imbalance, and by accurately appraising all four performance components.

Key components of debriefing

Debriefing allows athletes to see the bigger pre-performance picture, and a more detailed and focused post-performance picture. Initially, debriefing was confined to brief coach-athlete discussions describing what happened and focusing on how athletes felt about what they had accomplished. Objective feedback – primarily provided by the coach – tended to concentrate on preventive measures to ensure improvement in subsequent performances. It was quickly realised that debriefing had more to offer than just precautionary effects (Hogg, 2002). Debriefing models, protocols and guidelines servicing individual sports steadily developed to suit sport specific needs.

Roth (2015) highlighted three essentials for a debriefing protocol (in aviation) as: 1) The ability to relive and mentally recall the performance experience. 2) The ability to reflect on one's effort and commitment when accurately evaluating outcomes. 3) The ability to learn, gather, absorb, and apply data that create a new vision, and transport the performance to the next level. Macquet et al. (2015) added that debriefing in a team sport setting should also: 4) foster athlete-coach trust relationships, and 5) improve the team's cognitive abilities. Middlemas et al. (2018) stressed 6) the need for team members to enjoy a full psychological recovery.

Macquet et al. (2015) studied the process of debriefing elite athletes during major competition in five different team sports. They focused on a qualitative analysis of the debriefing processes used by Head Coaches during national competitions to determine the precise tasks involved in a team debriefing exercise while also identifying the leadership style favoured by the nine Head Coaches. They posited that debriefing teams is about: 1) Establishing what happened exactly – emphasising the likely *causes* for performance success or failure. 2) Learning and sharing knowledge from data analyses (mainly *objective* and highly technical video feedback). 3) Exchanging observations that help to form a meaningful and immediate vision for future competition.

Debriefing team sport athletes competing at national or international levels is not a simple process. It is normally conducted under an intense time pressure, is obligated to generate practical and transparent information regarding performance improvements and is deemed necessary because of the implications attached to each country maintaining its expected competitive standing – one that assures future government funding or generates additional corporate sponsorship. Aspiring athletes are expected to willingly, responsibly and accountably reflect on the performance outcomes, while coaches identify tasks to be undertaken by the team support staff, and to meticulously prepare and present their debriefing conclusions so the team continues to function effectively.

Debriefing: Theoretical underpinnings

Debriefing has strong theoretical connections to several psychological theories, notably to *Attributional Theory* (Weiner, 1986), to *Self-Determination Theory* (Deci & Ryan, 1985), and to *Self-Efficacy Theory* (Bandura, 1997).

Attributions are explanations athletes give as to why they succeed or fail. These reasons influence subsequent motivations and behaviours. Weiner (1986) identified four common attributions – ability, effort (internal), the degree of task difficulty, and luck (external). Coaches should be aware of the attributional styles of their athletes – how they react to the happenings around them when performing under pressure, whether their responses are positive or negative, and how events, situations, and people affect their chances of achieving success. Athletes either perceive the causes for success or failure to lie within themselves (*internal factors – ability and effort*) or relating to the environment or situation (*external factors – task difficulty and luck*). Athletes who are more *internal* believe they are responsible and in control of the performance process, whereas athletes who are more *external* attribute their performance outcomes to outside forces diminishing responsibility for their actions. This unfolds in the debriefing process and helps increase the likelihood of athletes using more internal and controllable attributions.

Self-Determination Theory posits that athletes are motivated by the urge toward self-mastery and competence. They perceive themselves capable of meeting the task demands. Athletes are *intrinsically* motivated to pursue challenging goals by a sense of accomplishment, personal autonomy, and determination (Deci & Flaste, 1996). Other athletes are *extrinsically* motivated by rewards and recognition. They possibly experience less control over their efforts because they feel the burden of having to succeed placed on them by outside forces.

For the intrinsically motivated athlete the structured debriefing protocol empowers them to make any necessary changes and accentuates their feelings of competency, autonomy, and relatedness along with the urgent need to set meaningful short-term goals (Deci & Ryan, 2000).

Coaches enhance feelings of self-determination by encouraging their athletes to appraise and gain insights into their performance results and to assume full responsibility for their efforts. The approach should be 'athlete-centered'. Athletes must be sufficiently self-motivated to take control of their post-performance learning, and be actively involved in any future planning, preparation, and goal setting.

Self-efficacy is a term used to describe a person's or teams' belief in their ability to produce the desired results under specific conditions. *Self-Efficacy Theory* refers to whether or not athletes believe they can accomplish the task and achieve their stated goals. However, if the conditions change, the athletes' beliefs in their competency to accomplish a certain level of performance might change too. Self-efficacy is susceptible to change in four ways: 1) In relation to the performance itself – as repeated success increases self-efficacy, while repeated failure diminishes it. 2) Through vicarious experiences – watching others doing well or poorly can affect one's own self-efficacy. 3) By verbal persuasion or encouragement from the coach or significant others which can boost self-efficacy. 4) In feelings of emotional arousal or in how highly or lowly athletes are activated to perform. Research suggests that some athletes recognise their excessively high activation states to be beneficial to their performance, while others might experience disruptive negative anxiety states – e.g., fear of a poor result or loss of self-motivation (Hagger et al., 2001).

Coaches should recognise that self-efficacy is increased, or at least safeguarded, by a carefully constructed debriefing exercise. Debriefing is more than a casual dialogue about WHAT went well and what did not. It is an uncomfortable exercise that demands inner shovelling to confront one's vulnerability or to fortify one's courage to take calculated risks. While self-awareness is heightened debriefing may also endanger fragile levels of self-efficacy and self-confidence, especially when the performance is poor.

The importance of feedback and self-reflection

Performance efforts require an exchange of information about the results i.e., *feedback*. The ability to communicate feedback is a critical component of the debriefing procedure. At first, athletes need to acknowledge their own feelings and assimilate their own *subjective or intrinsic feedback* regarding their performance efforts before absorbing any *objective or extrinsic feedback* prepared and presented by the coach. Knowledge about how well the athlete performed and knowledge about the results should be integrated so they initiate cognitive understanding and learning. Feedback is positively presented, involving praise and encouragement, or negatively accentuated, if the performance is poor, and is accompanied by sensitive questioning, facilitating heightened self-awareness (Chow & Luzzeri, 2019). Knowledge acquired should create a strategy for further action. Feedback is an essential part of the mechanics of skill acquisition, perfecting the technical component of performance. Some athletes crave feedback, and not solely for skill development, but for its positive influence on their competencies, satisfaction, and autonomous motivation to make immediate changes to their behaviours. Feedback should always be challenging rather than threatening, and emphasise empowerment skills – i.e. autonomy, a sense of belonging in the team setting, and an acute awareness of one's competencies.

Coaches' feedback confirms whether athletes are technically performing up to expectation or not. They need to deliver feedback from a strength-based approach ascertaining how athletes might make use of their strengths to compensate for weaknesses. Negative feedback can focus on their knowledge and skills (which are more changeable) rather than on any special talents. Feedback increases perceptual awareness and provides detail to help athletes reach their expectations while teaching them to attribute their performance successes or disappointments to a lower or higher degree of effort and commitment (Dweck, 2006).

Feedback does not always produce results or changes, but *reflection* can instigate an immediate response from athletes who understand what must be undertaken to improve their performance efforts. *Self-reflection* is a spiritual component of performance (Mumford, 2016), a key factor in expert learning, referring to the extent to which individual and team athletes are able to 1) appraise their performance and determine WHAT they have learned from a particular effort, and 2) HOW they can envision and effectively integrate this knowledge into subsequent action.

Reflection is linked to the mental skill of self-awareness and requires monitoring without judgement. Positive reflective thinking produces significant change in the athlete's cognitions, emotions, and behaviours, and immediately kick starts the mental and emotional recovery process. Research indicates that elite athletes tend to readily engage in self-reflection. Athletes should be encouraged to use their powers of reasoning early on in their development (Jonker et al., 2010). Reflective athletes are more likely to improve the technical, physical, tactical, mental, and emotional components of performance more effectively when following a systematic debriefing procedure.

Coaches should encourage gifted athletes to reflect on their competitive efforts. Journalising helps to articulate their reflective thoughts. It is toxic for athletes to let their inner dialogue fester for any length of time on poor performances. Negative thinking only delays the recovery process. Reflection is taught by engaging in carefully designed self-reflective exercises, and performance debriefing is one such exercise. Following an effective debriefing protocol, athletes can discover new and meaningful information that emanates from the performance experience itself.

Appraising the performance – asking the right questions

Debriefing involves feedback, reflection, and performance appraisal. What does the athlete think about in the post-performance setting? Typically, when asked to evaluate their performance efforts, athletes allow their inner self-critic to lead the conversation. This is counter-productive thinking leading to a diminished sense of self. Accurate performance evaluations are best garnered by sensitive *questioning* rather than by coaches *telling* elite athletes what they need to do. Asking the right questions allows athletes to answer for themselves and boost their autonomy. Debriefing invites self-inspection, teases out mistakes, recognises possibilities, and commits athletes to appropriate action.

The right questions should relate to the four performance components, prompting deeper thoughts as to how they actually performed, what were the exact consequences of their efforts, and what might be adjusted or changed. Hogg (1995) discovered that too many questions did not yield a definitive pathway for meaningful action. Hogg (in press) reduced the number of debriefing questions to four. His four-by-four model (see Figure 5.3 later) is fairly rigid allowing for a methodical reflective approach rather than one that invites uncontrolled thinking or reasoning. The four selected questions were reached after conducting debriefing sessions with individual and team athletes at all levels of ability and across a number of different sports. They are:

1. What did I do well?
2. What did I do not so well?
3. What can I do better?
4. How can I accomplish this (or do better)?

These questions encourage athletes and coaches to pin point precisely which aspects of the performance are solid, and which are faulty.

First, athletes must maintain a positive outlook on their performance efforts by focusing on what they did well. There are many positives in any performance that can boost the athlete's feelings and stabilise their self-efficacy and self-confidence. Athletes should start by debriefing their strengths and their correct actions under pressure before attending to their weaknesses. By highlighting their strong points first, coaches can help them to stay focused on what they do well.

Second, unregulated mental chatter has no place in the debriefing process. Athletes need to identify mistakes, address them, and refrain from relentlessly questioning their competencies and values. If the performance is lacking, athletes must not allow their inner dialogue to trigger self-doubt, or retain feelings of uncertainty or fear, or entertain negative emotional states (disappointment, embarrassment, frustration, or even anger). There is urgency to move on.

Third, athletes should genuinely care about what they can do better, maintaining confidence levels if the performance was successful, or rebuilding it, if the performance failed to reach expectation. Accurate recall and self-reflection effects self-efficacy, emotional states, and self-talk patterns (Allen et al., 2010). In this context using mindfulness-based stress reduction should be considered, as it is said to provide more veridical perception, reduce negative affect and improve vitality and coping (Grossman et al., 2004). A sub-question for reflection is: what opportunities for improvement do I realistically have?

Finally, athletes need to repair things satisfactorily both for the short- and long-term by determining and utilising the self-reflective tools that are available. They should preview the upcoming performance requirements, be prepared to make corrections in training, and inject new meaning into their goal pursuits.

The responses to the four questions disclose why athletes did or did not meet their performance expectations, facilitate their physical and mental recovery, teach responsibility and accountability for performance outcomes, and help them move on without further brooding.

Coaches should make a habit of asking the athletes at the end of quality training to accurately evaluate how they performed and what they learned. Coaches need to develop their debriefing skills, and to recognise the emotional hurdles to straddle related to the athlete's age and stage of growth and development.

The design of a debriefing protocol

Debriefing should follow a designed protocol in terms of its delivery. Lederman (1992) identified seven structural elements to a debriefing process. These common factors as they relate to a sporting context are: 1) The debriefer – the head coach or delegate. 2) Those who have to be debriefed – individual or team athletes and staff. 3) The experience itself – a significant performance that requires analysis and appraisal. 4) The impact of the experience – the competition effects on the athlete(s). 5) The recollection – recall and reflection of performance data. 6) The report – dissemination of information to all involved. 7) The timing – duration between event and debrief.

There are several constraints that shape a debriefing protocol (resources, experience, competencies, team dynamics etc.), and the coach must navigate these skillfully. A stepwise approach to debriefing individual sport athletes was suggested by Hogg (2002) and is summarised in Figure 5.1. These steps can be modified to suit athlete and coach preferences and cater to the sport specific environment.

Individual sport athletes need to: 1) Buy into the debriefing process and exhibit complete trust in it. 2) Provide themselves with subjective feedback by answering the four key questions, either as part of their warm-down protocol, or at later time. 3) Share performance information and establish a strong coach-athlete trust relationship. Without two-way communication and a solid rapport, it is difficult to accomplish an effective performance evaluation (Mageau & Vallerand, 2010). 4) Empower themselves to self-regulate debriefing skills by aiming to generate meaningful responses that reflect positive values, attitudes, and intrinsic motivational levels. 5) Revisit their self-motivation and re-adjust their cognitions based on what inspires or activates them to perform well.

Team sport athletes can also follow a team debriefing protocol which is more difficult to conduct because of team size and complexity. The extent of the debriefing protocol depends on the competitive structure – whether the team is engaged in weekly games requiring analysis, or in a knockout tournament when debriefs are in closer proximity. Team debriefing is conducted either as a collective group or in terms of positional play (Middlemas et al., 2018). Reliance rests heavily on video feedback.

Macquet et al. (2015) studied team debriefing from a coaching perspective. They posited team debriefing is primarily concerned with: 1) Analyzing the performance accurately, highlighting what happened exactly, and recognising the causes for success or failure. 2) Learning and sharing knowledge from data analyses and observations that helps to form a future vision. 3) Fostering and improving the athlete-coach trust relationship. 4) Ensuring a full psychological recovery.

Macquet et al. (2015) concluded effective team debriefing requires a two-step approach involving specific tasks. First, a *preparation* step driven by what is currently occurring in the competition and inclusive of all areas of support. Second, a *presentation* step involving the post-performance sharing of pertinent information to team members and staff in order to facilitate preparations for subsequent competitive efforts. Head Coaches require a well-established philosophical viewpoint behind their choice of leadership style whether their approach is transactional or transformational or both. Relying on their findings, a stepwise approach to debriefing teams is suggested in Figure 5.2.

Team athletes need to: 1) Self-reflect during warming down activities to ascertain their contribution to the team effort. 2) Provide input focusing on the causes for the team's success or short fall. 3) Give themselves subjective feedback supported by data (video playback). 4) Discuss actions to be taken to ensure corrections are in place before the next performance. 5) Determine how these

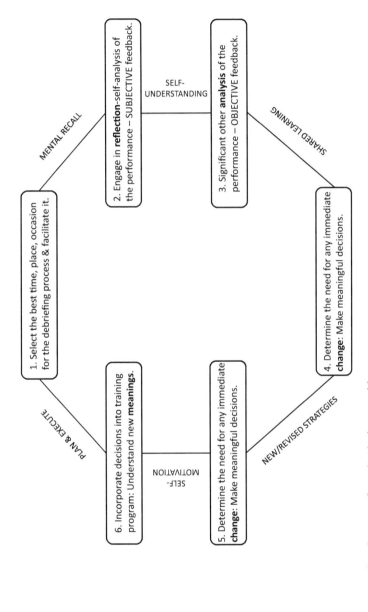

Figure 5.1 Debriefing steps for individual sport athletes.

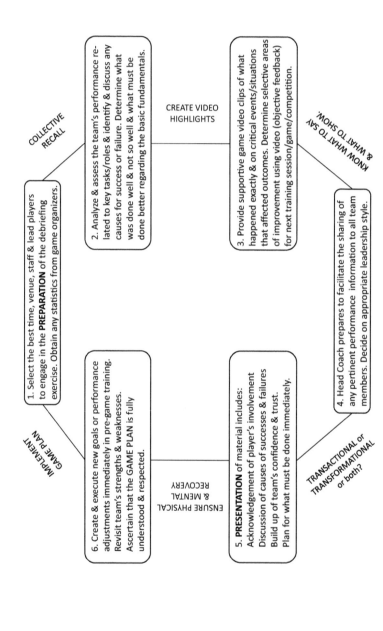

COLLECTIVE
RECALL

CREATE VIDEO
HIGHLIGHTS

KNOW WHAT TO SAY
& WHAT TO SHOW.

IMPLEMENT
GAME PLAN

ENSURE PHYSICAL
& MENTAL
RECOVERY

TRANSACTIONAL or
TRANSFORMATIONAL
or both?

1. Select the best time, venue, staff & lead players to engage in the **PREPARATION** of the debriefing exercise. Obtain any statistics from game organizers.

2. Analyze & assess the team's performance related to key tasks/roles & identify & discuss any causes for success or failure. Determine what was done well & not so well & what must be done better regarding the basic fundamentals.

3. Provide supportive game video clips of what happened exactly & on critical events/situations that affected outcomes. Determine selective areas of improvement using video (objective feedback) for next training session/game/competition.

4. Head Coach prepares to facilitate the sharing of any pertinent performance information to all team members. Decide on appropriate leadership style.

5. **PRESENTATION** of material includes: Acknowledgement of player's involvement Discussion of causes of successes & failures Build up of team's confidence & trust. Plan for what must be done immediately.

6. Create & execute new goals or performance adjustments immediately in pre-game training. Revisit team's strengths & weaknesses. Ascertain that the GAME PLAN is fully understood & respected.

Figure 5.2 Debriefing steps for team sport athletes.

adjustments are tactically implemented. 6) Establish agreement on purposeful short-term goals to pursue in quality training and be accomplished before the next competition.

Coaches need to increase or maintain the right level of collective energy among team members, and to generate enthusiasm without making odious comparisons or creating a threatening or humiliating atmosphere. Team debriefings can instigate discussions that positively facilitate team cohesiveness (Pain & Harwood, 2009).

Examining debriefing studies across disciplines, Tannenbaum and Cerasoli (2013) clarified four essential elements that define and differentiate debriefing from other interventions. These are: 1) *Active self-learning* – participants engage in forms of self-discovery rather than relying solely on objective feedback. 2) *Developmental intent* – the primary intent is to learn and improve the four performance components. 3) *A specific event* – reflection, feedback, and performance analysis address a significant competitive event. Feedback is directed at the strengths and weaknesses of the individual or the team. 4) *Multiple information sources* – there is input from team personnel, participants, and at least one external data source (video). Personal observations are best recorded using specifically designed debriefing sheets (Figure 5.3).

Head coaches determine the design of the debriefing session with crystal clear learning objectives which are either established beforehand or emerge as the debrief evolves.

Debriefing and performance improvement

Testing for a link between the debriefing procedure and any performance improvement would prove to be intrusive, time consuming, and difficult to manage. McArdle et al. (2010) attempted to examine the debriefing process and found it difficult to make a direct link between debriefing and performance improvement because too many other factors are involved.

A recent meta-analysis of 46 debriefing studies claims that debriefing does improve performance (Tannenbaum & Cerasoli, 2013). However, the debriefing protocol following an elite performance must be intently focused, specifically structured, and regularly delivered with consistency. Debriefing improves knowledge, skills, and competencies. It helps athletes to realise difficult performance objectives and to avoid costly mistakes.

Tannenbaum and Cerasoli (2013) found evidence for the following hypotheses: 1) Individuals and teams utilising debriefing protocols are more effective than those who do not. 2) Debriefing sessions are effective when levels of competency, focus, and measurement are aligned. They further examined three characteristics believed to improve the quality of a debriefing session – viz., facilitation, a high level of structure, and the help of multi-media aids. However, the data did not allow for any clear conclusions, so further research is needed. In particular, a positive influence of multi-media aids could not be confirmed.

PERFORMANCE DEBRIEFING exercise. Name: _____   Date: _____   Competition: _____   Target time: sub 2.21.00

QUESTIONS	TECHNICAL/SKILL	PHYSICAL/PHYSIOLOGICAL	TACTICAL/STRATEGIC	MENTAL/EMOTIONAL
1. WHAT did I do well?	Kept hips high for first 100m & felt streamlined. Kick was stronger off walls. Used controlled breathing pattern. Breathing every 2 strokes for 150m. Felt smooth for 1st. 100m.	Stroke felt very strong for first 75m. Good push out the back. Controlled my hand entry. Sufficient strength to accelerate through the pull for 125-150m.	I tried to keep my split 50 times even to hit my 200m target time: 50m = 31.00 100m = 36.00 (1:07.00) 150m = 36.70 200m = 36.03 (1:12.73) Final time: 2: 19.73	Pleased with my 200 Fly time at this stage of training – know I can do better with increased training. I did try to think more both pre-race & post-race to get myself into a good mental state – felt positive.
2. WHAT did I not do well?	Started to drop my hips on last 75m – & too much undulation on last 50m. Head too high starting at last turn. Felt hands slipping outwards on front end of the stroke. Lost strong hand exit at 150m.	Started to slip entry & finish of pull at 125. Not fit enough yet. Elbows started dropping. Hand deceleration @ 125m. Need to work on underwater technique at turns. Head too high on breakouts. Last 100m physically hard! Kick changed from 2 beat to 1.5	Worked on stroke count but did not hold what I hoped to do – was erratic & not strong enough at this stage of seasonal training. Last 100m - I was slipping & stroke count increased.	I hate to admit – but I could have warmed up with greater mental purpose. I needed longer – was rushed & failed to get in what I normally do so I am totally ready. Did not feel in the best mental space.
3. WHAT can I do better?	Maintain a higher body position throughout 200m & use strong/even downbeat leg kick. Timing of the leg kick – at hand entry & hand press to finish stroke. Aim not to rush the stroke on 2nd. 100m. More control.	Need stronger hands to hold water. More wrist work in gym on weights & pulleys. Got to think PRESS at end of stroke. Need stronger leg kick on 2 beat for total swim. Added time to best time, but hit under target time for this meet.	Need to work on breathing pattern - breathing every 2 strokes for whole race or 2:1:1.for last 50m if necessary. Hold stroke count to not more than 2 stroke increase per 50m – try 22-24-26 in quality training sets.	Prepare well – with a plan for every race – not rely on what I did last season. Be sure to execute the plan rather than worry or doubt. Need to look at cue word to motivate myself to push myself hard on 3rd. 50m.
4. HOW can I accomplish this?	Got to work hard in training to maintain even paced 50m repeats @ 35-36 secs. Improve fav set 16x50 Fly on 60. Work at 2nd 100m pace time @ sub 1.12.0. Stroke length & speed on fly single arm drills.	Keep head down for 2-3 strokes at breakouts. Timing of leg kick. Keep working at arm strength in gym – weights & pulley exercises. Work harder at specific fly arm drills – I must concentrate more in fly training sets.	Remember to keep head in line rather than lifting too high to breathe. Execute wall turns at speed so there is no loss of momentum. Head down for 2-3 strokes at breakouts.	Work more purposefully on visualizing my 200m fly race & add specific detail over time & practice. Establish & try some more cue words to help with my concentration especially at the 150m.

Mark on a scale of 1 – 10   Performance Satisfaction Scale:
Your degree of satisfaction.

1		5		10
Not at all satisfied				Extremely satisfied

Result: 200m Fly* 2:19.73. I give this swim a 7 on the PSS.

Figure 5.3 Performance debriefing exercise.
Note: PSS = Performance Satisfaction Scale.

Benefits of using a debriefing protocol

Bohl (1991) and Mitchell (1983, 1988) highlighted the benefits of conducting debriefing procedures following disasters or traumatic incidents – notably a reduction in negative emotions and a quick return to normal functioning. Debriefing injects renewed energy into training so that the pursuit of excellence remains exciting and motivates athletes to participate in planning future performances. Tackling failures exposed in the debriefing process is critical for success.

Debriefing is a vital testing system encouraging athletes to accurately identify any gaps between their real and imagined talent, and to take immediate action that will improve their future performances. Debriefing provides new learning and challenges that refresh lack-luster performances encouraging athletes to stand back, examine options, and apply an appraisal-reappraisal technique to trigger their emotional recovery (Lazarus, 2000).

Some cautions

History suggests that performance break-throughs begin with multiple failures. Athletes must redefine failure and success – what it means to them and how they can endure and handle it. Learning from mistakes and finding solutions will eradicate internal and external fears. Success does not happen in an instant. It requires lengthy application and willingness to persevere, and mental toughness, courage, and resilience in the post-performance setting. Grit is a key factor driving long term success (Duckworth, 2016).

There is a place for empathy when coping with performance disappointments. Failure precipitates emotional distresses and raises defensive barriers. Self-compassion, introduced into the psychology literature by Neff (2003), is an additional construct focusing on self-kindness, while providing emotional safety in the face of disappointment, and recognising failure to be both a human and a shared experience (Mosewich et al., 2013).

Recent research suggests self-compassion has a place in sport (Mosewich et al., 2019), and likely in the debriefing process. Ceccarelli et al. (2019) found that athletes with higher levels of self-compassion enjoyed better adaptive psychological and physiological responses to failed performance than those with lower self-compassion. Wilson et al. (2019), looked at self-compassion and mental toughness, and most athletes thought the two were compatible and worked in a 'zipper effect'. However, some athletes might perceive self-compassion to be the opposite of mental toughness.

Finally, parents engage in 'debriefing' their children's sport performances with the intent of being supportive influences. They need to understand the composition of the debriefing process, and to safeguard their child's intrinsic motivation, performance enjoyment, and satisfaction. Coaches should educate parental groups about balanced and honest feedback without negative comment (Elliott & Drummond, 2017). Little is known about the acceptable behaviour of sport parents in the post-performance setting, though research indicates that female athletes especially welcome positive comments rather than overly critical feedback (Knight et al., 2011).

Leadership implications for the coach

How the debriefing protocol is defined and facilitated is under the responsibility of the head coach. There are many styles of leadership. *Transformational leaders* motivate athletes to exceed their self-interests for the greater good. They are attentive to the self-worth and confidence needs of team members – whether actively playing or patiently awaiting their turn. They serve as mentors encouraging athletes to recognise the causes of poor performances, and make necessary corrections by questioning and challenging their personal goals. They address any emotional needs of athletes who feel mentally stressed (Bass et al., 2003).

Transactional leaders tend to acknowledge and reward their athletes' efforts when they do well, and recognise inadequacies when behaviours are inappropriate. They maintain control over athletes providing direction especially when there are time constraints. This style is employed by coaches when presenting a detailed appraisal of team efforts. Instead of encouraging athletes to find their own solutions, coaches present practical ways for athletes to reach their goals while still remaining open to input.

According to Bass (1999) and Macquet et al. (2015) the best coaches are both transformational and transactional leaders and use debriefing to highlight experiential knowledge, objective, corrective feedback, and a future vision for team members (including substitutes, who may contribute to the team's success if they embrace the role they are asked to play).

Coaches and athletes need a compatible view of what happened in the performance. This understanding allows them to focus on those elements of the performance requiring discussion and immediate correction. Coaches should help to initiate a self-reflective mindset, actively assist performance closure, and create expectations around new efforts. At the conclusion of a debriefing exercise, athletes should know WHAT is expected of them in the next training session, and HOW they can accomplish it. Debriefing guidelines for individual and team sports are summarised in Figure 5.4.

When debriefing in individual sports, coaches should be aware that athletes can be overwhelmed by internal or external feedback, have difficulty accepting it, or unwilling to make changes intuitively or practically.

In team sports, debriefing is concerned with assessing outcomes of their own game efforts rather than those of the opposition. Data learned is presented to all team members in an organised fashion and with the help of video feedback. Focus can fall on three to four critical issues requiring collaboration of the team unit. Athletes may have different interpretations of the game results depending on their competency levels or their perception of the role they

Pre-performance:

General considerations: – for both TEAM & INDIVIDUAL SPORTS:

Pre-performance:

❑ Design & provide a debriefing model or structure to suit your sport & prepare your agenda very carefully.
❑ Educate your athletes about the debriefing process, its importance & benefits, its structure & focus, your role as coach & theirs as athletes.
❑ Highlight the significance of mental recall, honest reflection, & both subjective & objective feedback & the need to gain new insights into the performance.
❑ Explain the need to accurately answer the 4 debriefing questions.
❑ Create a psychologically healthy environment that seeks the causes for success or failure without assigning blame, one that encourages all athletes to share their experiences, & to freely discuss ways to turn learning opportunities into meaningful action.
❑ Aim to conduct the debriefing session close to the competitive event to facilitate accurate memory & recall.
❑ Always allow sufficient time for the debriefing exercise, clarify any constraints, & look for willingness & commitment from all athletes to be involved in the protocol.

Post-performance:

❑ Check whether objectives were met & encourage athletes to engage in internal feedback without being overly self-critical.
❑ Recognize that every athlete makes mistakes – the idea is not to repeat them unnecessarily.
❑ Always admit to your own errors & frame all mistakes as learning opportunities.
❑ Be sure that you & your athletes are on the same page & are prepared to collaborate fully.
❑ Be sure you are exhibiting the very attributes that you are looking for in your athletes when analyzing performance outcomes & gathering performance data.
❑ Be sure to clarify any Dos & Don'ts to avoid unnecessary missteps.
❑ Contribute your own feedback once the athletes have expressed their perspectives.

Specific considerations for: INDIVIDUAL SPORTS:

Post-performance:

❑ Acknowledge the need for a growth mindset rather than accepting reluctance to cooperate when analyzing post performance outcomes.
❑ Stress the need for self-discovery & a willingness to change or adjust behaviours speedily.
❑ When giving objective feedback following competition or quality training, develop good interpersonal skills – inviting questions & seeking information rather than just telling your athletes the way you see the outcomes.
❑ Explain patiently what individual challenges must be done better & what action steps need to be taken immediately.
❑ Indicate & discuss any lessons learned & what needs to be integrated into the next training session or into the overall competitive plan.
❑ Spend 5-10 minutes on the debriefing protocol with each athlete following competition & fill in any knowledge gaps.
❑ Target any barriers or hindrances to be overcome swiftly.
❑ Keep a sense of humour.

Specific consideration for TEAM SPORTS:

Post-performance preparation & presentation:

❑ Following a poor team performance focus on what went wrong & not on who to blame for letting it happen.
❑ Encourage all team members to share their thoughts & feelings first & before you present yours.
❑ Be aware of fruitless discussion & redirect conversation to issues that are in the control of the team.
❑ Make time for the formal team briefing/debriefing sessions (20-45 mins) in a suitable venue free from distractions.
❑ Address ambiguities that could cause stress & extra work or hardship on simple tasks.
❑ Be sure team members are aware of what is set in stone & what is negotiable when it come to making agreements on future actions.
❑ Prepare the debrief agenda concentrating on everything the team must now do & be sure to enter an agreement & a clear understanding.
❑ Present high tech video playback as objective feedback & aim to be your strong self in front of the team.
❑ Always stress the significance of teamwork & cooperation to ensure performance improvement.

Figure 5.4 Debriefing guidelines for the Head Coach.

played (Macquet & Stanton, 2014). In team debriefing, players are uncomfortable crystalising a defeat especially when they can identify the culprit as the one who – e.g., failed to score in the penalty shoot out. Failure must not be addressed by blaming others, making excuses, or pretending it did not happen.

Getting everyone on the same page requires a functional debriefing structure whose agenda minimises any misunderstandings or fruitless discussion (Macquet,

2013), and creates expectations that match how well athletes are currently stretching themselves in training.

Conclusion and recommendations for practice

Debriefing is a resource that helps athletes overcome their vulnerability and involves them in developing PLANS to improve subsequent training and competition. Experienced athletes should: 1) reference and re-examine previous performance efforts, 2) learn to autonomously make decisions about deliberate practice, 3) handle any adversity during competition, 4) be open to new data, and 5) cope with any emerging negative emotions or mood states when underperforming. Focus is on evaluating the positive or negative facts of the athlete's performance rather than on their feelings.

Athletes must reimagine any changes that will transform their future performances, be willing to investigate any exposed mistakes, recognise the gaps between the results they expected and those they achieved. They can now determine how these gaps might be effectively bridged.

The athlete's mindset is driven by a desire for success. Those with a *fixed mindset* will ignore their mistakes since they believe they cannot measurably change anything – so why bother? Those with a *growth mindset* view failure as an important aspect of learning and developing, and actively seek to make creative changes or take enlightened risks (Dweck, 2006). Debriefing generates new data, engages squarely with failure, and excites the imagination to push personal boundaries into performance triumphs. Figure 5.3 presents an individual sport debriefing exercise sheet completed by an adolescent female 200m butterfly swimmer following the first meet of the swim season (Hogg, in press). Other tools are available to help athletes learn from their efforts and plan for the future – e.g., Post Event Reflection Sheet (Chow & Luzzeri, 2019), and Holder's Performance Evaluation Sheet (Holder, 1997).

Questions remain and room exists to broaden the understanding and appreciation for debriefing skills and protocols, while pursuing research of any technical advances in the collection and assessment of performance data unique to the sport (McClusky, 2014). Future research can better explain factors that moderate the effectiveness of debriefing protocols, interventions, tools, and visual aids. Research can address how data is best delivered to all athletes both in individual and team functioning, the effects of leadership styles, the delivery and reception of meaningful feedback, and how performance and well-being outcomes are interrelated. Finally, is debriefing helped or hindered by coaching cultural norms or differences?

Debriefing is a focused exercise that allows athletes to see the bigger performance picture and plan for future success. Without an organised protocol there is limited reflection or reporting to generate learning and understanding of what was done well or not so well. Habitual quality practice in training or competition encourages debriefing skills to become more automatic.

Debriefing helps athletes to reflect on intended actions, identify limitations, consolidate knowledge and competencies, fix systematic problems, and discuss crucial areas of their performance that require immediate improvement. Tannenbaum and Cerasoli (2013) provide empirical support and a solid evidentiary basis for the effectiveness of both individual and team debriefing protocols. However, it is important to further explore, define, and validate the structure, role and efficiency of debriefing skills, to rigorously test the best protocols in selected sports, and to ensure that athletes strengthen their core values through accurate self-reflection and evaluation, while continuing to experience success, enjoyment, and a healthy recovery.

References

Allen, M. S., Jones, M. V., & Sheffield, D. (2010). The influence of positive reflection on attributions, emotions, and self-efficacy. *The Sport Psychologist*, *24*(2), 211–226.

Bandura, A. (1997). *Self-efficacy: The exercise of control*. Freeman.

Bass, B. M. (1999). Two decades of research and development in transformational leadership. *European Journal of Work and Organizational Psychology*, *8*(1), 9–32.

Bass, B. M., Avolio, B. J., Jung, D. I., & Berson, Y. (2003). Predicting unit performance by assessing transformational and transactional leadership. *Journal of Applied Psychology*, *88*(2), 207–218.

Bohl, N. (1991). The effectiveness of brief psychological interventions in police officers after critical incidents. In J. Reese, J. Horn, & C. Dunning (Eds.), *Critical incidents in policing. Revised* (pp. 31–38). U.S. Government Printing Office.

Boud, D., Keogh, R., & Walker, D. (1985). *Using experience for learning*. Open University Press.

Ceccarelli, L. A., Guiliano, R. J., Glazebrook, C. M., & Strachan, S. M. (2019). Self-compassion and psycho-physiological recovery from recalled sport failure. *Frontiers in Psychology*, *10*, 1564. https://doi.org/10.3389/fpsyg.2019.01564

Chow, C. M., & Luzzeri, M. (2019). Post event reflection: A tool to facilitate self-awareness, self-monitoring and self-regulation in athletes. *Journal of Sport Psychology in Action*, *10*(2), 106–118.

Deci, E. L., & Flaste, R. (1996). *Why we do what we do: Understanding self-motivation*. Penguin Books.

Deci, E. L., & Ryan, R. M. (1985). *Intrinsic motivation and self-determination in human behavior*. Plenum.

Deci, E. L., & Ryan, R. M. (2000). The "what" and "why" of goal pursuits: Human needs and the self-determination of human behavior. *Psychological Inquiry*, *11*(4), 227–268.

Duckworth, A. (2016). *Grit – The power of passion and perseverance*. Vermillion.

Dweck, C. S. (2006). *Mindset: The new psychology of success*. Random House.

Elliott, S. K., & Drummond, M. J. N. (2017). Parents in youth sport: What happens after the game? *Sport, Education and Society*, *22*(3), 391–406.

Eppich, W. J., Hart, D., & Huffman, J. L. (2021). Debriefing in emergency medicine. In C. Strother, Y. Okuda, N. Wong, & S. McLaughlin (Eds.), *Comprehensive healthcare simulation: Emergency medicine* (pp. 33–46). Springer.

Fanning, R. M., & Gaba, D. M. (2007). The role of debriefing in simulation-based learning. *Simulation in Healthcare*, *2*(2), 115–125.

Garden, A. L., LeFevre, D. M., Waddington, H. L., & Weller, J. M. (2015). Debriefing after simulation-based non-technical skill in healthcare: A systematic review of effective practice. *Journal of Anaesthesia and Intensive Care Medicine, 43*(3), 300–308.

Grossman, P., Niemann, L., Schmidt, S., & Walach, H. (2004). Mindfulness-based stress reduction and health benefits: A meta-analysis. *Journal of Psychosomatic Research, 57*(1), 35–43.

Hagger, M. S., Chatzisarantis, N., & Biddle, S. J. (2001). The influence of self-efficacy and past behavior on the physical activity intentions of young people. *Journal of Sports Science, 19*(9), 711–725.

Harris, B. (1988). A history of debriefing in social psychology. In J. G. Morawski (Ed.), *The rise and experimentation in American psychology* (pp. 188–212). Yale University Press.

Hogg, J. M. (1995). *Mental skills for swim coaches*. Sport Excel Publishing.

Hogg, J. M. (1998). The post-performance debriefing process: Getting your capable track and field athletes to the next level of performance. *New Studies in Athletics, 13*(3), 49–56.

Hogg, J. M. (2002). Debriefing: A means to increasing recovery and subsequent performance. In M. Kellmann (Ed.), *Enhancing recovery: Preventing underperformance in athletes* (pp. 181–197). Human Kinetics.

Hogg, J. M. (in press). *Mental preparation for successful swimming performance: A workbook to help swim coaches deliver a mental skills training program*. InstaPrint.

Holder, T. (1997). A theoretical perspective of performance evaluation. In R. J. Butler (Ed.), *Sport psychology in performance* (pp. 68–86). Butterworth-Heinemann.

Jonker, L., Elferink-Gemser, M. T., de Roos, I. M., & Visscher, C. (2010). Differences in self-regulatory skills among talented athletes: The significance of competitive level and type of sport. *Journal of Sport Sciences, 28*(8), 901–908.

Knight, C. J., Neely, K. C., & Holt, N. L. (2011). Parental behaviors in team sports: How do female athletes want parents to behave? *Journal of Applied Sport Psychology, 23*(1), 76–92.

Lazarus, R. S. (2000). Cognitive-motivational-relational theory of emotion. In Y. L. Hanin (Ed.), *Emotions in sport* (pp. 39–63). Human Kinetics.

Lederman, L. C. (1992). Debriefing: Toward a systematic assessment of theory and practice. *Simulation & Gaming, 23*(2), 145–160.

Macquet, A.-C. (2013). Getting them on the same page: A method to study the consistency of head coaches' and athletes' situation understanding during training sessions and competitions. *The Sport Psychologist, 27*(3), 292–295.

Macquet, A.-C., & Stanton, N. A. (2014). Do the coach and athlete have the same picture of the situation? Distributed situation awareness in an elite sport context. *Applied Ergonomics, 45*(3), 724–733.

Macquet, A.-C., Ferrand, C., & Stanton, N. A. (2015). Divide and rule: A qualitative analysis of the debriefing process in elite team sports. *Applied Ergonomics, 51*, 30–38.

Mageau, G. A., & Vallerand, R. J. (2010). The coach-athlete relationship: A motivational model. *Journal of Sport Sciences, 21*(11), 883–904.

McArdle, S., Martin, D., Lennon, A., & Moore, P. (2010). Exploring debriefing in sports: A qualitative perspective. *Journal of Applied Sport Psychology, 22*(3), 320–332.

McClusky, M. (2014). *Faster, higher, stronger: How sport science is creating a new generation of super athletes and what we can learn from them*. Hudson Street Press.

Meyer, H. (2001). Psychological debriefing: Theory, practice and evidence. *Journal of the American Medical Association, 286*(5), 604–605.

Middlemas, S., Croft, H. G., & Watson, F. (2018). Behind closed doors: The role of debriefing and feedback in a professional rugby team. *International Journal of Sport Science and Coaching, 13*(2), 201–212.

Mitchell, J. T. (1983). When disaster strikes … The critical incident stress debriefing process. *Journal of Emergency Medical Services, 8*(1), 36–39.

Mitchell, J. T. (1988). Stress. The history, status and future of critical incident stress debriefings. *Journal of Emergency Medical Services, 13*(11), 46–47, 49–52.

Mosewich, A. D., Crocker, P., Kowalski, K. C., & DiLongis, A. (2013). Applying self-compassion in sport: An intervention with women athletes. *Journal of Sport and Exercise Psychology, 33*, 103–123.

Mosewich, A. D., Ferguson, L. J., McHugh, T. F., & Kowalski, K. C. (2019). Enhancing capacity: Integrating self-compassion in sport. *Journal of Sport Psychology in Action, 10*(4), 235–243.

Mumford, G. (2016). *The mindful athlete: Secrets to pure performance.* Parallax Press.

Murphy, J. D., & Duke, W. M. (2011). *The debrief imperative.* Fast Pencil Inc.

Neff, K. (2003). Self-compassion: An alternative conceptualization of a healthy attitude toward oneself. *Self and Identity, 2*(2), 85–101.

Pain, M., & Harwood, C. G. (2009). Team building through mutual sharing and open discussion on team functioning. *The Sport Psychologist, 23*(4), 523–542.

Reyes, D. L., Tannenbaum, S. I., & Salas, E. (2018). Team development: The power of debriefing. *People and Strategy, 41*(2), 46–51.

Roth, W. M. (2015). Cultural practices and cognition in debriefing: The case of aviation. *Journal of Cognitive Engineering and Decision Making, 9*(3), 263–278.

Rudolph, J. W., Simon, R., Raemer, D. B., & Eppich, W. J. (2008). Debriefing as formative assessment: Closing performance gaps in medical education. *Academic Emergency Medicine, 15*(11), 1010–1016.

Sundheim, D. (2013). *Taking smart risks: How sharp leaders win when stakes are high.* McGraw Hill.

Tannenbaum, S. I., & Cerasoli, C. P. (2013). Do team and individual debriefs enhance performance? A meta-analysis. *Human Factors, 55*(1), 231–245.

Weiner, B. (1986). *An attributional theory of motivation and emotion.* Springer.

Wilson, D., Bennett, E. V., Mosewich, A. D., Faulkner, G. E., & Crocker, P. R. E. (2019). The "zipper effect": Exploring the relationship of mental toughness and self-compassion among Canadian elite women athletes. *Psychology of Sport and Exercise, 40*, 61–70.

6 Engaging in creative behaviours and activities as a well-being and recovery approach

Veronique Richard, V. Vanessa Wergin, and John Cairney

An embodied and embedded perspective on creativity

Creativity can be defined as a process that both explores and expands the area of possibility for individuals, groups, and society. It should not be reduced to a product or a trait (e.g., a creative person) but rather is defined by the expanded zone of possibility that creative actions build on and open for self and others (Glăveanu, 2021). Furthermore, creativity can be conceived as embodied, which implies that brain and body are intrinsically coupled (Gallagher, 2015) and embedded within the environment (Malinin, 2019). Drawing on these conceptions, the *Creative Potential System model* (Richard et al., 2021) stipulates that actively engaging with creative environments and activities challenges individuals' systems to allow the expansion of cognitive, affective, physical, and social resources. This enriched repertoire broadens one's perception of affordances (i.e., possibility of actions), increasing the likelihood of meaningful and agentic actions. In other words, cultivating the possible (Bruner, 1960), through creative actions and activities, may open a door for individuals to explore beyond the immediacy of their reality. With these conceptions of creativity in mind, it is reasonable to question how the expansion of the possible contributes to human flourishing. Specifically, the current chapter reviews the literature on the impacts of engaging in creative activities and behaviours on well-being and recovery to suggest novel approaches and research questions.

Creativity and well-being

There are multiple, and sometimes seemingly oppositional, ways to approach and explore the relationship between creativity and well-being as defined by "the realisation of one's unique potential through physical, mental, emotional, and spiritual development in relationship to self, others, and the environment"

Richard, V., Wergin, V. V., & Cairney, J. (2024). Engaging in creative behaviours and activities as a well-being and recovery approach. In M. Kellmann & J. Beckmann (Eds.), *Fostering Recovery and Well-being in a Healthy Lifestyle: Psychological, Somatic, and Organizational Prevention Approaches* (pp. 92–102). Routledge.

DOI: 10.4324/9781003250654-8

(Gordon & O'Toole, 2015, p. 335). For instance, following the so-called 'mad-genius hypothesis', creativity is associated with various psychopathologies (Simonton, 2014) and thus, well-being could be viewed as compromised by creative productivity or diverse forms of creative expression. Alternatively, well-being can be positively impacted by creative expression and work (see Acar et al., 2021, for details). A recent meta-analysis revealed that a positive relationship between well-being and creativity prevails, with the greatest effect found between the engagement in creative activities/behaviours and well-being (Acar et al., 2021).

Creative activities and behaviours

The expression of one's creative potential needs not to be directed toward revolutionising the 'world' in order to have personal benefits. According to Richards (2007), mundane moments of insights or engaging in creative hobbies daily can impact positive functioning. Following this assumption, Conner et al. (2018) examined the relationship between the time spent engaging in everyday creative activities (e.g., coming up with novel or original ideas; expressing oneself in an original and useful way), positive and negative affect, and flourishing in 658 young adults using a 13-day daily diary method. Findings revealed that investing more time in creative behaviours and activities is associated with increased emotional well-being (i.e., positive affect and flourishing) on the following day and that this gain in well-being in turn is linked with creative activities on the same day. In line with these findings, scholars suggest that creative activities are promising intervention strategies to foster well-being (Conner et al., 2018; Forgeard & Eichner, 2014; Lomas, 2016).

A more deliberate engagement in creative activities may also contribute to well-being. Amongst the broad array of activities that may be classified as 'creative', the relationship between the engagement in creative arts and well-being has gained traction in recent years. For instance, growing research on the use of art therapy – "the creative process of art making to improve and enhance the physical, mental, and emotional well-being of individuals of all ages" (Forgeard & Eichner, 2014, p. 144) – confirms its effectiveness to reduce symptoms associated with mental ill health such as depression (Jenabi et al., 2023), trauma-related disorders (Morison et al., 2022), and anxiety disorders (Lu et al., 2021). Nevertheless, scholars believe that there is still an untapped potential for the role of creative arts in the promotion of well-being that goes beyond alleviating disorder and distress (Forgeard & Eichner, 2014; Lomas, 2016).

Namely, in 2019 the World Health Organization (WHO) conducted a scoping review questioning the role of the arts in improving health and well-being. Findings revealed that an engagement with the arts can be effective in promoting both physical and mental health (Fancourt & Finn, 2019). Building on this review, Shim et al. (2021) studied the impact of the arts and humanities interventions on the flourishing of healthy populations. They found that interventions using music, visual arts, theatre, or a combination of multiple art forms significantly impact participants' emotional and social well-being as well as positive sense of self. Furthermore, to successfully implement an art intervention, they highlighted the importance of establishing a safe and supportive climate that allows peer interactions and is tailored to participants' needs. For instance, silk painting was used as an 'arts for health' activity and its impact on nurses' health and well-being was investigated (Karpavičiūtė & Macijauskienė, 2016). Different from art therapy sessions, 'arts for health' activities aimed at allowing nurses to engage with the art of silk painting, express their creativity, relax, and socialise with other nurses in the group. After 10 weeks, the nurses practicing silk painting significantly improved their emotional well-being and vitality/energy, while reducing their general fatigue compared to a group of nurses that maintained their regular professional activities. These results are in line with major cohort studies conducted in the United States and United Kingdom between 2017 and 2022, showing significant evidence for the role of creative arts in improving health and well-being over the lifespan (Fancourt et al., 2023).

Potential mechanisms explaining the creative expression and well-being relationship

In an effort to explain the relationship between the engagement with the arts and humanities and well-being outcomes, Tay et al. (2018) proposed four mechanisms: immersion, embeddedness, socialisation, and reflectiveness. First, *immersing* oneself in an artistic experience has the power to capture one's attention, triggering a wide variety of sensory and emotional states resulting in a feeling of being 'carried away'. This phenomenon may, for instance, impact neural activities (Vessel et al., 2012), leading to positive affective changes supporting superior well-being (Tay et al., 2018). Being *embedded* in ones' creative craft may promote flourishing. Namely, the complete connection between mind-body and environment required by dance-based activities has been associated with subjective well-being (Malkina-Pykh, 2015), self-esteem as well as coping effectiveness (Quiroga Murcia et al., 2010). Accordingly, engaging in creative pursuit may broaden individuals' *social roles and diversify and proliferate identities* within communities and cultures. This can have a protective effect, especially in the context of stress where "[m]ultiple identities can enhance resiliency, as individuals can draw on these different identities when a life event or transition affects one's identity" (Tay et al., 2018, p. 218). Finally, because of its multiple modes of engagement, the creative arts present various *self-reflective possibilities* that can facilitate emotional processing when one is faced with adversity.

Following their cohort studies, Fancourt et al. (2023) also developed a theoretical framework to explain how creative arts impact health and well-being using complexity sciences. Because creative activities involve complex and dynamic interactions, well-being outcomes may be achieved through intertwined psychological, biological, social, and behavioural mechanisms of action. For example, engaging with creative group activities may simultaneously stimulate individuals' capacity to regulate emotions (i.e., psychological), lower their cortisol level (i.e., biological), and increase their connectivity with others (i.e., social), leading to the emergence of health outcomes such as an enhanced sense of fulfillment (i.e., well-being component). Another central aspect of complexity theory is the notion that, when challenged, complex systems as a whole self-organise and adapt to the environment to facilitate the emergence of new order (Poutanen, 2013). According to the *Creative Potential System model* (Richard et al., 2021) introduced earlier, engaging in creative activities involves dealing with ambiguity, novelty, and unexpectency, and might therefore challenge the intrinsic dynamic of a system. To deal with increased levels of system entropy, self-organisation processes are activated. Self-organisation processes may help a system "changing from unorganized to organized" or "changing from a bad organization to a good one" (Ashby, 1962, p. 267). In the latter instance, the system will undergo phase transitions (e.g., bifurcation route, shift route, or metastability) and spontaneously organise into novel and functional states better adapted to the environment (see Kelso, 2001, 2012 for more details on self-organising dynamical systems).

Combining these two mechanistic hypotheses, it could be argued that the *immersive*, *embedded*, *social*, and/or *reflective* nature of creative activities (Tay et al., 2018) activate a unique combination of psychological, biological, social, and behavioural systems supporting adaptation processes (Fancourt et al., 2023). While these adaptation processes may lead to skill expansion, they could also promote the system's recovery from stressors, as discussed next.

Creative expression as a recovery method?

Recovery can be defined as "the compensation of deficit states of an organism (e.g., fatigue or decrease in performance) and, according to the homeostatic principle, a reestablishment of the initial state" (Kellmann, 2002, p. 6). While recovery can be achieved by a break from stress, it can also be achieved by a change of stress. In other words, activities that interfere with distinctive physiological and psychological systems may optimise recovery (Kellmann, 2002). Hence, in disciplines that, for instance, involve the acquisition of highly specialised motor skills, the recruitment of analytical or convergent thinking, or the adoption of a narrow focus, creative activities can promote a system shift that activates movement versatility, intuition, broad focus, or divergent thinking. Hereby the frequently solicited system rests while other systems are taking over in order to optimise recovery.

Sport provides a salient example of how this might operate. Although athletes are frequently admired for their capacity to take varied, rare, and flexible decisions leading to outstanding victories (e.g., tactical creativity; Kempe & Memmert, 2018) or for their capacity to adapt in a unique and original way to a specific environment (e.g., movement creativity; Bar-Eli et al., 2008), sport training does not regularly integrate creative activities. In fact, the acquisition of expertise in sport often involves hyper-specialisation requiring athletes to engage in hours of prescribed movement repetition (Richard et al., 2023).

This regiment can negatively impact athletes' energy levels (Cresswell & Eklund, 2007; Hughes & Leavey, 2012), highlighting the importance of recovery in this context (Kellmann et al., 2018). Drawing on the assumption that alternating systems may lead to recovery (Kellmann, 2002), integrating creative activities may be an additional way to balance the repetitive load of sport training. For instance, after an intense technical training, athletes could be offered to cool down using creative movement activities, reflecting on their practice through drawing or painting, or even connecting with their teammates through improvisation games. Hereby, the stress caused by the physical and mental demands of repetitive training could be reduced, while the creative system is stimulated, igniting the growth of other skills (e.g., affective and social) needed to achieve excellence in sport.

While this has yet to be empirically tested in sport, the role of creative activities in the recovery process has been shown effective in the workplace. For instance, Eschleman et al. (2014) reported positive associations between creative activity and recovery experiences as measured by employees' perception of mastery, control, detachment, and relaxation. They argue that creative activity generates resources that help workers recover from the experience of stress at work and perform better as a result. The performance related outcomes can be explained by creativity being transferred from the creative activity to the job.

In this vein, the serious engagement of scientists in an 'integrated network of enterprise', i.e. "the ability to explore a wide range of apparently unrelated activities and to connect the knowledge and skills gained" (Root-Bernstein et al., 2008, p. 56) was found to be associated with scientific success defined by Nobel prize awards (Root-Bernstein et al., 2008). Specifically, biographies of Nobel laureates demonstrate that they were more likely to be seriously engaged in various forms of arts and crafts than any other groups of scientists. While authors argue that arts and crafts may have helped successful scientists broaden their perception of the world, engagement in creative activities may also have contributed to their recovery by stimulating alternative systems. After a day focusing on numbers, formulas, or cells, stimulating the mind differently by playing music, sculpting, or painting, may have relaxed certain cognitive functions while igniting others. This complex yet rich 'mind gym' over an extensive period of time may have contributed to the scientists' creative achievements.

This last assumption highlights the potential reciprocal relationship between recovery and creativity. In addition to the positive effect of creative expression on recovery, recovery seems to also foster creative potential. Relaxing leisure time-activities, such as dancing or Hatha yoga, have been shown to improve originality (Bollimbala et al., 2022), while recovery through vacation and/or travel appears to improve creativity in terms of cognitive flexibility but not in terms of originality (de Bloom et al., 2014). Syrek et al. (2021) find that vacations have a time delayed effect on employees' creativity, whereby employees generally feel less creative when returning from a recovering holiday due to the workload they are confronted with during their first days. The authors do, however, report increased creativity in employees two weeks after their return from holidays.

It appears to be important that employees stay cognitively attached to their job during their leisure time for positive effects on creativity to occur (de Jonge et al., 2012). In line with this, Weinberger et al. (2018) emphasise the importance of recovery, and efficient sleep in particular, for creativity in entrepreneurs. Those entrepreneurs who reflect on problem solving outside of working hours, are found to be more creative compared to their older peers who tend to mentally switch off from work during their free time. These findings highlight the importance of cognitive attachment to work during off-time (Balk, this volume, Chapter 4). By positively reflecting on work, entrepreneurs engage in thinking about work related problems during their free time and therefore recover while also increasing their creativity when returning to the job (Binnewies et al., 2009).

In sum, if engaging in creative activities fosters recovery and recovery in turn increases creative potential and well-being, this dynamic cycle has the potential to maintain itself once creative or recovering activities are initiated. It may thus be relevant to introduce creative practices to further enhance recovery and establish a creativity-recovery cycle, providing individuals with more resources to face challenging and stressful situations, especially in high performance environments. The high demands and expectations that these environments impose on individuals could for example be balanced by the integration of creative activities as a recovering routine to regulate emotions. We know that emotions as well as their regulation on an individual (Campo et al., 2017) and interpersonal level (Tamminen & Crocker, 2013) play a major role for performance outcomes in difficult performance situations. Interestingly, pretend play, a type of role play designed for children, has been found to be positively related to creativity and emotion regulation (Hoffmann & Russ, 2012). Thus, including creative practices, such as role play, to debrief difficult performance situations may help individuals better understand and process their own emotions as well as others' emotions while acquiring new creative strategies to regulate themselves and others in these situations.

Conclusion and recommendations for practice

Supporting creative behaviours and integrating creative activities into high performance environments may require a paradigm shift. Specifically, we must move away from the assumption that engaging in a greater quantity of very specialised and focused training or practice is all it takes to achieve excellence (e.g., deliberate practice; Ericsson et al., 1993). Not only this assumption is flawed (Macnamara et al., 2016), we argue here that allowing high performers such as musicians, surgeons, athletes, scientists, etc., to experience a variety of enriching and meaningful activities could promote their well-being and recovery, in turn impacting performance.

A first crucial step towards this shift from quantity to quality of experience involves increasing stakeholders' awareness of the benefits of designing creativity supportive environments to promote well-being and recovery.

Because organisations frequently experience time-pressure, increasing stake-holders awareness of the most beneficial creative activities to support well-being and recovery is likely going to accelerate the inclusion of creative practices in daily routines (Eschleman et al., 2014). This chapter provides a foundation to build on for such educative campaigns.

The progressive and consistent integration of creative activities is also para-mount to support a successful paradigm shift. To start, targeting 'moments' in everyday life and daily routines that are sometimes underutilised, such as breaks between tasks, can present great integration opportunities. For instance, Rasmussen and Østergaard (2016) developed strategies for stimulating creativity in youth sport by initiating training session with *energisers* in an environment free of judgement where mistakes were welcomed. Energisers are enriched movement activities that encourage individuals to try all sorts of ideas and to move in as many novel ways as possible. In this vein, beginning the integration of creative strate-gies into daily routines is indicated and once creative approaches are adopted, they should not be treated as an appendix (Rasmussen et al., 2022). To fully capture the benefits of these approaches on well-being and recovery, creativity supportive environments, allowing spaces for the exploration and expression of novel ideas, have to be purposefully designed. This can be facilitated by aligning the creative activities to organisations' values and goals. For instance, an organi-sation valuing risk taking could organise a monthly gathering where everyone is invited to share creative solutions to unresolved performance problems. Encouraging people to come up with bold ideas may lead to enhanced ideational risk taking, promoting creative expression and potentially well-being.

Beyond the integration of creative 'moments' within the daily environment, we also emphasised the positive roles of creative arts in promoting and sustaining well-being in this chapter. Building on the literature reviewed, we argue that uniting art with other high performance communities could present relevant mutual benefits. Namely, art communities could offer accessible 'extra-curricular' creative activities tailored to individual abilities, needs, interests etc., whereas high performance communities could share their expertise to support artists who want to push the limits of their performance in various directions. While this is an intriguing idea, we are cognisant of the complexity that such collaborations may present in the initial stages of the paradigm shift. Therefore, a more accessi-ble solution could be to encourage individuals in high performance contexts to pursue other activities outside of their area. In many societies, individuals prac-tice arts during their childhood and youth, as they are part of early educational programs. However, due to a lower likelihood of employability, arts are less rep-resented in higher education (Pollard & Wilson, 2014). Similarly, many youth athletes are pursuing artistic activities (e.g., music, arts, theatre) parallel to their sport involvement. Regrettably, once they are identified as athletically 'talented', the increased training requirements can become an 'all-consuming' experience leading athletes to relinquish other aspects of their identity (Douglas & Carless, 2009; Hughes & Leavey, 2012; Van Slingerland, 2021). Drawing on the immer-sion, embeddedness, socialisation, and reflectiveness mechanisms discussed above

(Tay et al., 2018), encouraging individuals to maintain their artistic identity during adulthood – even if their engagement with the art is recreational – could be an accessible solution to support their well-being and recovery.

Because research linking creative expression, recovery, and well-being is still in its infancy, many research questions arise from this chapter. Specifically, a crucial question to answer empirically concerns the relationship between creative expression, well-being, and recovery. Are they all intertwined in a complex pattern or is there a hierarchical relationship linking them? For instance, could recovery be a mediator or a moderator to the relationship between creative expression and well-being and is this latter relationship bi-directional? More applied research testing different creative interventions must be conducted to answer these questions. Once a creative intervention is established, we suggest organisations and academics to team up to monitor the impact of such transformations on the cognitive, affective, physical, and social repertoire expansion over time. Longitudinal and holistic tracking methods could enhance our understanding of the mechanisms underlying the relationship between creative engagement and well-being and recovery parameters. Similarly, future research should examine differences in well-being and recovery states of individuals devoting time to engage with art compared to those focusing solely on their area of performance. This would provide evidence to support the benefits of diversification beyond a discipline (Richard et al., 2023).

Creativity is about expanding the possible. Whether it is through daily actions or purposeful engagement with creative crafts, being or becoming creative opens options for self-discovery. Broadening individuals' cognitive, affective, physical, and social repertoire through creativity may foster their desire to explore beyond and find solutions that suit them. Because there is no one-size-fits-all recipe to achieve a state of well-being and restfulness, it is probably best to empower people with the capacity to create their own.

References

Acar, S., Tadik, H., Myers, D., Sman, C., & Uysal, R. (2021). Creativity and well-being: A meta-analysis. *The Journal of Creative Behavior, 55*(3), 738–751.

Ashby, W. R. (1962). Principles of the self-organizing system. In H. V. Foerster & J. G. W. Zopf (Eds.), *Principles of self-organization: Transactions of the University of Illinois Symposium* (pp. 255–278). Pergamon Press.

Bar-Eli, M., Lowengart, O., Tsukahara, M., & Fosbury, R. D. (2008). Tsukahara's vault and Fosbury's flop: A comparative analysis of two great inventions. *International Journal of Innovation Management, 12*, 21–39.

Binnewies, C., Sonnentag, S., & Mojza, E. J. (2009). Feeling recovered and thinking about the good sides of one's work. *Journal of Occupational Health Psychology, 14*(3), 243–256.

Bollimbala, A., James, P. S., & Ganguli, S. (2022). Grooving, moving, and stretching out of the box! The role of recovery experiences in the relation between physical activity and creativity. *Personality and Individual Differences, 196*, 111757. https://doi.org/10.1016/j.paid.2022.111757

Bruner, J. S. (1960). *The process of education.* Harvard University Press.

Campo, M., Sanchez, X., Ferrand, C., Rosnet, E., Friesen, A., & Lane, A. M. (2017). Interpersonal emotion regulation in team sport: Mechanisms and reasons to regulate teammates' emotions examined. *International Journal of Sport and Exercise Psychology,* *15*(4), 379–394.

Conner, T. S., Deyoung, C. G., & Silvia, P. J. (2018). Everyday creative activity as a path to flourishing. *The Journal of Positive Psychology, 13*(2), 181–189.

Cresswell, S. L., & Eklund, R. C. (2007). Athlete burnout: A longitudinal qualitative study. *The Sport Psychologist, 21*(1), 1–20.

de Bloom, J., Ritter, S., Kühnel, J., Reinders, J., & Geurts, S. (2014). Vacation from work: A 'ticket to creativity'?: The effects of recreational travel on cognitive flexibility and originality. *Tourism Management, 44,* 164–171.

de Jonge, J., Spoor, E., Sonnentag, S., Dormann, C., & Van Den Tooren, M. (2012). "Take a break?!" Off-job recovery, job demands, and job resources as predictors of health, active learning, and creativity. *European Journal of Work and Organizational Psychology, 21*(3), 321–348.

Douglas, K., & Carless, D. (2009). Abandoning the performance narrative: Two women's stories of transition from professional sport. *Journal of Applied Sport Psychology, 21*(2), 213–230.

Ericsson, K. A., Krampe, R. T., & Tesch-Roemer, C. (1993). The role of deliberate practice in the acquisition of expert performance. *Psychological Review, 100,* 363–406.

Eschleman, K. J., Madsen, J., Alarcon, G., & Barelka, A. (2014). Benefiting from creative activity: The positive relationships between creative activity, recovery experiences, and performance-related outcomes. *Journal of Occupational and Organizational Psychology, 87*(3), 579–598.

Fancourt, D., Bone, J., Bu, F., Mak, H., & Bradbury, A. (2023). *The impact of arts and cultural engagement on population health: Findings from major cohort studies in the UK and USA 2017–2022.* UCL.

Fancourt, D., & Finn, S. (2019). *What is the evidence on the role of the arts in improving health and well-being? A scoping review. Health Evidence Network synthesis report.* World Health Organization.

Forgeard, M. J. C., & Eichner, K. V. (2014). Creativity as a target tool for positive intervention. In A. C. Parks & S. M. Schueller (Eds.), *The Wiley Blackwell handbook of positive psychological interventions* (pp. 135–154). John Wiley & Sons, Ltd.

Gallagher, S. (2015). How embodied cognition is being disembodied. *The Philosophers' Magazine, 68,* 96–102.

Glăveanu, V. P. (2021). *The possible: A sociocultural theory.* Oxford University Press.

Gordon, J., & O'Toole, L. (2015). Learning for well-being: Creativity and inner diversity. *Cambridge Journal of Education, 45*(3), 333–346.

Hoffmann, J., & Russ, S. (2012). Pretend play, creativity, and emotion regulation in children. *Psychology of Aesthetics, Creativity, and the Arts, 6*(2), 175–184.

Hughes, L., & Leavey, G. (2012). Setting the bar: Athletes and vulnerability to mental illness. *British Journal of Psychiatry, 200*(2), 95–96.

Jenabi, E., Bashirian, S., Ayubi, E., Rafiee, M., & Bashirian, M. (2023). The effect of the art therapy interventions on depression symptoms among older adults: A meta-analysis of controlled clinical trials. *Journal of Geriatric Psychiatry and Neurology, 36*(3), 185–192.

Karpavičiūtė, S., & Macijauskienė, J. (2016). The impact of arts activity on nursing staff well-being: An intervention in the workplace. *International Journal of Environmental Research and Public Health, 13*(4), 1–17.

Kellmann, M. (2002). Underrecovery and overtraining: Different concepts – Similar impact? In M. Kellmann (Ed.), *Enhancing recovery: Preventing underperformance in athletes* (pp. 3–24). Human Kinetics.

Kellmann, M., Bertollo, M., Bosquet, L., Brink, M., Coutts, A. J., Duffield, R., Erlacher, D., Halson, S. L., Hecksteden, A., Heidari, J., Kallus, K. W., Meeusen, R., Mujika, I., Robazza, C., Skorski, S., Venter, R., & Beckmann, J. (2018). Recovery and performance in sport: Consensus statement. *International Journal of Sports Physiology and Performance*, *13*(2), 240–245.

Kelso, J. A. S. (2001). Self-organizing dynamical systems. In N. J. Smelser & P. B. Baltes (Eds.), *International encyclopedia of the social & behavioral sciences* (pp. 13844–13850). Elsevier.

Kelso, J. A. S. (2012). Multistability and metastability: Understanding dynamic coordination in the brain. *Philosophical Transactions of the Royal Society B: Biological Sciences*, *367*, 906–918.

Kempe, M., & Memmert, D. (2018). "Good, better, creative": The influence of creativity on goal scoring in elite soccer. *Journal of Sports Sciences*, *36*, 2419–2423.

Lomas, T. (2016). Positive art: Artistic expression and appreciation as an exemplary vehicle for flourishing. *Review of General Psychology*, *20*(2), 171–182.

Lu, G., Jia, R., Liang, D., Yu, J., Wu, Z., & Chen, C. (2021). Effects of music therapy on anxiety: A meta-analysis of randomized controlled trials. *Psychiatry Research*, *304*, 114137. https://doi.org/10.1016/j.psychres.2021.114137

Macnamara, B. N., Moreau, D., & Hambrick, D. Z. (2016). The relationship between deliberate practice and performance in sports: A meta-analysis. *Perspectives on Psychological Science*, *11*(3), 333–350.

Malinin, L. H. (2019). How radical is embodied creativity? Implications of 4E approaches for creativity research and teaching. *Frontiers in Psychology*, *10*, 2372. https://doi.org/10.3389/fpsyg.2019.02372

Malkina-Pykh, I. G. (2015). Effectiveness of rhythmic movement therapy: Case study of subjective well-being. *Body, Movement and Dance in Psychotherapy*, *10*(2), 106–120.

Morison, L., Simonds, L., & Stewart, S.-J. F. (2022). Effectiveness of creative arts-based interventions for treating children and adolescents exposed to traumatic events: A systematic review of the quantitative evidence and meta-analysis. *Arts & Health*, *14*(3), 237–262.

Pollard, V., & Wilson, E. (2014). The "entrepreneurial mindset" in creative and performing arts higher education in Australia. *Artivate*, *3*(1), 3–22.

Poutanen, P. (2013). Creativity as seen through the complex systems perspective. *Interdisciplinary Studies Journal*, *2*, 207–221.

Quiroga Murcia, C., Kreutz, G., Clift, S., & Bongard, S. (2010). Shall we dance? An exploration of the perceived benefits of dancing on well-being. *Arts & Health*, *2*(2), 149–163.

Rasmussen, L. J. T., Glăveanu, V. P., & Østergaard, L. (2022). "The principles are good, but they need to be integrated in the right way": Experimenting with creativity in elite youth soccer. *Journal of Applied Sport Psychology*, *34*(2), 294–316.

Rasmussen, L. J. T., & Østergaard, L. D. (2016). The creative soccer platform: New strategies for stimulating creativity in organized youth soccer practice. *The Journal of Physical Education, Recreation & Dance*, *87*, 9–19.

Richard, V., Cairney, J., & Woods, C. T. (2023). Holding open spaces to explore beyond: Toward a different conceptualisation of specialisation in high-performance sport. *Frontiers in Psychology*, *14*, 1089264. https://doi.org/10.3389/fpsyg.2023.1089264

Richard, V., Holder, D., & Cairney, J. (2021). Creativity in motion: Examining the creative potential system and enriched movement activities as a way to ignite it. *Frontiers in Psychology*, *12*, 690710. https://doi.org/10.3389/fpsyg.2021.690710

Richards, R. (2007). *Everyday creativity and new views of human nature: Psychological, social, and spiritual perspectives.* American Psychological Association.

Root-Bernstein, R., Allen, L., Beach, L., Bhadula, R., Fast, J., Hosey, C., Kremkow, B., Lapp, J., Lonc, K., Pawelec, K., Podufaly, A., Russ, C., Tennant, L., Vrtis, E., & Weinlander, S. (2008). Arts foster scientific success: Avocations of Nobel, National Academy, Royal Society, and Sigma Xi members. *Journal of Psychology of Science and Technology, 1,* 51–63.

Shim, Y., Jebb, A. T., Tay, L., & Pawelski, J. O. (2021). Arts and humanities interventions for flourishing in healthy adults: A mixed studies systematic review. *Review of General Psychology, 25*(3), 258–282.

Simonton, D. K. (2014). The mad-genius paradox: Can creative people be more mentally healthy but highly creative people more mentally ill? *Perspective on Psychological Science, 9*(5), 470–480.

Syrek, C. J., de Bloom, J., & Lehr, D. (2021). Well recovered and more creative? A longitudinal study on the relationship between vacation and creativity. *Frontiers in Psychology, 12,* 784844. https://doi.org/10.3389/fpsyg.2021.784844

Tamminen, K. A., & Crocker, P. R. E. (2013). "I control my own emotions for the sake of the team": Emotional self-regulation and interpersonal emotion regulation among female high-performance curlers. *Psychology of Sport and Exercise, 14*(5), 737–747.

Tay, L., Pawelski, J. O., & Keith, M. G. (2018). The role of the arts and humanities in human flourishing: A conceptual model. *The Journal of Positive Psychology, 13*(3), 215–225.

Van Slingerland, K. (2021). *Design, implementation, and evaluation of a sport-focused mental health service delivery model within a canadian centre for mental health and sport* [Doctoral dissertation, University of Ottawa, Canada]. uO Research. http://hdl.handle.net/10393/42792

Vessel, E., Starr, G. G., & Rubin, N. (2012). The brain on art: Intense aesthetic experience activates the default mode network. *Frontiers in Human Neuroscience, 6,* 66. https://doi.org/10.3389/fnhum.2012.00066

Weinberger, E., Wach, D., Stephan, U., & Wegge, J. (2018). Having a creative day: Understanding entrepreneurs' daily idea generation through a recovery lens. *Journal of Business Venturing, 33*(1), 1–19.

7 "Use it right"

The relationship between digital media and recovery

Jahan Heidari and Michael Kellmann

The role of digital media in the modern society

Digital media have established themselves as a vital part of many people's lives and play a role in various areas of individual functioning such as the organisation of everyday routines and schedules or the interaction with friends and colleagues (Reyna et al., 2018). Depending on the definition, digital media include electronic devices such as laptops, smartphones, or tablets as well as ways of communication such as text messages, e-mails and, in particular, social media.

The digital devices serve as a medium for users to access the Internet or to consume and exchange digital content like series, movies, or music (Guinibert, 2022; Guse et al., 2012). Quantifying the extent of digital media use is extremely difficult, as a result of the complexity and diversity of practices that can be considered digital media activity. Kemp (2022) provides an overview of various indicators of digital media activity and reports that, as of January 2022, 67.1% of the world's population are unique mobile phone users, while 58.4% are active social media users. For the mobile phone users, that percentage includes an increase of 1.8% compared to 2021, whereas the percentage of active social media users registers a considerable growth of 10.1% compared to January 2021. Kemp (2022) also analyzed the daily usage time of digital media of individuals in the 16–64 age range. The time spent using the Internet amassed to an average of 6h 58min each day with social media activities accounting for 2h 27min of daily use. The emergence and steady growth of social media is underlined by calculations and projections regarding the number of global social network users between 2017 to 2025. In 2017, 2.86 billion global users were recorded, while the number is projected to increase to 4.41 billion global users in the year 2025 (Dixon, 2022).

When having a closer look at the demographic characteristics of the digital media users, a rather consistent finding reported across different countries and

Heidari, J., & Kellmann, M. (2024)."Use it right": The relationship between digital media and recovery. In M. Kellmann & J. Beckmann (Eds.), *Fostering Recovery and Well-being in a Healthy Lifestyle: Psychological, Somatic, and Organizational Prevention Approaches* (pp. 103–114). Routledge.

DOI: 10.4324/9781003250654-9

cultural contexts is a higher usage of digital media and particularly social media in the younger population, especially in the age group between 20 and 29 years. This refers not only to the general population, but also to the demographic of adolescent athletes (Fiedler et al., 2023). A total of 14.1% of all female users and 18.1% of all male users are in the age range of 20–29 years and mark the largest subgroup with respect to the total group of active social media users (Kemp, 2022). This finding aligns to findings from Germany with regard to the online presence where 92% of the individuals between 18 and 33 years indicate to be online every day (Techniker Krankenkasse, 2021). Taken all these data together, it can be clearly stated that digital media, and social media as an important facet, have permeated many areas in our lives and are serving a variety of motives and purposes.

Luchman et al. (2014) conducted a study with young Americans and developed a model to categorize motives of social media usage. The two overarching dimensions derived from the study were *content-specific* and *fun-related* motives which were deemed applicable to social media networks in general. Each network or site can be associated with an intersection between these dimensions. For example, *Instagram* was put into the subcategory *socially-driven fun* as it was rated as low-content-specific and high-fun-focused.

On a more specific level for the adult population, motives of social media use were classified into four sections as it is done with the modified version of the *Motivation for Twitter Use Measure* (Lee & Kim, 2014) by transferring it to social media in general (Schivinski et al., 2020). These four dimensions are *surveillance* (e.g., "To discover the pressing issues of our society"), *network expansion* (e.g., "To provide information about my interests to others"), *intrapersonal motive* (e.g., "To forget the complications of everyday life"), and *relationship maintenance* (e.g., "To contact friends and family") which cover the different nature and extent of potential usage motives. Attempts to scientifically and quantitatively assess the variety of underlying motives are an ongoing topic in research as shown by the emergence of instruments such as the Scale of Motives for Using Social Networking Sites (Pertegal et al., 2019) or the Motivations for Social Media Use Scale (Rodgers et al., 2021). While, the plethora of digital media and its integration into everyday life leads to a complex array of motives, digital media also affects the well-being of individuals in different ways.

Consequences of digital media for well-being

Findings on the relationship between digital media and well-being are mixed and the impact of digital media on well-being depends on a variety of variables, such as the purpose of the usage. Liu et al. (2019) conducted a meta–analysis focusing on the associations between digital communication media and psychological well-being. Digital communication media was found to enhance well-being when used as a facilitator for social interactions regarding significant relationships but had a detrimental effect on well-being when social media networks were only passively consumed and browsed through. Explanations for the positive effects when used actively were ascribed to the increase in happiness and self-esteem when receiving positive feedback to one's posts. The negative effects were interpreted through the fact that the time invested in browsing was lost to actually engage with important others. Additionally, negative feelings could arise when socially comparing one's life to the positively skewed social media content online. Twenge and Campbell (2019) summarised the data from three large-scale datasets examining adolescent's media use and psychological well-being and used facets such as happiness and depression to operationalise psychological well-being in their study. The overall result across the sample indicated that more time on digital media was associated with lower well-being. Specifically, usage times of more than five hours a day were linked to the lowest levels of well-being, thereby indicating a detrimental consequence of heavy digital media use. Interestingly, the light users with less than one hour per day reported the highest levels of well-being, even higher than nonusers. This implies an exposure-response model without detailing the type of activity and content that has been consumed (Twenge & Campbell, 2019). Some overlap of these tendencies were also reported by Twigg et al. (2020) in their longitudinal study which, among other aspects, looked at the influence of social media use on life satisfaction (e.g., experience of positive emotions) in UK children aged between 10 and 15 years. Again, heavy use with more than four hours a day was related to lower life satisfaction, with low to moderate use seemingly not having an impact. The interaction results between gender and social media use indicate more pronounced negative associations between high social media use and life satisfaction for girls than boys.

A specific and pivotal domain of well-being in light of digital media use in children and adolescents is sleep. Lund et al. (2021) summarised the results of 49 studies with children and adolescents in the 0–15 years age range. Usage of digital media in terms of electronic devices was linked to shorter sleep duration and partly associated with reduced sleep quality and delayed bedtime. This adds to the knowledge of associations between digital media use and well-being in children and adolescents and emphasises potential starting points of interventions (e.g., reduction of usage time, focus on gender differences). While the majority of studies on digital media and well-being are conducted with children, adolescents, and younger adults, some research has focused on the demographic of older adults (Simons et al., 2023). This goes along with a shift of perspective. For younger individuals, a bias towards studying potential detrimental effects of too much use appears to be present. For older individuals, digital media can serve as an entrance ticket to increased well-being through more social inclusion and a reduction of loneliness.

Recovery as essential component of well-being

Within the abundant research regarding well-being, recovery has emerged as a vital puzzle piece when it comes to the investigation of associations between health and performance in various settings such as elite sports (Heidari et al., 2019; Kellmann et al., 2018). Recovery can be specified as:

an inter- and intraindividual multilevel (e.g., psychological, physiological, social) process in time for the re-establishment of personal resources and their full functional capacity. Recovery includes a broad range of physiological processes like sleep, motivated behaviour (like eating and drinking) and goal-oriented components (like relaxation or meeting friends). Recovery activities can be passive or active and in many instances recovery is achieved indirectly by activities, which stimulate recovery processes like active sports.

(Kallus, 2016, p. 42)

Recovery can be effective on different levels. First, a buffering effect of recovery regarding external and internal stressors in terms of the prevention of negative developments needs to be noted. Second, recovery consists of the restoration of resources after episodes of stress to re-establish a state of balance from a psychophysiological level. Recovery can be achieved through several mechanisms such as a reduction of stress, the modification of stress loads, the appraisal of stress, and a complete break from stress. It is not a linear process being easily applicable to all individuals and situations but rather describes a cumulative, subjective, and continuing development impacted by previous activities or events (Kellmann et al., 2018). Potential recovery activities can be categorised into passive, active, and pro-active approaches. Passive methods could consist of massages, sauna, cryotherapy, or with regard to digital media, watching a TV series on the tablet. During passive interventions, physiological as well as psychological reactions and restoration processes are initiated and aim to rebuild pre-task performance states. Active recovery could again target physiological and psychological restoration and could involve moderate exercise to eliminate the results of fatigue through physical activity. Psychologically, doing a Yoga program via YouTube to detach from the stress of the day could be listed as an example. In case recovery includes a purposeful, self-initiated, and self-determined action, it falls into the category of pro-active recovery which has the highest fit between individual needs and need satisfaction (Heidari et al., 2019; Kellmann et al., 2018). While it appears to be quite simple to balance stress and recovery on a theoretical level, the threat of detrimental developments in terms of increased stress and insufficient recovery is eminent. Holistic recovery and stress management depends on the analysis and inclusion of all factors that impact performance and well-being, such as training (e.g., frequency, intensity), lifestyle (e.g., sleep, nutrition, digital media), health status (e.g., infections), or the social environment (e.g., family, colleagues). A continuous exposition to dysfunctional demands and habits (e.g., excessive social media time) may overwhelm the resources of individuals and could affect the physiological and psychological health and well-being negatively in terms of back pain (Heidari et al., 2018), burnout (Gustafsson et al., 2017), or mental health (Schneiderman et al., 2005). When considering the diversity of stressors present in today's society, digital media has emerged as relatively new factor which needs to be added to the equation of stress and recovery. In a daily routine that is already very busy, permanent digital accessibility and the pressure to contribute digital content (e.g., via Instagram) act as additional stressors.

Findings on stress, recovery, and digital media

Despite a growing number of investigations to assess associations between digital media and recovery, the majority of studies have focused on psychological stress in the context of digital media (Reinecke et al., 2017). Therefore, to provide an overview of the research landscape regarding the three topics of stress, recovery, and digital media, a two-step approach has been chosen to delineate the findings of this section of the chapter. First, the term *digital stress* and its four underlying components will be outlined. These components will then be linked and put into perspective with research on *media-induced recovery* according to the four components of recovery (i.e., *mastery, control, detachment, relaxation*) which were defined by Sonnentag and Fritz (2007). *Digital stress* describes stress as a consequence of specific aspects of social media use and consists of the four components *connection overload, availability stress, Fear of Missing Out*, and *approval anxiety* (Reinecke et al., 2017). *Connection overload* as a facet of *digital stress* can be classified as a resource-consuming phenomenon and can occur as a result of an imbalance between the amount of available information and the individual capacity to process and deal with the information (Steele et al., 2020). *Availability stress* describes distress stemming from the individual perception to be digitally approachable and respond to the messages, posts, etc. from others within their own social media network (Thomée et al., 2010; Wolfers & Utz, 2022). The third component of *Fear of Missing Out* is substantiated by significant research especially in the demographic of adolescents and young adults and defines the phenomenon of distress resulting of actual or perceived social impact of being absent from digital situations or interactions of a rewarding nature within the peer group (Bloemen & De Coninck, 2020; Steele et al., 2020). Finally, *digital stress* entails the facet of *approval anxiety* which means that individuals experiencing this kind of stress are dealing with states of doubt and insecurity regarding others' responses and reactions to one's social media activity (Marengo et al., 2021).

It becomes evident that the use of digital media can be accompanied by several stressors emerging from various mechanisms associated with it. However, when considering social media in the context of the stress-coping process according to the model of Wolfers and Utz (2022), a more salutogenic perspective on digital media also needs to be taken into account and can be subsumed under media-induced recovery as a means of preventing digital stress or dealing with digital stress. Several experimental studies draw a more nuanced picture of recovery associated with the type of media activity and one's usage. Aspects such as interactivity and involvement appear to initiate media-induced recovery as shown by the study of Reinecke et al. (2011). The participants in the study were assigned to interactive media (i.e., playing a video game), non-interactive media (i.e., watching a video clip), and a non-media control condition. Individuals in the interactive condition reported significantly higher mastery and control experiences while involvement also resulted as a significant predictor of media-induced recovery. Another characteristic which has emerged as beneficial within the relationship between media and recovery is the affective note of the consumed media content.

Janicke et al. (2018) investigated the association between watching positive and personally relevant YouTube videos and recovery experiences in the workplace. Personally relevant videos predicted mastery recovery experiences, while positive affect predicted psychological detachment and relaxation experiences. These results implied the overall potential of such videos for workplace recovery. Another investigation focusing on the role of content valence was conducted by Rieger, Reinecke, and Bente (2017). Participants were first confronted with a straining task and were subsequently assigned to three different conditions, namely a movie clip with positive affective valence, a movie clip with negative affective valence, and a control condition with no media exposure. Both media conditions affected recovery experiences. While the positive video impacted relaxation and psychological detachment, the negatively connoted video increased involvement and energetic arousal (i.e., the continuum from sleepiness to vigilance).

When considering specific types of media such as video games or smartphone use on recovery experiences, both Reer and Quandt (2020) as well as Rieger, Hefner, and Vorderer (2017) report various pathways between involvement with such media and markers of well-being and recovery. Reer and Quandt (2020) reported various positive functions of video games for users such as escaping negative real-life situations, stress, and the perception of control and autonomy while interacting with others with similar interests. Rieger, Hefner, and Vorderer (2017) focused on smartphone use on recovery experiences and found mixed results. While the facet of relaxation was lower in smartphone users, the aspects of autonomy and control appeared to be positively affected. A potential caveat to the outlined recovery research is the gap between investigations in laboratory settings and the transferability of the results to real life as described by Reinecke and Hofmann (2016). Higher levels of exhaustion after straining days of work were associated with negative feelings of guilt and when engaging in digital behaviour. Media use was then considered as procrastination, although research on the relationship between ego depletion and media use suggests that using digital media in a state of depleted self-control resources could actually restore self-control capacities and could therefore serve as a form of recovery experience (Tice et al., 2007). Based on the illustration of the findings on media use, digital stress, and media-induced recovery, practical starting points for health-promoting media use will be presented.

Suggestions for the beneficial use of digital media for recovery

In order to illustrate the potential of digital media for recovery enhancement, the transtheoretical model will be used as a theoretical framework and guideline to outline the process of media-induced recovery (Prochaska & DiClemente, 2005). The aim is to delineate a pathway from perceiving digital media as mainly resource-providing instead of resource-consuming (Sonnentag et al., 2017; Sonnentag & Zijlstra, 2006). The transtheoretical model has been applied in a variety of settings (e.g., smoking cessation, career transitions in elite youth athletes and serves as an applicable model due to its comprehensibility and practical relevance (Park et al., 2012; Robinson & Vail, 2012). It consists of five phases, namely pre-contemplation, contemplation, preparation, action, and maintenance. To start with the phase of pre-contemplation, individuals using digital media in this phase do not consider digital media as a tool to promote recovery. Their usage patterns may be focused on maintaining the status quo without thinking about the potential consequences with individuals displaying a lack of awareness of the resource-consuming nature of their media use (Canadian Paediatric Society, 2019; Steele et al., 2020). In the contemplation stage, individuals may have perceived some unpleasant outcomes and effects on their well-being as a result of too much digital media (e.g., reduced happiness) and are starting to weigh the pros and cons of their media usage behaviour (Twenge, 2019). It is important to notice that media usage should not be considered detrimental per se. Rather, the pro-active use of certain digital activities and the knowledge of the type of activities which provide individuals with positive emotions need to be mapped out (Reer & Quandt, 2020). Strategies to promote media-induced recovery in the stage of contemplation could therefore consist of educational elements regarding digital media and the respective pros (e.g., connecting with friends worldwide) and cons (e.g., passively consuming social media content) that are perceived individually while pointing out the benefits of consciously monitoring the individual digital activity. A shift from contemplating digital media as a resource-consuming towards a resource-providing behaviour should be initiated (Sonnentag et al., 2017; Sonnentag & Zijlstra, 2006).

Considering the stage of preparation, individuals might have started to track their digital media activity and are starting to obtain a more detailed picture of their media-related behaviour. Ideally, this monitoring process will be combined with mood tracking using respective apps (e.g., Daylio; Chaudhry, 2016) in order to gain an understanding of the relationship between the type and volume of digital media consumption and one's well-being. Ideas on how to establish such a monitoring routine can be found in publications in the sport context (Heidari et al., 2019). Another pivotal step in this stage to foster media-induced recovery consists of the identification of as many obstacles as possible (e.g., fear of missing out, availability stress) which stand in the way of recovery (Reinecke et al., 2017). Dealing with these obstacles and setting concrete and attainable goals in terms of small steps should be encouraged and the developed strategies such as screen time limits, disabling push notifications, or the pro-active use of social media for meaningful social interactions (Morris & Cravens Pickens, 2017; Throuvala et al., 2019; Vanden Abeele et al., 2022) should be prepared for their practical implementation (e.g., checklist entailing the three main goals). Within the action phase, the deliberations of the preparation phase are put into practice. This phase is described as relatively volatile and can be accompanied by relapses in terms of a more resource-consuming than resource-providing usage of digital media.

Actual interventions in practical settings to engage in digital media in a recovery-promoting manner should connect to existing research underlining the potential of stress management and mindfulness apps to promote media-induced recovery (Chittaro & Vianello, 2016). Depending on individual preferences, mobile or video games or scheduled interactions with significant others could also serve as strategies to restore depleted resources (Ostic et al., 2021). Digital media might also be blended with offline activities by using health and fitness apps to increase recovery through physical activity (Sullivan & Lachman, 2017). As long as these experiences go along with positive emotions and tangible changes, the stage of maintenance and routine can be reached. When putting these changes of the perception and behaviour towards digital media into practice, it should be noted that inter- and intraindividual preferences (e.g., games vs. chats, daily events) need to be taken into account in order to permanently convert digital media consumption into a resource-providing activity (Collins et al., 2019; Kallus, 2016).

Conclusion and recommendations for practise

Examining the use of social media in relation to recovery can provide helpful insights into the individual motives and psychophysiological effects on users. Findings on the associations between media usage, stress, and recovery paint a multi-faceted picture of their positive and negative impact depending on differing variables. Interactivity and involvement have been shown to work as positive factors to promote media-induced recovery since they target the facets of mastery and control within the model of Sonnentag and Fritz (2007). These psychological underpinnings should be used to tailor practical interventions where individuals can exchange digitally about their recovery strategies and are able to design specific recovery strategies to foster involvement. When considering the aspects of relaxation and detachment, positive affect while consuming media content emerged as an important puzzle piece to facilitate recovery. Transferring these findings to the substantial body of research on the recovery concept of Kellmann et al. (2018), the way to develop the ability to use media in a recovery enhancing manner is to pro-actively and reflectively engage in media-related behaviour depending on intraindividual needs. This approach ideally starts with a phase of self-monitoring digital media consumption and well-being, and the deduction of strategies and content in support of individual recovery (e.g., listening to NBA podcasts). In this case, media-induced recovery is pro-actively started, contains positive valence, and includes the facets of relaxation, possibly detachment, and control. These theoretical underpinnings need to be substantiated by (daily life) research in the field and should be extended to various demographics. Digital media will remain an integral part of our lives, so we might as well aim to use them in a recovery promoting manner.

References

Bloemen, N., & De Coninck, D. (2020). Social media and fear of missing out in adolescents: The role of family characteristics. *Social Media + Society*, 6(4), 2056305120965517. https://doi.org/10.1177/2056305120965517

Canadian Paediatric Society. (2019). Digital media: Promoting healthy screen use in school-aged children and adolescents. *Paediatrics & Child Health*, 24(6), 402–408.

Chaudhry, B. M. (2016). Daylio: Mood-quantification for a less stressful you. *Mhealth*, 2(8), 34. https://doi.org/10.21037/mhealth.2016.08.04

Chittaro, L., & Vianello, A. (2016). Evaluation of a mobile mindfulness app distributed through on-line stores: A 4-week study. *International Journal of Human-Computer Studies*, 86, 63–80.

Collins, E., Cox, A., Wilcock, C., & Sethu-Jones, G. (2019). Digital games and mindfulness apps: Comparison of effects on post work recovery. *JMIR Mental Health*, 6(7), e12853. https://doi.org/10.2196/12853

Dixon, S. (2022). *Number of global social network users 2017-2025*. Retrieved December 21, 2022 from https://www.statista.com/statistics/278414/number-of-worldwide-social-network-users/

Fiedler, R., Heidari, J., Birnkraut, T., & Kellmann, M. (2023). Digital media and mental health in adolescent athletes. *Psychology of Sport and Exercise*, 67, 102421. https://doi.org/10.1016/j.psychsport.2023.102421

Guinibert, M. (2022). Defining digital media as a professional practice in New Zealand. *Kōtuitui: New Zealand Journal of Social Sciences Online*, 17(2), 185–205.

Guse, K., Levine, D., Martins, S., Lira, A., Gaarde, J., Westmorland, W., & Gilliam, M. (2012). Interventions using new digital media to improve adolescent sexual health: A systematic review. *Journal of Adolescent Health*, 51(6), 535–543.

Gustafsson, H., DeFreese, J. D., & Madigan, D. J. (2017). Athlete burnout: Review and recommendations. *Current Opinion in Psychology*, 16, 109–113.

Heidari, J., Beckmann, J., Bertollo, M., Brink, M., Kallus, K. W., Robazza, C., & Kellmann, M. (2019). Multidimensional monitoring of recovery status and implications for performance. *International Journal of Sports Physiology and Performance*, 14(1), 2–8.

Heidari, J., Mierswa, T., Hasenbring, M., Kleinert, J., Levenig, C., Belz, J., & Kellmann, M. (2018). Recovery-stress patterns and low back pain: Differences in pain intensity and disability. *Musculoskeletal Care*, 16(1), 18–25.

Janicke, S. H., Rieger, D., Reinecke, L., & Connor, W. (2018). Watching online videos at work: The role of positive and meaningful affect for recovery experiences and well-being at the workplace. *Mass Communication and Society*, 21(3), 345–367.

Kallus, K. W. (2016). Stress and recovery: An overview. In K. W. Kallus & M. Kellmann (Eds.), *The Recovery-Stress Questionnaires: User manual* (pp. 27–48). Pearson Assessment.

Kellmann, M., Bertollo, M., Bosquet, L., Brink, M., Coutts, A. J., Duffield, R., Erlacher, D., Halson, S. L., Hecksteden, A., Heidari, J., Kallus, K. W., Meeusen, R., Mujika, I., Robazza, C., Skorski, S., Venter, R., & Beckmann, J. (2018). Recovery and performance in sport: Consensus statement. *International Journal of Sports Physiology and Performance*, 13(2), 240–245.

Kemp, S. (2022, January 26). *Digital 2022: Global overview report*. Retrieved December 21, 2022 from https://datareportal.com/reports/digital-2022-global-overview-report

Lee, E.-J., & Kim, Y. W. (2014). How social is Twitter use? Affiliative tendency and communication competence as predictors. *Computers in Human Behavior*, 39, 296–305.

Liu, D., Baumeister, R. F., Yang, C.-C., & Hu, B. (2019). Digital communication media use and psychological well-being: A meta-analysis. *Journal of Computer-Mediated Communication, 24*(5), 259–273.

Luchman, J. N., Bergstrom, J., & Krulikowski, C. (2014). A motives framework of social media website use: A survey of young Americans. *Computers in Human Behavior, 38,* 136–141.

Lund, L., Solvhoj, I. N., Danielsen, D., & Andersen, S. (2021). Electronic media use and sleep in children and adolescents in western countries: A systematic review. *BMC Public Health, 21*(1), 1598. https://doi.org/10.1186/s12889-021-11640-9

Marengo, D., Montag, C., Sindermann, C., Elhai, J. D., & Settanni, M. (2021). Examining the links between active Facebook use, received likes, self-esteem and happiness: A study using objective social media data. *Telematics and Informatics, 58,* 101523. https://doi.org/10.1016/j.tele.2020.101523

Morris, N., & Cravens Pickens, J. D. (2017). "I'm not a gadget": A grounded theory on unplugging. *The American Journal of Family Therapy, 45*(5), 264–282.

Ostic, D., Qalati, S. A., Barbosa, B., Shah, S. M. M., Galvan Vela, E., Herzallah, A. M., & Liu, F. (2021). Effects of social media use on psychological well-being: A mediated model. *Frontiers in Psychology, 12,* 678766. https://doi.org/10.3389/fpsyg.2021.678766

Park, S., Tod, D., & Lavallee, D. (2012). Exploring the retirement from sport decision-making process based on the transtheoretical model. *Psychology of Sport and Exercise, 13*(4), 444–453.

Pertegal, M.-Á., Oliva, A., & Rodríguez-Meirinhos, A. (2019). Development and validation of the Scale of Motives for Using Social Networking Sites (SMU-SNS) for adolescents and youths. *PLoS One, 14*(12), e0225781. https://doi.org/10.1371/journal.pone.0225781

Prochaska, J., & DiClemente, C. (2005). The transtheoretical approach. In J. C. Norcross & M. R. Goldfried (Eds.), *Handbook of psychotherapy integration* (2nd ed., pp. 147–171). Oxford University Press.

Reer, F., & Quandt, T. (2020). Digital games and well-being: An overview. In R. Kowert (Ed.), *Video games and well-being: Press start* (pp. 1–21). Springer.

Reinecke, L., Aufenanger, S., Beutel, M. E., Dreier, M., Quiring, O., Stark, B., Wölfling, K., & Müller, K. W. (2017). Digital stress over the life span: The effects of communication load and internet multitasking on perceived stress and psychological health impairments in a German probability sample. *Media Psychology, 20*(1), 90–115.

Reinecke, L., & Hofmann, W. (2016). Slacking off or winding down? An experience sampling study on the drivers and consequences of media use for recovery versus procrastination. *Human Communication Research, 42*(3), 441–461.

Reinecke, L., Klatt, J., & Krämer, N. C. (2011). Entertaining media use and the satisfaction of recovery needs: Recovery outcomes associated with the use of interactive and noninteractive entertaining media. *Media Psychology, 14*(2), 192–215.

Reyna, J., Hanham, J., & Meier, P. (2018). The Internet explosion, digital media principles and implications to communicate effectively in the digital space. *E-Learning and Digital Media, 15*(1), 36–52.

Rieger, D., Hefner, D., & Vorderer, P. (2017). Mobile recovery? The impact of smartphone use on recovery experiences in waiting situations. *Mobile Media & Communication, 5*(2), 161–177.

Rieger, D., Reinecke, L., & Bente, G. (2017). Media-induced recovery: The effects of positive versus negative media stimuli on recovery experience, cognitive performance, and energetic arousal. *Psychology of Popular Media Culture, 6*(2), 174–191.

Robinson, L. M., & Vail, S. R. (2012). An integrative review of adolescent smoking cessation using the Transtheoretical Model of Change. *Journal of Pediatric Health Care*, *26*(5), 336–345.

Rodgers, R. F., McLean, S. A., Gordon, C. S., Slater, A., Marques, M. D., Jarman, H. K., & Paxton, S. J. (2021). Development and validation of the Motivations for Social Media Use Scale (MSMU) among adolescents. *Adolescent Research Review*, *6*(4), 425–435.

Schivinski, B., Brzozowska-Woś, M., Stansbury, E., Satel, J., Montag, C., & Pontes, H. M. (2020). Exploring the role of social media use motives, psychological well-being, self-esteem, and affect in problematic social media use. *Frontiers in Psychology*, *11*, 617140. https://doi.org/10.3389/fpsyg.2020.617140

Schneiderman, N., Ironson, G., & Siegel, S. D. (2005). Stress and health: Psychological, behavioral, and biological determinants. *Annual Review of Clinical Psychology*, *1*, 607–628.

Simons, M., Reijnders, J., Janssens, M., Lataster, J., & Jacobs, N. (2023). Staying connected in old age: Associations between bonding social capital, loneliness and well-being and the value of digital media. *Aging & Mental Health*, *27*(1), 147–155.

Sonnentag, S., & Fritz, C. (2007). The Recovery Experience Questionnaire: Development and validation of a measure for assessing recuperation and unwinding from work. *Journal of Occupational Health Psychology*, *12*(3), 204–221.

Sonnentag, S., Venz, L., & Casper, A. (2017). Advances in recovery research: What have we learned? What should be done next? *Journal of Occupational Health Psychology*, *22*(3), 365–380.

Sonnentag, S., & Zijlstra, F. R. H. (2006). Job characteristics and off-job activities as predictors of need for recovery, well-being, and fatigue. *Journal of Applied Psychology*, *91*(2), 330–350.

Steele, R. G., Hall, J. A., & Christofferson, J. L. (2020). Conceptualizing digital stress in adolescents and young adults: Toward the development of an empirically based model. *Clinical Child and Family Psychology Review*, *23*(1), 15–26.

Sullivan, A. N., & Lachman, M. E. (2017). Behavior change with fitness technology in sedentary adults: A review of the evidence for increasing physical activity. *Frontiers in Public Health*, *4*, 289. https://doi.org/10.3389/fpubh.2016.00289

Techniker Krankenkasse. (2021). *Schalt mal ab, Deutschland* [Swith off, Germany]. Retrieved December 21, 2022 from https://www.tk.de/resource/blob/2099616/630d3a2e429edc359f15fd8225dcd45c/2021-studie-schalt-mal-ab-data.pdf

Thomée, S., Dellve, L., Härenstam, A., & Hagberg, M. (2010). Perceived connections between information and communication technology use and mental symptoms among young adults – A qualitative study. *BMC Public Health*, *10*(1), 66. https://doi.org/10.1186/1471-2458-10-66

Throuvala, M. A., Griffiths, M. D., Rennoldson, M., & Kuss, D. J. (2019). Motivational processes and dysfunctional mechanisms of social media use among adolescents: A qualitative focus group study. *Computers in Human Behavior*, *93*, 164–175.

Tice, D. M., Baumeister, R. F., Shmueli, D., & Muraven, M. (2007). Restoring the self: Positive affect helps improve self-regulation following ego depletion. *Journal of Experimental Social Psychology*, *43*(3), 379–384.

Twenge, J. M. (2019). More time on technology, less happiness? Associations between digital-media use and psychological well-being. *Current Directions in Psychological Science*, *28*(4), 372–379.

Twenge, J. M., & Campbell, W. K. (2019). Media use is linked to lower psychological well-being: Evidence from three datasets. *Psychiatric Quarterly*, *90*(2), 311–331.

Twigg, L., Duncan, C., & Weich, S. (2020). Is social media use associated with children's well-being? Results from the UK Household Longitudinal Study. *Journal of Adolescence*, *80*, 73–83.

Vanden Abeele, M. M. P., Halfmann, A., & Lee, E. W. J. (2022). Drug, demon, or donut? Theorizing the relationship between social media use, digital well-being and digital disconnection. *Current Opinion in Psychology*, *45*, 101295. https://doi.org/10.1016/j.copsyc.2021.12.007

Wolfers, L. N., & Utz, S. (2022). Social media use, stress, and coping. *Current Opinion in Psychology*, *45*, 101305. https://doi.org/10.1016/j.copsyc.2022.101305

Part III

Somatic prevention approaches

8 Psychological relaxation techniques to enhance recovery in sports

Michael Kellmann, Maximilian Pelka, and Jürgen Beckmann

Introduction

Stress and recovery have been discussed extensively in the context of sport performance settings (Kellmann & Beckmann, 2022; Kellmann et al., 2018, 2023). The term stress is used to describe a process caused by a load or demand beyond the level of normal functioning characterised by homeostatic dysregulation (Kellmann & Kallus, 2016). It has long been recognised that exposure to severe bio-psycho-social stressors (i.e., noise, pain, family, finances, social relationships, etc.) negatively affects a person's health status (Tennant et al., 1985). Even short-term imbalances between stress and recovery could already lead to critical disadvantages (Bengtsson et al., 2013). Consequences of these imbalances such as increased fatigue, poor concentration, disturbed mood, and altered eating and sleeping patterns are often associated with short-term decrements of performance (Jakowski et al., 2023). Additionally, muscular tension, anxiety, and subsequent heightened arousal impair athletic performance. Learning self-regulation skills to improve recovery is therefore paramount for sustaining or improving well-being and athletic performance (Beckmann, 2023).

To mobilise performance reserves during competition, an athlete needs to be sufficiently activated. However, arousal levels can develop too quickly and become dysfunctional. Through specific psycho-regulative procedures from sport psychological training, athletes can be taught self-regulation skills, which enable them to achieve an optimal state of activation in training and competition, i.e., appropriate levels of mental and/or physical excitement. Self-regulation training is not only aimed at changing performance-impairing physical activation, but also at eliminating irrelevant thoughts, which could cause confusion and affect concentration negatively (Beckmann et al., 2023). Furthermore, it is aimed at eliminating a motor performance-impairing self-focus (Mesagno & Beckmann, 2017). The perception of increased physical activation can trigger irrelevant and

Kellmann, M., Pelka, M., & Beckmann, J. (2024). Psychological relaxation techniques to enhance recovery in sports. In M. Kellmann & J. Beckmann (Eds.), *Fostering Recovery and Well-being in a Healthy Lifestyle: Psychological, Somatic, and Organizational Prevention Approaches* (pp. 117–130). Routledge.

DOI: 10.4324/9781003250654-11

debilitating thoughts ("I am nervous"). In sport performance, it is essential that athletes avoid the occurrence of such potentially performance-impairing reactions. If such reactions still occur, they should be able to deal with them. Systematic relaxation techniques can play a central role in those processes.

A prerequisite for optimal performance in sports is, in addition to relaxing, being able to systematically activate oneself or being able to modify activation/arousal states. For many years it has been assumed that optimal performance is expected at a moderate activation/arousal state of athletes (Andreassi, 2007). According to this assumption, if the activation level is too low, performance-relevant components cannot be retrieved, possibly due to the lack of competition activation. If levels are too high, optimal performance is not to be expected due to the accompanying muscular tension and tightness. The decisive factor in that process is not the physical arousal itself, but the cognitive processes triggered by it (Beckmann & Rolstad, 1997), such as irrelevant thoughts.

Since the optimal arousal for performance can vary interindividually from one sport to another (Beckmann & Elbe, 2015) there are individual characteristics of optimal activation. This is also referred to as the *Individual Zones of Optimal Functioning* model (IZOF; Hanin, 1997). To achieve an optimal level of competition activation, athletes should be able to relax or to activate themselves dependent on the context. In many psychological techniques, the ability to relax is a prerequisite for their successful execution (Birrer & Morgan, 2010), e.g., imagery requires a relaxed state. In addition, relaxation is an important basis for many other sport psychological intervention and training programmes (Beckmann & Elbe, 2015).

Altogether, there are three general fields of application for relaxation training: 1) recovery, 2) self-regulation for optimal activation, 3) pre-requisite for psychological skills training. This chapter will primarily deal with the function of relaxation as a recovery tool to support performance as well as well-being.

Relaxation as a recovery tool

Relaxation serves many different functions in managing a variety of health conditions. In clinical practise, the value of relaxation as a supportive method has been shown repeatedly (Petermann, 2020). In sports, Kellmann and Beckmann (2020) point out that relaxation techniques are primarily used with the following four aims: First, in the long-term, a greater serenity with regard to the onerous training and competition situation should be established. This should be combined with building up expectations to be able to regulate oneself effectively in these situations. The second, short-term aim points towards disturbing thoughts that are to be removed in the immediate preparation for competition and during it to achieve and keep full focus. However, the necessary competition activation must not be reduced. Third, relaxation supports regeneration after training and competition, especially in the case of injuries. Finally, relaxation is the basis for the training of further self-regulation skills, such as imagery, similar to systematic desensitisation in behavioural therapy.

From these aims it can be derived that the function of relaxation techniques as a recovery tool in sport is threefold: Being 1) a strategy to develop inner balance, 2) a regeneration accelerator, and 3) a self-regulation tool. Kudlackova et al. (2013), Keilani et al. (2016), and Pelka et al. (2016) reported that the most used techniques are progressive muscle relaxation, systematic breathing, hypnosis, eastern meditation, and imagery.

Relaxation as a means of developing inner balance

Looking at the long-term effects of training, relaxation techniques can be used to develop the personality of an athlete in the sense of increasing his/her inner balance. The athlete learns to focus on, and at the same time solve, problems of his/her specific sport. Practising relaxation techniques should start at the beginning of the preparation for a season and then should be taken over to the entire preparation period.

In addition to the elimination of tension and the support of regeneration, direct body-related goals are the sensitisation for, and focus on, one's own body and its physical processes. Being aware of one's body can support the movement sequences, which are practised. In addition, a feeling for tensed and relaxed muscles should be developed. The acquisition of relaxation skills should lead towards the ability to self-regulate one's own physical and psychological state.

At the same time, athletes should develop greater serenity, which allows them to accept unexpected – in particular, unfavourable – conditions. In golf, for example, it is said that the golfer should develop humility. This is connected to the fact that perceptual thresholds increase against disturbing internal and external stimuli. There should also be an affective equilibrium, so athletes are no longer sitting in an emotional 'rollercoaster', i.e., the feeling of excitement after a success is no longer acknowledged with absolute dejection in a subsequent failure/loss. This should also increase the ability to concentrate.

Last but not least, the serenity that develops through relaxation training also contributes to the improvement of general well-being. The positive overall feeling with a lack of negative affect reduces a defencive attitude and creates access to one's own strengths and own resources (Kuhl, 2001).

Relaxation as a regeneration accelerator

Recovery processes in elite sports also serve to restore the individual operational conditions and well-being after training and competition (Kellmann & Beckmann, 2022; Kellmann et al., 2018; Loch et al., 2019). In today's high-performance sport environments training is scheduled twice or even three times a day (training camp). Outside of training camps, demands from school, university, and/or work as well as personal relationships affect an athlete and all of which must be paid tribute within a limited overall time budget. With systematically practised relaxation techniques, the probability of successfully using the scarce resource 'time' after training or in short breaks within a day is increased. Therefore, the somatotropic and psychotropic effects of relaxation can have the function of a 'regeneration accelerator'. Relaxation between training sessions accelerates the natural recovery process and allows for more intensive and increased training loads (Pelka et al., 2017). Furthermore, the authors argue that recovery after stress is more rapid with the aid of relaxation techniques compared to passive recovery. Regeneration processes play a decisive role in the event of rising fatigue, with regard to restoring the ability to act after stress.

If regeneration is not possible and stress (physical and psychological) accumulates, underrecovery or overtraining are possible consequences (Meeusen & De Pauw, 2022). However, if recovery is used appropriately, high stress levels can be tolerated, and it does not have to be negative to be highly stressed (Kellmann, 2002). In the context of this chapter, relaxation is thus classified as a purposeful recovery strategy.

Relaxation as a method of self-regulation

Prior to competition, relaxation has two important functions that can be actively controlled by the athlete. Many – sometimes even experienced – athletes report that they cannot sleep properly two to three nights before an important competition (Erlacher, 2019; Erlacher et al., 2011). This reduced sleep quality and quantity can be detrimental to physical performance. This happens either directly through lack of recovery or indirectly through the fact that an athlete, after bad sleep, doubts whether she/he is still able to perform at all (Caia et al., 2022; Ehrlenspiel et al., 2018). In these situations, the deliberate creation of a relaxation state could lead to a stopping of rumination. Using relaxation as 'sleep assistance' is a functional aid to react to disturbing cognitions and support overnight recovery.

On the day of the competition, athletes experience different levels of activation, depending on their experience and self-regulation ability. As stated earlier, a certain level of activation is necessary to provide athletic performance. Therefore, in the sense of a contraindication, there should be no relaxation training on the competition day, as otherwise the necessary activation could be lost. The use of systematic relaxation techniques (e.g., progressive muscle relaxation, or autogenic training) is only possible and useful if athletes have learned to reactivate themselves properly. For some athletes, however, relaxation as a strategy is a prerequisite to build up the concentration necessary for performing in competition.

If athletes do not possess relaxation and/or mobilisation skills, the relaxation response could be triggered through imagery, especially on competition days. Initially, it is possible to initiate the elicitation of the relaxation response through systematic breathing. Besides that, and as a matter of principle, athletes should always try to relax briefly while preparing for competition so that 'uncontrollable' activation tips could be prevented. The same also applies to the time period right before competition. For example, in rowing, boats usually lie at the start at least ten minutes before competition. During these ten minutes, most athletes try to build up concentration for the race through a ritualised process with smaller tasks to avoid irrelevant cognitions. If these still occur, a relaxation response should be triggered through visualising a relaxing image, which then should lead to an increase in concentration and focus on the competition.

Recently, self-regulation has also been increasingly discussed in the context of embodied cognition (MacIntyre et al., 2019). It is assumed that cognition, emotion, and physical processes are closely related. Linked to that, a very simple technique has proven to be effective. Dynamically squeezing the left hand for 10 to 15 seconds results in so-called 'high alpha' (10–12Hz) waves spreading across the brain, which relaxes and inhibits disturbing thoughts (Cross-Villasana et al., 2015). Because of the higher connectivity of the right hemisphere, this self-relaxing technique only works when the left hand is pressed. Several studies have shown that this technique can prevent choking under pressure (Beckmann et al., 2013, 2021).

Procedure

In sport psychological consultation, relaxation is an important topic (Birrer & Morgan, 2010). Primarily, the focus lies on the current concern of the athlete and how to stabilise or optimise performance in a specific context. However, it is frequently the case that a missing key variable is relaxation. Thus, further tests, e.g., questionnaires, or (semi-) structured interviews, are carried out to assess how the athlete usually uses relaxation and whether a relaxation response can be elicited in a targeted manner. In recent years, interest in systematic relaxation techniques has increased (Kudlackova et al., 2013). Responses to the various techniques (e.g., systematic breathing, progressive muscle relaxation, autogenic training, hypnosis) are individually different and have different areas of application in sports. Therefore, together with the athlete, the sports psychologist should define the procedure to be learned and explain the background information and possible effects. The selection of the appropriate technique is then based on previous experience, type of sport, and the specific problem in combination with the clients' preference.

The structure of relaxation training in sports is derived from Vaitl (2020) and consists of an introductory phase, which is followed by relaxation induction and the actual development of the relaxation response. In addition, imagery can be integrated at the end of the development of the relaxation response. In this specific situation, the athlete puts herself/himself into a relaxing and positive situation and links this relaxing state to a self-selected image. Linking a relaxation state and an image is intended to create a firm 'connection', so that optimally an athlete's image elicits a relaxation response (Martin et al., 1999). The procedure is completed by bringing participants back from the relaxation state to a conscious, wakeful, and relaxed state. After every session, a debriefing should be scheduled to assess whether there were difficulties or if modifications should be made (Hogg, this volume, Chapter 5). The ultimate goal is that athletes use relaxation techniques independently.

Techniques

Relaxation techniques used in sports are manifold and include, amongst others, autogenic training, biofeedback, progressive muscle relaxation, systematic breathing, and hypnosis (Kudlackova et al., 2013; Pelka et al., 2016; Weinberg & Gould, 2010). Other widely used strategies in recovery settings are music and power naps (Jones et al., 2017; Pelka et al., 2017; Terry et al., 2020). The following paragraphs exemplarily display three strategies which support the recovery process.

Hypnosis

Basically, hypnosis induces a state of trance that does not greatly differ from the trance brought about by autogenic training. Thus, hypnotic inductions are primarily associated with relaxation, sedation, and well-being. The hypnotherapist will address the person: "As you sit here, and as you, despite the environment or just because of the noise you hear, focus more and more on the words you hear, you perhaps notice that you would like to close your eyes…". This is a way of inducing a state of trance, which might be deepened by saying, "With each exhalation you become more relaxed, with each breath you get deeper into trance". Hypnosis has been applied in sports for a relatively long time and has helped athletes to improve training and performance (Straub & Bowman, 2016). Ligget (2000) advocates self-hypnosis in sports. This can only be recommended after several sessions with a professional hypnotherapist because in trance, psychological problems that were well suppressed until now might enter consciousness and the athlete might not be able to handle this. However, if after a number of sessions with a hypnotherapist, the likelihood of those problems turning up is considerably low, self-hypnosis may be an option. One trance induction technique that could be used is the '5, 4, 3, 2, 1 technique' (Dolan, 1991). It is a type of meditative technique. The client is told to fix their focus on a specific point. Then five things that can be seen in the client's peripheral vision are stated. Next, five things that can be heard are addressed. Then five things that can be sensed are stated. In the next round, four things that can be seen, heard, and sensed are stated. With every round the number of things perceived is reduced by one. After having addressed only one thing that is seen, one thing that is heard, and one thing that is felt usually a state of trance is reached. The client may now close their eyes. After arriving at a stage of mild trance (deep trance is not required) forms of imagination can be used such as 'safe place', 'improving concentration', etc. The client can be asked to imagine a safe place in which they felt relaxed and stable on a somatic level, a situation in which the body felt vital, resilient, and fully comfortable. The client is instructed to indulge completely in this situation, to feel it in every cell of their body, and to fully revive the positive feelings. While basking in the situation, the hypnotherapist asks the client to give a name for their safe place. The client is told that they can go to this place whenever they need to go there to relax and build confidence.

Many of the objectives to be achieved through imagery can also be addressed through hypnosis. The difference to mental skill training lies in the induction of a state of trance in hypnosis that attempts to arrive at changes at the unconscious level.

Music

Almost every athlete spends some time before, between, and/or after competition or training with self-selected music from portable devices. In addition to widespread use, there is no strategy which is as tailor-made to one's preferences as music. Recent studies have shown that music affects attention, emotions, and regulation of emotions, and has an influence on increased work readiness and performance, as well as on reducing inhibitions. Compared to systematic relaxation techniques, music is often regarded as a naïve strategy, but in the end, it is, as already indicated, one of the most popular and attractive strategies. Many findings also show effects of music on a variety of performance-related parameters (Karageorghis, 2017). According to Karageorghis and Priest (2012), music can be regarded as a legal stimulant or sedative.

Terry et al. (2020) reported in their meta-analytical review that music was associated with significant beneficial effects on affective valence, physical performance, perceived exertion, and oxygen consumption. In physiological terms, increases or decreases of the respiratory rate or heart rate, are potential responses to rhythmic components of music. The physiological processes are the same as in recovery. It was postulated that music induces relaxation through the influence on automatic and central nervous processes (Gillen et al., 2008). On one hand, the anxiolytic effect of music is manifested through the suppressive effect on the sympathetic nervous system, i.e., reducing adrenergic activity and neuromuscular arousal. On the other hand, music triggers the limbic system to release endorphins, which play a decisive role in the enhancement of well-being. It has already been shown that music can attract attention from incriminating events to more pleasant and soothing thoughts, and thereby reducing symptoms of anxiety and pain (MacDonald et al., 2003; Nilsson, 2008; Seers & Carroll, 1998). Among the few researchers who have assessed the efficacy of music as recovery from exercise, Jones et al. (2017) found that fast-tempo, positively-valanced music (applied during recovery periods) induces a more pleasant experience in a high-intensity interval training setting. In summary, relaxation and music are both associated with decreased heart rate, systolic blood pressure, and norepinephrine production (Szmedra & Bacharach, 1998). A further similarity is the reduction of muscle tension followed by increased blood flow and faster lactate decomposition.

Progressive muscle relaxation

One of the most used techniques in sports is progressive muscle relaxation (Kudlackova et al., 2013). A reason could be that athletes are already familiar with relaxing and activating their muscles during the training process. Therefore, this technique is supposed to be the most 'physical' of the relaxation procedures. The change of tension and relaxation during the exercise is so familiar to the athletes that they usually have no difficulty in relaxing while following the instructions (see Table 8.1 for modified instructions).

Consequently, progressive muscle relaxation is usually preferred over other procedures. However, it should also be considered that not all athletes react similarly to each technique. Regular feedback loops are an important feature of the learning process during the relaxation process, if necessary, to: a) modify the procedure; or b) select another technique. A detailed description of a progressive muscle relaxation session is provided in the following section.

Modification of a standard procedure

If learning relaxation techniques in a systematic way is not possible, e.g., for time-related reasons, we recommend the use of progressive muscle relaxation with subsequent imagery. Essentially, progressive muscle relaxation, which is predominantly used in sport, follows the structure of a standard procedure (Bernstein & Borkovec, 1973; Hamm, 2020). For athletes, it is useful to use a shortened form as they are already familiarised with the change between relaxed and tensed muscles through their physical training. A progressive muscle relaxation version, preferred by us, is aimed at eight muscle groups and systematic breathing. From our applied experience it seems to be helpful that after an introductory concentration phase, the programme starts with the facial muscles. This order supports building up concentration for the entire phase in the beginning of the procedure (Table 8.1).

In the first three sessions the muscle groups are repeatedly tensed and relaxed (three times). In order to be economic, some muscle groups are grouped together during sessions four to six, i.e., muscle groups are then activated simultaneously. These groups are then tensed and relaxed twice. In the seventh to ninth sessions, the grouped muscles are tensed and relaxed only once. In addition, the instruction is shortened from the seventh session on, i.e., only the muscle groups are announced and the athlete controls tension and relaxation time himself/herself.

In the beginning, the sport psychologist informs the athlete about the course, mechanisms, and possible effects of progressive muscle relaxation. In addition, attention is drawn to practise effects, i.e., time to elicit a relaxation response is reduced following repeated execution. Furthermore, the athletes receive the instruction that they should execute the relaxation technique highly concentrated and should not fall asleep (which still happens to many during the first sessions).

Conclusion and recommendations for practise

Relaxation techniques should be integrated as an essential part of an athletes' training regimen. They should be practised before or between training and/or practice sessions, so that athletes are still able to engage in them in a state of

Table 8.1 A procedure for relaxation induction with progressive muscle relaxation and subsequent imagination (based on Bernstein et al., 2007).

Initiation: Reduction of exaggerated expectations and fears
• Background information about mechanisms and effects of progressive muscle relaxation
• Practise effects
• Aim: Highly concentrated execution without falling asleep

Relaxation induction: Shifting attention to a (passive) receptive, inwardly-directed orientation; reduction of sensory input
• Taking a seat (cabman's relaxing position) or laying on the floor (mat)
• Instruction to rest, starting to focus (setting up concentration)

Developing relaxation: Staying in an intermediate state between wakefulness and sleep

order	muscles	instruction	frequency (session number)		
			1–3	4–6	7–9
(1)	forehead	frowning	3×	2×	1×
(2)	around nose, cheeks, and chin	pull a face	3×	2×	1×
(3)	shoulders and neck	raise shoulders	3×	2×	1×
(4)	arms	tense upper arm and forearm (right and left)	3×	2×	1×
(5)	fingers	make a fist (right and left)	3×	2×	1×
(6)	focus on breathing	inhale (4s), hold breath (1–2s) and exhale slowly (6–8s)	3×	3×	3×

Instruction: "The entire upper body is relaxed now, let the relaxation flow into your legs".

order	muscles	instruction	1–3	4–6	7–9
(7)	thighs	tense both thighs	3×	2×	1×
(8)	calves	pull your toes towards your head (while your legs remain on the floor)	3×	2×	1×
(9)	toes	roll your toes	3×	2×	1×

(*Continued*)

Table 8.1 (Continued)

Linking relaxation to a self-selected picture (imagery)

- Instruction: "The whole body is relaxed [...] head, upper body and legs. Now imagine a situation in which you feel comfortable. [...] For some it is staying at the beach, for others a clearing in the forest, or a completely different situation. [...] Take such a situation and try to imagine everything as detailed as possible. [...] Feel the warmth on your skin, hear the voices around you, and experience relaxation. [...] Imagine the colours and experience your environment precisely. [...] Devote yourself fully to the situation... [...]".

Retrieval

- Instruction: "Please follow my instruction while I will soon count backwards from ten to one. [...] 10, 9, 8, 7, 6 (move your muscles slowly), 5, 4, 3 (stretch and move a little bit more), 2, 1 (open your eyes, you are awake now, focused and relaxed)".

Debriefing

- Ask if and how the relaxation has worked, and if yes which disturbances have occurred, and which sensations have been encountered.

concentration. Essentially, an efficient provision of relaxation competence requires a long-term perspective. Adopting such a long-term systematic practise approach (Beckmann & Elbe, 2015) is accompanied by various positive side effects. Relaxation could serve as a regeneration accelerator and is particularly helpful in case athletes tend to be nervous prior to competition ('starting fever') and/or cannot sleep or slept badly in the night before competition. Additionally, relaxation marks a prerequisite for the execution of mental training (e.g., imagery). However, practising relaxation techniques in their detailed version on the competition day is contraindicated, because it could jeopardise the necessary activation for competition.

In the beginning of a long-term approach, systematic breathing should be introduced and practised. Systematic breathing is administered at this point, as it is one of the simplest approaches to relaxation and, additionally, an integral part of every other relaxation technique. Thereby, the exhalation should be deliberately prolonged compared to the inhalation (Pelka et al., 2017). After exhaling, a short pause follows, after which the inhalation automatically starts again. If an understanding of the actual physiological mechanisms of relaxation is necessary, it can be conveyed via biofeedback in this phase. Through the use of biofeedback (as technical support) ordinarily unavailable internal physiological processes can be made visible for the athlete in a meaningful, rapid, precise, and consistent form (Zaichkowsky & Fuchs, 1988). This is followed by the introduction of progressive muscle relaxation (about eight to ten sessions) with the goal of achieving sensitisation for the body/muscles. The last episode of the training programme would consist of autogenic training with a focus on three basic exercises (heaviness, warmth, respiration) aiming at long-term psychotropic effects. Thereafter, autogenic training and progressive muscle relaxation may remain an integral part of the training regimen. The composition and development of the training schedule strongly depend on previous experiences and individual preferences. Additionally, like practising their physical skills, it is important that athletes practise their psychological skills such as relaxation techniques and routines on a daily basis.

References

Andreassi, J. L. (2007). Concepts in psychophysiology. In J. L. Andreassi (Ed.), *Psychophysiology – Human behavior and physiological response* (pp. 16–42). Psychology Press.

Beckmann, J. (2023). Self-regulation of recovery. In M. Kellmann, S. Jakowski, & J. Beckmann (Eds.), *The importance of recovery for physical and mental health: Negotiating the effects of underrecovery* (pp. 53–69). Routledge.

Beckmann, J., Beckmann-Waldenmayer, D., & Wolf, S. A. (2023). Self-regulation in competitive sports. In J. Schüler, M. Wegner, H. Plessner, & R. C. Eklund (Eds.), *Sport psychology* (pp. 491–512). Springer Nature.

Beckmann, J., & Elbe, A.-M. (2015). *Sport psychological interventions in competitive sports.* Cambridge Scholars Publishing.

Beckmann, J., Fimpel, L., & Wergin, V. V. (2021). Preventing a loss of accuracy of the tennis serve under pressure. *PLoS One 16*(7), e0255060. https://doi.org/10.1371/journal.pone.0255060

Beckmann, J., Gröpel, P., & Ehrlenspiel, F. (2013). Preventing motor skill failure through hemisphere – Specific priming. Cases from choking under pressure. *Journal of Experimental Psychology. General, 142*, 679–691.

Beckmann, J., & Rolstad, K. (1997). Aktivierung, Selbstregulation und Leistung: Gibt es so etwas wie Übermotivation? [Activation, self-regulation and performance: Is there anything like over-motivation?]. *Sportwissenschaft, 27*(1), 23–37.

Bengtsson, H., Ekstrand, J., & Hägglund, M. (2013). Muscle injury rates in professional football increase with fixture congestion: An 11-year follow-up of the UEFA Champions League injury study. *British Journal of Sports Medicine, 47*(12), 743–747.

Bernstein, D. A., & Borkovec, T. D. (1973). *Progressive relaxation training. A manual for the helping professions*. Research Press Company.

Bernstein, D. A., Carlson, C. R., & Schmidt, J. F. (2007). Progressive relaxation. In P. M. Lehrer, R. L. Woolfolk, & W. E. Sime (Eds.), *Principles and practice of stress management* (pp. 88–124). The Guilford Press.

Birrer, D., & Morgan, G. (2010). Psychological skills training as a way to enhance an athlete's performance in high-intensity sports. *Scandinavian Journal of Medicine and Science in Sports, 20*, 78–87.

Caia, J., Kelly, V. G., Driller, M. W., & Halson, S. L. (2022). The role of sleep in the performance of elite athletes. In M. Kellmann & J. Beckmann (Eds.), *Recovery and well-being in sport and exercise* (pp. 131–151). Routledge.

Cross-Villasana, F., Gröpel, P., Doppelmayr, M., & Beckmann, J. (2015). Unilateral left-hand contractions produce widespread depression of cortical activity after their execution. *PloS One, 10*(12), e0145867. https://doi.org/10.1371/journal.pone.0145867

Dolan, Y. (1991). *Resolving sexual abuse: Solution-focused therapy and Ericksonian hypnosis for adult survivors*. W.W. Norton.

Ehrlenspiel, F., Erlacher, D., & Ziegler, M. (2018). Changes in subjective sleep quality before a competition and their relation to competitive anxiety. *Behavioral Sleep Medicine, 16*(6), 553–568.

Erlacher, D. (2019). *Sport und Schlaf* [Sport and sleep]. Springer.

Erlacher, D., Ehrlenspiel, F., Adegbesan, O. A., & Galal El-Din, H. (2011). Sleep habits in German athletes before important competitions or games. *Journal of Sports Sciences, 29*(8), 859–866.

Gillen, E., Biley, F., & Allen, D. (2008). Effects of music listening on adult patients' pre-procedural state anxiety in hospital. *International Journal of Evidence-Based Healthcare, 6*(1), 24–49.

Hamm, A. (2020). Progressive Muskelentspannung [Progressive muscle relaxation]. In F. Petermann (Ed.), *Entspannungsverfahren* (6th ed., pp. 150–168). Beltz.

Hanin, Y. L. (1997). Emotions and athletic performance: Individual Zones of Optimal Functioning model. *European Yearbook of Sport Psychology, 1*, 29–72.

Jakowski, S., Kiel, A., Kullik, L., & Erlacher, D. (2023). Sleep to heal and restore: The role of sleep in the recovery and regeneration process. In M. Kellmann, S. Jakowski, & J. Beckmann (Eds.), *The importance of recovery for physical and mental health: Negotiating the effects of underrecovery* (pp. 141–153). Routledge.

Jones, L., Tiller, N. B., & Karageorghis, C. I. (2017). Psychophysiological effects of music on acute recovery from high-intensity interval training. *Physiology and Behavior, 170*, 106–114.

Karageorghis, C. I. (2017). *Applying music in exercise and sport.* Human Kinetics.

Karageorghis, C. I., & Priest, D.-L. (2012). Music in the exercise domain: A review and synthesis (Part I). *International Review of Sport and Exercise Psychology, 5*(1), 44–66.

Keilani, M., Hasenohrl, T., Gartner, I., Krall, C., Furnhammer, J., Cenik, F., & Crevenna, R. (2016). Use of mental techniques for competition and recovery in professional athletes. *Wiener Klinische Wochenschrift, 128*(9–10), 315–319.

Kellmann, M. (2002). Underrecovery and overtraining: Different concepts – Similar impact? In M. Kellmann (Ed.), *Enhancing recovery: Preventing underperformance in athletes* (pp. 3–24). Human Kinetics.

Kellmann, M., & Kallus, K. W. (2016). The Recovery-Stress Questionnaire for Athletes. In K. W. Kallus & M. Kellmann (Eds.), *The Recovery-Stress Questionnaires: User manual* (pp. 86–131). Pearson Assessment.

Kellmann, M., & Beckmann, J. (2020). Sport und Bewegung [Sport and Movement]. In F. Petermann (Ed.), *Entspannungsverfahren* (6th ed., pp. 346–355). Beltz.

Kellmann, M., & Beckmann, J. (Eds.). (2022). *Recovery and well-being in sport and exercise.* Routledge.

Kellmann, M., Bertollo, M., Bosquet, L., Brink, M., Coutts, A. J., Duffield, R., Erlacher, D., Halson, S. L., Hecksteden, A., Heidari, J., Kallus, K. W., Meeusen, R., Mujika, I., Robazza, C., Skorski, S., Venter, R., & Beckmann, J. (2018). Recovery and performance in sport: Consensus statement. *International Journal of Sports Physiology and Performance, 13*(2), 240–245.

Kellmann, M., Jakowski, S., & Beckmann, J. (Eds.). (2023). *The importance of recovery for physical and mental health: Negotiating the effects of underrecovery.* Routledge.

Kudlackova, K., Eccles, D. W., & Dieffenbach, K. (2013). Use of relaxation skills in differentially skilled athletes. *Psychology of Sport and Exercise, 14*(4), 468–475.

Kuhl, J. (2001). *Motivation und Persönlichkeit: Interaktionen psychischer Systeme* [Motivation and personality: Interactions of psychological systems]. Hogrefe.

Ligget, D. R. (2000). *Sport hypnosis.* Human Kinetics.

Loch, F., Ferrauti, A., Meyer, T., Pfeiffer, M., & Kellmann, M. (2019). Resting the mind – A novel topic with scarce insights. Considering potential mental recovery strategies for short rest periods in sports. *Performance Enhancement & Health, 6*, 148–155.

MacDonald, R. A., Mitchell, L. A., Dillon, T., Serpell, M. G., Davies, J. B., & Ashley, E. A. (2003). An empirical investigation of the anxiolytic and pain reducing effects of music. *Psychology of Music, 31*(2), 187–203.

MacIntyre, T. E., Madan, C. R., Brick, N. E., Beckmann, J., & Moran, A. P. (2019). Imagery, expertise, and action: A window into embodiment. In M. L. Cappuccio (Ed.), *The MIT Press handbook of embodied cognition and sport psychology* (pp. 625–650). MIT Press.

Martin, K. A., Moritz, S. E., & Hall, C. R. (1999). Imagery use in sport: A literature review and applied model. *The Sport Psychologist, 13*, 245–368.

Mesagno, C., & Beckmann, J. (2017). Choking under pressure: Theoretical models and interventions. *Current Opinion in Psychology, 16*, 170–175.

Meeusen, R., & De Pauw, K. (2022). Overtraining – What do we know? In M. Kellmann & J. Beckmann (Eds.), *Recovery and well-being in sport and exercise* (pp. 51–62). Routledge.

Nilsson, U. (2008). The anxiety- and pain-reducing effects of music interventions: A systematic review. *AORN Journal, 87*(4), 780–807.

Pelka, M., Heidari, J., Ferrauti, A., Meyer, T., Pfeiffer, M., & Kellmann, M. (2016). Relaxation techniques in sports: A systematic review on acute effects on performance. *Performance Enhancement and Health, 5*(2), 47–59.

Pelka, M., Kölling, S., Ferrauti, A., Meyer, T., Pfeiffer, M., & Kellmann, M. (2017). Acute effects of psychological relaxation techniques between two physical tasks. *Journal of Sports Sciences, 35(3)*, 216–223.

Petermann, F. (2020). Entspannungsverfahren [Relaxation techniques]. In F. Petermann (Ed.), *Entspannungsverfahren* (6th ed., pp. 19–44). Beltz.

Seers, K., & Carroll, D. (1998). Relaxation techniques for acute pain management: A systematic review. *Journal of Advanced Nursing, 27*, 466–475.

Straub, W. F., & Bowman, J. J. (2016). A review of the development of sport hypnosis as a performance enhancement method for athletes. *Journal of Psychology and Clinical Psychiatry, 6(6)*, 00378. https://doi.org/10.15406/jpcpy.2016.06.00378

Szmedra, L., & Bacharach, D. W. (1998). Effect of music on perceived exertion, plasma lactate, norepinephrine and cardiovascular hemodynamics during treadmill running. *International Journal of Sports Medicine, 19(1)*, 32–37.

Tennant, C., Langeluddecke, P., & Byrne, D. (1985). The concept of stress. *Australian and New Zealand Journal of Psychiatry, 19(2)*, 113–118.

Terry, P. C., Karageorghis, C. I., Curran, M. L., Martin, O. V., & Parsons-Smith, R. L. (2020). Effects of music in exercise and sport: A meta-analytic review. *Psychological Bulletin, 146(2)*, 91–117.

Vaitl, D. (2020). Neurobiologische Grundlagen der Entspannungsverfahren [Neuro-biological basics of relaxation techniques]. In F. Petermann (Ed.), *Entspannungsverfahren* (6th ed., pp. 47–64). Beltz.

Weinberg, R., & Gould, D. (2010). *Foundations of sport and exercise psychology*. Human Kinetics.

Zaichkowsky, L. D., & Fuchs, C. Z. (1988). Biofeedback applications in exercise and athletic performance. *Exercise and Sport Sciences Reviews, 16(1)*, 381–422.

9 Yoga for recovery and well-being in athletes

Selenia di Fronso, Maurizio Bertollo, and Claudio Robazza

Introduction

The practise of yoga originated in India over 5000 years ago and it has always been approached to reach and maintain physical and mental health (Brinsley et al., 2021). The word *yoga* derives from the Sanskrit root *yuj* which means 'to join' or 'to unite'. In fact, it is recognised that the practise of yoga leads to a union and to harmony between the mind and the body (di Fronso et al., 2021), reducing stress and restoring calm and inner peace. Nowadays, the word yoga refers to a range of comprehensive activities including holistic exercises, such as balance, stretching, breathing or meditation, which benefit people both mentally and physically (di Fronso & Bertollo, 2021). For this reason, yoga can be described as a multicomponent practise where physical activity is carefully combined with mental practise guided by a holistic philosophy of psychophysical well-being (Vergeer & Biddle, 2021). This fruitful combination leads to beneficial effects involving, for example, calming the mind, improving mindfulness skills, developing, and training body awareness and control (Vergeer, 2018). Furthermore, yoga can exert beneficial effects on postural stability (Ni et al., 2014), balance (di Fronso et al., 2021; Kadachha et al., 2016), sleep disorders, depression, pain perception (Wahbeh & Nelson, 2019), stress and muscle tension, and increase resilience and self-care (Anderson et al., 2017).

Despite being rooted mainly in eastern culture and values, yoga as a mindbody practise has become popular in western society; for example, from 2012 to 2016 the number of people practising yoga in the US increased by 50% (Yoga Alliance, 2016) and in the modern society yoga strongly characterises the landscape of classes offered in fitness clubs (Cartwright et al., 2020). Importantly, yoga practise is gaining increasing attention also in the sport domain (di Fronso et al., 2022). This growth and popularity are crucial clues to the importance yoga is assuming for recreationally active people and athletes' well-being. In this

di Fronso, S., Bertollo, M., & Robazza, C. (2024). Yoga for recovery and well-being in athletes. In M. Kellmann & J. Beckmann (Eds.), *Fostering Recovery and Well-being in a Healthy Lifestyle: Psychological, Somatic, and Organizational Prevention Approaches* (pp. 131–142). Routledge.

DOI: 10.4324/9781003250654-12

chapter, while addressing the topic of yoga strategies in the sport context, we first provide an overview of the yoga-based interventions for well-being in athletes of different levels (di Fronso et al., 2022; Grilli Cadieux et al., 2022). Second, we draw from the research on the interventions to improve sleep quality to describe the usefulness of yoga nidra practise for improving athletes' recovery and recovery-stress balance (di Fronso & Bertollo, 2021; Podlog et al., 2023). Finally, we discuss the utility of pranayama techniques and other restorative interventions for athletes' recovery and well-being (Brown & Gerbarg, 2005; La Forge, 2005). The three sections on yoga practise for athletes' well-being, sleep quality and recovery are closely intertwined and are believed to impact athletes' performance and health. Well-being and optimal recovery are part of a virtuous cycle that enables athletes to manage physical and mental stressors effectively (Kellmann et al., 2018; Podlog et al., 2023). Yoga strategies can induce physical and mental states that enhance athletes' well-being and boost recovery. In turn, optimal recovery can enhance the mental and physical well-being of athletes and ultimately lead to better performance.

Yoga interventions for well-being

One of the primary goals in sport and exercise psychology is the well-being of athletes (Grilli Cadieux et al., 2021). Fear of failure, dysfunctional anxiety, or emotional mismanagement can lead to detrimental consequences for athletic performance and increase psychological distress and depressive disorder (Al Majali & Ashour, 2020). Beyond cognitive-behavioural strategies (focused primarily on psychological skills training), acceptance- and awareness-based interventions (like mindfulness) can be used to deal with dysfunctional emotions of athletes (di Fronso et al., 2022; Grilli Cadieux et al., 2021) and improve their psychophysical well-being. These interventions can stimulate athletes' moment to moment awareness and encourage a better tolerance of their internal states such as negative thoughts and emotions (di Fronso et al., 2022).

Sharing similarities with mindfulness practise, yoga encourages athletes to become aware of and accept their internal states thereby promoting their well-being. Indeed, yoga can allow thoughts, emotions, and other sensations within the individual to come and go without struggling or experiencing the need to change them. Overall, there are several types of yoga characterised by different physical intensities and components potentially leading to multiple effects in athletes and performers (Table 9.1). These effects encompass not only improved strength, flexibility, agility (Bal & Kaur, 2009), and cardiorespiratory performance (Harinath et al., 2004), but also reduced negative mood, anxiety, and stress (di Fronso et al., 2022), and enhanced injury prevention (Arbo et al., 2020), recovery time and body awareness (Sharma, 2015). Hatha yoga is aimed to create a state of harmony between mind and body through the practise of asanas (postures) and pranayama (breathing techniques). It can be used to help athletes reduce physical and mental stress, gain body awareness, and make them accept their physical limits (Kabat-Zinn & Hanh, 2009). The word *hatha*, which

Table 9.1 The different types of yoga, their intensity, components, and effects.

Yoga Type	Intensity	Components	Effects
Hatha Yoga	From moderate to high	Asanas, breathing, meditation/ relaxation	Increased stamina and flexibility; reduced physical and mental stress; enhanced mindfulness and body awareness; acceptance of the own physical limits
Mindful Yoga	Moderate	Asanas, breathing, meditation/ relaxation	Improved awareness of present moment feelings, attention focus, intention, and non-judgmental attitude; reduced stress and negative emotions; improved positive emotions
Bali-Yoga	From moderate to high	Asanas, breathing, meditation/ relaxation	Enhanced mental health; reduced performance anxiety; improved mindfulness and coping skills
Yoga Nidra	Low	Breathing, meditation/ relaxation	Improved sleep quality, physical and mental relaxation, cognitive restructuring processes and emotional detachment

means forceful, refers to the goal of increasing stamina and flexibility through long practise of asanas (e.g., warrior poses), which are a range of physical exercises designed to build both physical and mental strength. For instance, Goodman et al. (2014) involved an entire NCAA division I athletic team in hatha yoga sessions. Athletes reported greater tolerance to negative experiences and enhanced mindfulness levels. Premkumar and Devi (2013) found that asanas, breathing techniques and meditation practise had a significant impact on state anxiety of high-level athletes. Recently, Arbo et al. (2020) piloted an adapted version of an evidence-based hatha yoga protocol (Brems, 2015) with student athletes and noticed the intervention was successful in mitigating athletes' perception of psychophysical stress including fatigue, muscle soreness, and injury proneness.

Similar beneficial effects can be obtained through the practise of mindful yoga, in which individuals cultivate mindful awareness of the body while they move, stretch, or hold a position. It is suggested that the practise of mindful yoga leads to substantial improvements in awareness of present moment feelings, attention focus, intention, and non-judgmental attitude (Russell & Arcuri, 2015). As part of a mindful sport performance enhancement programme, mindful yoga was found to be associated with a long-term change in sport anxiety in a follow-up study with professional archers, golfers, and runners (Thompson et al., 2011). Also, di Fronso et al. (2022) highlighted the positive effects of ten mindful yoga sessions, included in a mindfulness-based stress reduction programme, on perceived stress and functional psychobiosocial states in athletes competing at different levels (i.e., international, national, and regional) and recreationally active people. Specifically, while practising mindful yoga, the body (and a mindful contact with it) likely represented a valuable, positive resource and the place where athletes and recreationally active people experienced deep states of calmness and positive emotions.

In the multitude of interventions aimed to ameliorate the psychophysical states of athletes and other performers, Bali-yoga was recently proposed and tested (Grilli Cadieux et al., 2022). This yoga intervention, which takes its name from Madan Bali, one of the most famous yoga instructors, includes psychoeducational contents on the benefits of yoga and the psychophysiological features of athletic performance (e.g., reduced performance anxiety, increased concentration, and mindfulness), breathing techniques, meditation and relaxation executed right after each posture to stimulate 'bodily rejuvenation' in participants. Bali-yoga can be easily adapted to athletes or performers needs and training regimens (Anestin et al., 2017; Filho et al., 2016). Adopted among circus student-artists, it was found to enhance their mental health (Filho et al., 2016), mindfulness levels and coping skills, and decrease performance anxiety (Grilli Cadieux et al., 2022). These results are in line with previous research on the effects of contemplative techniques on performance anxiety of athletes (Kaufman et al., 2019). Guided relaxation, a key component in Bali-yoga, is believed to lead to a healthy recovery-stress balance, increased general well-being, reduced somatic symptoms, and improved ability to cope with pain (Willmarth et al., 2014). Moreover, despite Bali-yoga did not reduce perceived anxiety in the short term, the meditation component enhances the athletes' awareness of uncomfortable feelings of anxiety without avoiding or trying to suppress them, and therefore tends to improve the individuals' ability to manage emotions both within and outside the performance context (Glass et al., 2019).

Yoga nidra for sleep quality and recovery enhancement

Beyond more physical yoga styles, there are meditation-based practises like yoga nidra (YN), whose name literally means yoga sleep. As discussed by Podlog et al. (2023), the practise of YN, executed in supine position, naturally stimulates a hypnagogic state wherein an individual is physiologically asleep yet maintains an internal/external awareness (Saraswati et al., 2009; Sharpe et al., 2021). While there is a withdrawal from other senses and a detachment from most of the stimuli, during YN practise the auditory channel remains receptive so that participants stay aware of the guide's instructions. Conscious sleep differentiates YN from other meditation-based practises such as transcendental meditation or body scan (di Fronso & Bertollo, 2021). YN is also described as a complete and systematic method to induce physical and mental relaxation which includes cognitive restructuring processes, guided body awareness, visualisation and breathing exercises aimed to turn individuals inward, away from outer experiences

(Saraswati, 2009). In particular, cognitive restructuring processes are stimulated by one of the core components of a YN session, namely a personal resolution called Sankalpa, the Sanskrit word for 'intention'. This resolution is a simple, short, and positive sentence (e.g., "I am relaxed", "I am successful") which is repeated at the beginning and at the end of the session 'driving' the unconscious towards the desired state (Saraswati, 2009). For more detail on yoga nidra practise see Table 9.2.

Recently, there has been a growing interest in YN effects on perceived stress, posttraumatic stress disorder, well-being, quality of life, insomnia and chronic sleep disorder in students, workers, and veterans (for a detailed overview of these topics, see iRest, 2022). One hour of YN practise is judged as restorative and rejuvenating as four hours of ordinary sleep (Saraswati, 2009), thus it is frequently suggested in sleep lab protocols (Sharpe et al., 2021). Sufficient sleep is one of the most important strategies for enhancing recovery (Eccles et al., 2021; Kullik & Kiel, this volume, Chapter 10; Meeusen et al., 2013), managing fatigue and preserving athletes' well-being (di Fronso & Bertollo, 2021). Notwithstanding the utmost importance of sleep for recovery in sport, the psycho(socio)physiological stressors experienced by athletes may undermine an adequate amount of sleep (Vitale et al., 2021). Insufficient sleep leads to underrecovery and cognitive impairments such as attention depletion or concentration disruption (Simpson et al., 2017). Considering that stressors should be counterbalanced by specific recovery strategies (Pelka et al., 2016), and given the importance of sleep for recovery, the practise of YN is recommended (Podlog et al., 2023). The stimulation of the parasympathetic system through this practise can increase slow-wave sleep which is associated with both subjective and objective sleep quality (Werner et al., 2015). These are two crucial parameters to improve the recovery-stress balance in athletes (Loch et al., 2019). YN was also shown to increase archery performance by enhancing athlete's vigilance and training participation as a consequence of better physical and mental recovery (Datta et al., 2020). Furthermore, YN effects on sleep latency (Datta et al., 2017; Moszeik et al., 2022) might

Table 9.2 The different stages of a *yoga nidra* session.

1	**Sankalpa**: A resolution, an *intention* related to athletes' needs
2	**Rotation of consciousness**: Awareness to the different body parts
3	**Breath awareness**: Attention to the breathing without altering or forcing it
4	**Feelings and emotions**: Intense sensations are awakened and then 'removed'
5	**Visualisation★**: In this stage athletes should enter the hypnagogic state
6	**Ending**: Sankalpa is repeated and the participant slowly comes back to the reality

Note: Retrieved from di Fronso and Bertollo (2021, p. 2). *Sankalpa*: The Sanskrit word for 'intention' expressed as a simple, short, and positive sentence (e.g., "I am calm", "I am successful"); ★this part can be guided in detail (describing for example peaceful places) or be more open encouraging the participant (e.g., the athlete) to visualise personal functional places or moments. Stages 2, 3, and 4 are functional to relaxation and facilitate the hypnagogic state; sounds can be used to maintain active the auditory channel.

improve the athlete's 'sleepability' (i.e., the ability to nap on demand) and may be a fertile strategy to address any sleep difficulties or deficiencies (di Fronso & Bertollo, 2021). Also, YN combined with cognitive restructuring processes may stimulate emotional detachment and help regulate post-performance negative emotions (Balk & Englert, 2020). The practice of Sankalpa, which consists of repeating short positive sentences and intentions during a YN session, may indeed help reframe negative thinking and stimulate more positive emotions.

A YN session usually lasts approximately one hour. However, since time is a scarce resource – especially in sports venues and between training sessions – the practise can be shortened (e.g., 15-minute sessions), while still providing systematic physical and mental relaxation and restoration (Saraswati, 2009). YN could therefore be used as a regular training or competition recovery strategy to be executed between training sessions or competitions. During rest periods, YN may serve as a physical and mental recovery strategy to counteract the effects of multiple training bouts on a single day or consecutive competition bouts over a period of weeks or months. Importantly, due to the activation of the parasympathetic system, YN should not be practised too close to a competition to avoid excessive lowering of arousal levels. Also, YN 'naps', for example using taped instructions, can be used on trips while reaching training or competition venues (di Fronso & Bertollo, 2021). It is important to note that recovery is a highly individualised process, and therefore YN should be tailored according to individual sleep needs and requirements (Loch et al., 2019). For example, it should be avoided by individuals with hypersomnia problems and lack of alertness during the waking time of the day. However, more research is needed to ascertain the efficacy of an aware sleep state on sleep quality of athletes, especially those without daytime sleepiness issues.

Pranayama and other restorative interventions

As mentioned above, yoga can be described as a multicomponent strategy to reach, restore, and maintain a psychophysical well-being. Beyond postures, guided relaxation and meditation, breathing is one of the most important yoga components that has always characterised yoga practises. Yogic breathing techniques collectively take the name of *pranayama*. Pranayama is a Sanskrit name derived from the association of two words: 'prana', which means vital energy and breath of life, and 'yama', which means expansion, regulation, and control (Jayawardena et al., 2020). From a practical point of view, this name reflects the deliberate modifications of the breathing process, including rapid diaphragmatic breathing, slow and deep breathing, alternate nostril breathing, and breath retention (Joshi, 2006). Pranayama techniques incorporate four main phases of breathing: inhalation (*puraka*), exhalation (*rekaca*), internal breath retention (*antah kumbhaka*) and external breath retention (*bahih kumbhaka*) (Nivethitha et al., 2016). Pranayama has shown several positive effects on health when considered both together with other yoga components and on its own. These effects encompass ameliorate breathing function (Saxena & Saxena, 2009), improved cardiovascular health (Goyal et al., 2014), better cognition and reduced general stress (Dhruva et al., 2012). They were mainly observed in patients with cancer, respiratory and cardiovascular diseases (Jayawardena et al., 2020). Regarding the sport domain, pranayama offers athletes the opportunity to better learn how to purposefully 'quiet' the nervous system. For example, a deep exhalation during pranayama stimulates the vagus nerve which in turns triggers an intense state of relaxation. Moreover, research shows that pranayama can regulate the release of stress hormones (Lim & Cheong, 2015). Both these effects of pranayama can help athletes' lower anxiety levels and stay focused on the task at hand (La Forge, 2005). Of note, yogic breathing can also enhance stress-tolerance and mood (Brown & Gerberg, 2005) and, if used regularly after performance, can promote adequate physical and mental recovery.

Guided meditation is another important yoga component that contributes to individuals' well-being; similar to pranayama, it can be used alone (Varghese et al., 2018). A guided meditation intervention for athletes that is gaining increasing attention for research and applied purposes is body scan (di Fronso et al., 2022). In body scan practise, people focus their attention sequentially and non-judgementally on different body parts and bodily sensations, thereby training their acceptance of body feelings and self-regulation skills. Body scan is therefore proposed as a further useful strategy to increase feeling states that are functional to the recovery and psychophysical well-being of athletes and to cope with anxiety. Coimbra et al. (2021) recently found that a ten-minute routine using the body scan technique reduced mental fatigue induced by competition in volleyball players. These authors recommend this kind of intervention for the recovery and attenuation of fatigue in athletes. Similar to body scan, Jacobson's (1930) progressive muscle relaxation can specifically 'teach the body' to recognise and eliminate feelings of tension. To this purpose, this technique requires progressively tensing and relaxing small muscle groups in a prescribed order (Newmark & Bogacki, 2005). It is suggested as a mind to muscle strategy to help athletes reach a more complete relaxation and facilitate both performance and recovery-stress-balance (Kellmann et al., this volume, Chapter 8; Pelka et al., 2016). However, while there is consistent research showing the positive effects of relaxation on performance, more research is needed to shed light on the effects of the above-mentioned interventions for recovery in sport, as well as to better understand their mechanisms, who are the best 'responders' and what are the best practises.

Conclusion and recommendations for practice

In this chapter, we have addressed yoga interventions for athletes' recovery and well-being, including hatha yoga, mindful yoga, Bali-yoga, and yoga nidra, and highlighted their benefits. For example, we emphasised the importance of yoga nidra for sleep regulation, which is crucial for recovery and well-being. We also discussed the utility of asanas to reduce stress, to help athletes accept physical limits and negative thoughts and to build physical and mental strength. Finally, we explained how yoga components beyond asanas (i.e., pranayama, guided meditation, and relaxation) used alone or in more structured interventions could contribute to athletes' recovery and well-being.

Overall, the interventions described are expected to improve interoceptive awareness skills including identifying, accessing, and appraising internal bodily signals, which are considered as key components for emotion regulation (di Fronso et al., 2022), and consequently for psychophysical well-being and recovery in sport. Also, training interoceptive awareness skills may contribute to prevent or counteract bodily signals typical of non-functional overreaching/ overtraining syndrome (Meuseen et al., 2013). These are two conditions of performance decrement not followed by supercompensation, the first characterised by 3 to 4 weeks and the latter characterised by a bit longer period of reduced performance capacity (Carrard et al., 2022). Furthermore, while physical relaxation (e.g., muscle relaxation) can help cope with competitive anxiety, mental relaxation (e.g., meditation) can benefit general anxiety regulation (Grilli Cadieux et al., 2022). However, both mental and physical relaxation are fundamental to the relationship between well-being and recovery. Indeed, muscle relaxation alleviates muscle tension and physical stress typical of trainings and competitions. Physical relaxation translates in mental relaxation, positive feelings, and improved well-being, which facilitate recovery and recovery-stress balance. In turn, mental relaxation and meditation help athletes deal with anxiety even outside of the sport context, thereby boosting general well-being and recovery processes. Accordingly, yoga practise and its multifarious components can provide athletes and performers with a tool that allows them to choose which aspects they want to integrate in their training routine, according to their current and idiosyncratic needs.

From a practical perspective, the following suggestions are made to better integrate yoga into the sport context. For example, overdoing physically demanding yoga practises could overstrain the athlete, lead to pain and fatigue in the muscles and joints involved in movement execution, increase the risk of injuries, and impair recovery and well-being. Yoga is not a competitive practice, and everyone should reach and maintain yoga poses at their own pace. Moreover, to achieve the beneficial effects of hatha yoga or Bali-yoga, it is not necessary to perform extreme asanas, but rather simpler ones executed with mindful presence. An experienced instructor with both theoretical and practical knowledge is recommended. According to di Fronso and Bertollo (2021), "not only athletes but also practitioners may try to broaden their horizons and learn new mind-body techniques strengthening their holistic approach to sports coaching" (p. 3).

Yoga can be practised before competition (e.g., using breathing techniques) to alleviate pre-performance anxiety and enhance concentration, as well as after performance (e.g., using yoga nidra) to reduce body tension and arousal level, and to improve recovery and sleep. Providing athletes with one or more yoga sessions a week would be crucial in instilling awareness of the benefits of yoga. This would facilitate athletes' understanding of their own needs and a more fruitful use of yoga techniques.

References

Al Majali, S. A., & Ashour, L. M. (2020). The negative consequences of poor emotion management (anger, anxiety and frustration) on the brain and body. *Journal of Talent Development and Excellence, 12*(2s), 3410–3419.

Anderson, R., Mammen, K., Paul, P., Pletch, A., & Pulia, K. (2017). Using yoga nidra to improve stress in psychiatric nurses in a pilot study. *The Journal of Alternative and Complementary Medicine, 23*(6), 494–495.

Anestin, A. S., Dupuis, G., Lanctôt, D., & Bali, M. (2017). The effects of the Bali Yoga Program for breast cancer patients on chemotherapy-induced nausea and vomiting: Results of a partially randomized and blinded controlled trial. *Journal of Evidence-Based Complementary & Alternative Medicine, 22*(4), 721–730.

Arbo, G. D., Brems, C., & Tasker, T. E. (2020). Mitigating the antecedents of sports-related injury through yoga. *International Journal of Yoga, 13*, 120–129.

Bal, B. S., & Kaur, P. J. (2009). Effects of selected asanas in hatha yoga on agility and flexibility level. *Journal of Sport and Health Research, 1*(2), 75–87.

Balk, Y. A., & Englert, C. (2020). Recovery self-regulation in sport: Theory, research, and practice. *International Journal of Sports Science & Coaching, 15*, 273–281.

Brems, C. (2015). A yoga stress reduction intervention for university faculty, staff, and graduate students. *International Journal of Yoga Therapy, 25*, 61–77.

Brinsley, J., Girard, D., Smout, M., & Davison, K. (2021). Is yoga considered exercise within systematic reviews of exercise interventions? A scoping review. *Complementary Therapies in Medicine, 56*, 102618. https://doi.org/10.1016/j.ctim.2020.102618

Brown, R. P., & Gerbarg, P. L. (2005). Sudarshan Kriya yogic breathing in the treatment of stress, anxiety, and depression: Part II – Clinical applications and guidelines. *Journal of Alternative & Complementary Medicine, 11*(4), 711–717.

Carrard, J., Rigort, A.-C., Appenzeller-Herzog, C., Colledge, F., Königstein, K., Hinrichs, T., & Schmidt-Trucksäss, A. (2022). Diagnosing overtraining syndrome: A scoping review. *Sports Health, 14*(5), 6656–6673.

Cartwright, T., Mason, H., Porter, A., & Pilkington, K. (2020). Yoga practice in the UK: A cross-sectional survey of motivation, health benefits and behaviours. *BMJ Open, 10*, e031848. https://doi.org/10.1136/bmjopen-2019-031848

Coimbra, D. R., Bevilacqua, G. G., Pereira, F. S., & Andrade, A. (2021). Effect of mind-fulness training on fatigue and recovery in elite volleyball athletes: A randomized controlled follow-up study. *Journal of Sports Science & Medicine, 20*(1), 1–8. https://doi.org/10.52082/jssm.2021.1

Datta, K., Tripathi, M., & Mallick, H. N. (2017). Yoga nidra: An innovative approach for management of chronic insomnia – A case report. *Sleep Science and Practise, 1*, 1–11. https://doi.org/10.1186/s41606-017-0009-4

Datta, K., Kumar, A., & Sekar, C. (2020). Enhancement of performance in an elite archer after non-pharmacological intervention to improve sleep. *Medical Journal Armed Forces India, 76*, 338–341.

Dhruva, A., Miaskowski, C., Abrams, D., Acree, M., Cooper, B., Goodman, S., & Hecht, F. M. (2012). Yoga breathing for cancer chemotherapy-associated symptoms and quality of life: Results of a pilot randomized controlled trial. *Journal of Alternative Complementary Medicine, 18*, 473–479.

di Fronso, S., & Bertollo, M. (2021). The thin line between waking and sleeping in athletes: A call for yoga nidra in the sporting context. *Frontiers in Psychology, 12*, 654222. https://doi.org/10.3389/fpsyg.2021.654222

di Fronso, S., Robazza, C., Bondár, R. Z., & Bertollo, M. (2022). The effects of mindfulness-based strategies on perceived stress and psychobiosocial states in athletes and recreationally active people. *International Journal of Environmental Research and Public Health, 19*(12), 7152. https://doi.org/10.3390/ijerph19127152

di Fronso, S., Tamburrino, L., & Bertollo, M. (2021). The effects of hatha yoga and specific balance exercises in older adults living in nursing homes. *Sport Mont, 19*(1), 3–9.

Eccles, D. W., Caviedes, G., Balk, Y. A., Harris, N., & Gretton, T. W. (2021). How to help athletes get the mental rest needed to perform well and stay healthy. *Journal of Sport Psychology in Action, 12*, 259–270.

Filho, E., Aubertin, P., & Petiot, B. (2016). The making of expert performers at Cirque du Soleil and the National Circus School: A performance enhancement outlook. *Journal of Sport Psychology in Action, 7*(2), 68–79.

Glass, C. R., Spears, C. A., Perskaudas, R., & Kaufman K. A. (2019). Mindful sport performance enhancement: Randomized controlled trial of a mental training program with collegiate athletes. *Journal of Clinical Sport Psychology, 13*(4), 609–628.

Goodman, F. R., Kashdan, T. B., Mallard, T. T., & Schumann M. (2014). A brief mindfulness and yoga intervention with an entire NCAA Division I athletic team: An initial investigation. *Psychology of Consciousness: Theory, Research and Practise, 1*(4), 339–356.

Goyal, R., Lata, H., Walia, L., & Narula, M. K. (2014). Effect of pranayama on rate pressure product in mild hypertensives. *International Journal of Applied Basic Medical Research, 4*, 67–71.

Grilli Cadieux, E., Gemme, C., & Dupuis, G. (2021). Effects of yoga interventions on psychological health and performance of competitive athletes: A systematic review. *Journal of Science in Sport and Exercise, 3*(2), 158–166.

Grilli Cadieux, E., Richard, V., & Dupuis, G. (2022). Effects of Bali Yoga Program for athletes (BYP-A) on psychological state related to performance of circus artists. *International Journal of Yogic, Human Movement and Sports Sciences, 7*(1), 23–33.

Harinath, K., Malhotra, A. S., Pal, K., Prasad, R., Kumar, R., Kain, T. C., Rai, L., & Sawhney, R. C. (2004). Effects of hatha yoga and omkar meditation on cardiorespiratory performance, psychologic profile, and melatonin secretion. *Journal of Alternative and Complementary Medicine, 10*(2), 261–268.

iRest. (2022). *iRest Yoga Nidra Research*. Retreived December 16, 2023 from https://www.irest.us/research

Jacobson, E. (1930). *Progressive relaxation*. University of Chicago Press.

Jayawardena, R., Ranasinghe, P., Ranawaka, H., Gamage, N., Dissanayake, D., & Misra, A. (2020). Exploring the therapeutic benefits of pranayama (yogic breathing): A systematic review. *International Journal of Yoga, 13*(2), 99–110.

Joshi, K. S. (2006). *Yogic pranayama: Breathing for long life and good health*. Orient Paperbacks.

Kabat-Zinn, J., & Hanh, T. N. (2009). *Full catastrophe living: Using the wisdom of your body and mind to face stress, pain, and illness*. Delta.

Kadachha, D., Soni, N., & Parekh, A. (2016). Effects of yogasana on balance in geriatric population. *International Journal of Physiotherapy and Research, 4*(2), 1401–1407.

Kaufman, K. A., Glass, C. R., & Pineau, T. R. (2019). Mindful Sport Performance Enhancement (MSPE). In I. Ivtzan (Ed.), *Handbook of mindfulness-based programmes* (pp. 173–190). Routledge.

Kellmann, M., Bertollo, M., Bosquet, L., Brink, M., Coutts, A. J., Duffield, R., Erlacher, D., Halson, S. L., Hecksteden, A., Heidari, J., Kallus, K. W., Meeusen, R., Mujika, I., Robazza, C., Skorski, S., Venter, R., & Beckmann, J. (2018). Recovery and performance in sport: Consensus statement. *International Journal of Sports Physiology and Performance, 13*, 240–245.

La Forge, R. (2005). Aligning mind and body: Exploring the disciplines of mindful exercise. *ACSM's Health & Fitness Journal, 9*(5), 7–14.

Lim, S. A., & Cheong, K. J. (2015). Regular yoga practice improves antioxidant status, immune function, and stress hormone releases in young healthy people: A randomized, double-blind, controlled pilot study. *The Journal of Alternative and Complementary Medicine, 21*(9), 530–538.

Loch, F., Ferrauti, A., Meyer, T., Pfeiffer, M., & Kellmann, M. (2019). Resting the mind – A novel topic with scarce insights. Considering potential mental recovery strategies for short rest periods in sports. *Performance Enhancement & Health, 6*, 148–155.

Meeusen, R., Duclos, M., Foster, C., Fry, A., Gleeson, M., Nieman, D., Raglin, J., Rietjens, G., Steinacker, J., Urhausen, A., European College of Sport Science, & American College of Sports Medicine. (2013). Prevention, diagnosis and treatment of the overtraining syndrome: Joint consensus statement of the European College of Sport Science (ECSS) and the American College of Sports Medicine (ACSM). *Medicine and Science in Sport and Exercise, 45*, 186–205.

Moszeik, E. N., von Oertzen, T., & Renner, K. H. (2022). Effectiveness of a short yoga nidra meditation on stress, sleep, and well-being in a large and diverse sample. *Current Psychology, 41*, 5272–5286.

Newmark, T. S., & Bogacki, D. F. (2005). The use of relaxation, hypnosis, and imagery in sport psychiatry. *Clinics in Sports Medicine, 24*(4), 973–977.

Ni, M., Mooney, K., Richards, L., Balachandran, A., Sun, M., Harriell, K., Poutiampai, M., & Signorile, J. F. (2014). Comparative impacts of tai chi, balance training, and a specially-designed yoga program on balance in older fallers. *Archives of Physical Medicine and Rehabilitation, 95*(9), 1620–1628.

Nivethitha, L., Mooventhan, A., & Manjunath, N. K. (2016). Effects of various pranayama on cardiovascular and autonomic variables. *Ancient Science of Life, 36*, 2–7.

Pelka, M., Heidari, J., Ferrauti, A., Meyer, T., Pfeiffer, M., & Kellmann, M. (2016). Relaxation techniques in sports: A systematic review on acute effects on performance. *Performance Enhancement & Health, 5*(2), 47–59.

Premkumar, C. J., & Devi, C. U. (2013). Managing sports state anxiety with yoga among athletes – A probe into facts. *International Journal of Physical Education, Fitness and Sports, 2*(3), 41–44.

Podlog, L., Conti, C., di Fronso, S., & Bertollo, M. (2023). Underrecovery in elite athletes: Antecedents, implications and prevention strategies. In M. Kellmann, S. Jakowski, & J. Beckmann (Eds.), *The importance of recovery for physical and mental health: Negotiating the effects of underrecovery* (pp. 70–83). Routledge.

Russell, T. A., & Arcuri, S. M. (2015). A neurophysiological and neuropsychological consideration of mindful movement: Clinical and research implications. *Frontiers in Human Neuroscience, 9*, 282. https://doi.org/10.3389/fnhum.2015.00282

Saraswati, S. S. (2009). *Yoga nidra* (4th ed.). Yoga Publication Trust.

Saxena T., & Saxena, M. (2009). The effect of various breathing exercises (pranayama) in patients with bronchial asthma of mild to moderate severity. *International Journal of Yoga, 2*, 22–25.

Sharma, L. (2015). Benefits of yoga in sports – A study. *International Journal of Physical Education, Sports and Health, 1*(3), 30–32.

Sharpe, E., Lacombe, A., Butler, M. P., Hanes, D., & Bradley, R. (2021). A closer look at yoga nidra: Sleep lab protocol. *International Journal of Yoga Therapy, 31*(1), 20. https://doi.org/10.17761/2021-D-20-00004

Simpson, N. S., Gibbs, E. L., & Matheson, G. O. (2017). Optimizing sleep to maximize performance: Implications and recommendations for elite athletes. *Scandinavian Journal of Medicine & Science in Sports, 27*(3), 266–274.

Thompson, R. W., Kaufman, K. A., De Petrillo, L. A., Glass, C. R., & Arnkoff, D. B. (2011). One year follow-up of Mindful Sport Performance Enhancement (MSPE) with archers, golfers, and runners. *Journal of Clinical Sport Psychology, 5*(2), 99–116.

Varghese, M. P., Balakrishnan, R., & Pailoor, S. (2018). Association between a guided meditation practice, sleep and psychological well-being in type 2 diabetes mellitus patients. *Journal of Complementary and Integrative Medicine, 15*(4), 20150026. https://doi.org/10.1515/jcim-2015-0026

Vergeer, I. (2018). Participation motives for a holistic dance-movement practice. *International Journal of Sport and Exercise Psychology, 16*(2), 95–111.

Vergeer, I., & Biddle, S. (2021). Mental health, yoga, and other holistic movement practices: A relationship worth investigating. *Mental Health and Physical Activity, 21,* 100427. http://doi.org/10.1016/j.mhpa.2021.100427

Vitale, J. A., Nedelec, M., Skorski, S., & Lastella, M. (2021). The reciprocal relationship between sleep and stress in elite athletes. *Frontiers in Psychology, 12,* 797847. https://doi.org/10.3389/fpsyg.2021.797847

Wahbeh, H., & Nelson, M. (2019). iRest meditation for older adults with depression symptoms: A pilot study. *International Journal of Yoga Therapy, 29*(1), 9–17.

Werner, G. G., Ford, B. Q., Mauss, I. B., Schabus, M., Blechert, J., & Wilhelm, F. H. (2015). High cardiac vagal control is related to better subjective and objective sleep quality. *Biological Psychology, 106,* 79–85.

Willmarth, E., Davis, F., & Fitzgerald, K. (2014). Biofeedback and integrative medicine in the pain clinic setting. *Biofeedback, 42,* 111–114.

Yoga Alliance. (2016, November 15). *Yoga in America study conducted by yoga journal and yoga alliance reveals growth and benefits of the practice.* Retrieved April 13, 2023 from https://www.prnewswire.com/news-releases/2016-yoga-in-america-study-conducted-by-yoga-journal-and-yoga-alliance-reveals-growth-and-benefits-of-the-practice-300203418.html

10 Sleep well! A key strategy beyond sports

Lisa Kullik and Asja Kiel

Introduction

An essential and superior role in physiological and psychological recovery as well as in promoting health and general well-being is assigned to sleep. The importance is illustrated by the increasing number of studies on sleep over recent years. The key functions of sleep include recuperation processes, procedural learning, memory consolidation, brain stimulation, regulation of immune response, and metabolic processes (Siegel, 2005). In elite sports, adequate sleep behaviour is essential to optimise performance, prevent injuries, and enhance recovery (Kellmann et al., 2018; Walsh et al., 2021). The importance becomes clear, as in consequence of tight training and competition schedules in competitive sports the adequate scheduling of recovery can mean the difference between success and failure. Moreover, the role of sleep for health and regeneration is illustrated by the consequences of dysfunctional sleep behaviour, like the increasing risk of injury, mental disorders, or decreased performance (Fullagar et al., 2015; Kölling et al., 2019).

To enhance sleep and recovery, several recommendations exist. These insights of maintaining and establishing good sleep in athletes can also be transferred to other populations with demanding circumstances. An important step in improving sleep and benefit from it as a key recovery strategy is to develop an understanding of sleep as a conscious and adaptable phase. Therefore, it is necessary to consider individual preferences, characteristics like age, gender, and further genetic predispositions, living conditions, and environmental factors.

What characterises good sleep?

Approximately one-third of human life is spent asleep (Manfredini et al., 2023). While the exact functions of sleep are still not fully understood, sleep is considered and known to be of great importance for human well-being and

Kullik, L., & Kiel, A. (2024). Sleep well! A key strategy beyond sports. In M. Kellmann & J. Beckmann (Eds.), *Fostering Recovery and Well-being in a Healthy Lifestyle: Psychological, Somatic, and Organizational Prevention Approaches* (pp. 143–162). Routledge.

DOI: 10.4324/9781003250654-13

functioning as well as for physical, mental, and cognitive health (Cook & Charest, 2023; Manfredini et al., 2023). From a simplified behavioural perspective, sleep is defined as a passive and reversible state of reduced movement, no perception of and no response to environmental stimuli (Carskadon & Dement, 2011; Siegel, 2008). Simultaneously, sleep is a complex and multidimensional concept with multiple physiological processes preceding throughout the night (Chokroverty, 2010; Siegel, 2008). Further, sleep is regulated by circadian processes which will be described in more detail in the section on circadian rhythm and chronotype. During human sleep, two distinct main states are differentiated: Rapid eye movement (REM; stage R) and non-REM (NREM) sleep (Carskadon & Dement, 2011). NREM sleep is subdivided into three sleep stages N1–N3 according to the criteria of the American Academy of Sleep Medicine (Berry et al., 2012). Stage N1 is referred to as light sleep, N2 is termed deeper sleep, and N3 is described as the deepest NREM sleep stage also known as slow-wave sleep (SWS; Patel et al., 2022). While deep sleep is generally considered central for regenerative and repair processes, R sleep is essential for learning and memory consolidation processes (Patel et al., 2022; Peever & Fuller, 2017). However, recent research showed that SWS also plays a significant role in declarative memory consolidation (Rasch & Born, 2013). The two sleep states NREM and R recur in cycles, whereby one sleep cycle lasts for 90–110 minutes on average. A sleep cycle begins with successive NREM sleep stages from N1 to N3 followed by R sleep (Sullivan et al., 2021). There are approximately 4–6 sleep cycles per night in healthy adults with a high amount of deep sleep and less R sleep in the first third of the night followed by a continuous increase of R sleep and a concurrent decrease of deep sleep leading to R sleep prevailing in the last third of the night (Sullivan et al., 2021). Therefore, it is not only important to ensure an adequate sleep duration, but also to sleep for a sufficiently long time to ensure both an adequate amount of deep and R sleep. At a general level, NREM sleep accounts for the greatest share with 75 to 80% of total sleep and the remaining 20 to 25% of sleep are constituted by R sleep. Different sleep stages' amounts differ greatly and could be affected by different individual and environmental factors such as age, circadian rhythm, prior sleep loss, temperature extremes, substance use, or various diseases (Sullivan et al., 2021).

Especially due to the increase of wearables and commercial technologies to assess and monitor sleep, sleep duration seems to be one of the most obvious parameters to be considered when it comes to key characteristics of good sleep (Berryhill et al., 2020). The National Sleep Foundation made general recommendations on appropriate sleep durations across the lifespan (Hirshkowitz et al., 2015). The advised sleep duration decreases with increasing age. This can be illustrated with differing sleep duration recommendations for different age categories as listed in the section on sleep over the lifespan. The recommendations intend to ensure an adequate sleep duration regarding well-being and overall health as well as emotional, cognitive, and physical components of health (Hirshkowitz et al., 2015). It is important to consider the high individuality and individual variability of sleep patterns and sleep durations and hence to understand these recommendations as a benchmark and point of orientation to define a range from which there should be no strong derogations. This enables the detection and identification of discrepancies and strong deviations which can then be further assessed by means of validated sleep assessment tools (Fino & Mazzetti, 2019; Hirshkowitz et al., 2015).

The proportion of sleep stages can serve as one indicator of adequate and healthy sleep as different sleep stages have different functions as stated above. According to an expert panel of the National Sleep Foundation that postulated and published guidance on characteristics of healthy sleep and good sleep quality, several sleep architecture measures can be considered as benchmarks and indicators of sleep quality. These indicators are age specific as children's sleep and sleep needs differ from adult or older adult sleep (Ohayon et al., 2004). The corresponding recommendations on sleep stage distributions for different age groups are specified in the section on sleep over the lifespan.

When sleep architecture measures such as sleep stage distributions are used to determine the quality of sleep, the appropriateness of methods and instruments used to assess sleep architecture is essential to consider. The gold standard for assessing sleep architecture including sleep states and stages is polysomnography allowing for a complex and comprehensive analysis of sleep parameters including, among others, electroencephalogram, electrooculography, and electromyography (Fino & Mazzetti, 2019).

Further indicators for sleep quality include the time required to fall asleep (Sleep Onset Latency; SOL); wake after sleep onset (WASO) which describes the total duration of awake phases in the period from falling asleep to awakening in the morning and switching on the light; the number of awakenings with a duration of more than five minutes as well as sleep efficiency (SE) expressing the ratio between the total time actually spent asleep and the total time spent in bed (i.e., the time between switching off the lights in the evening to turning on the lights in the morning) in percent (Erlacher, 2019). Unlike the proportion of sleep stages, consistencies of indicators can be identified between the age groups. According to the National Sleep Foundation's sleep quality recommendations, a SOL of less than 30 minutes is considered as an appropriate indicator of good sleep quality in all age groups from infants to older adults; for the parameter of WASO the benchmark is also highly convergent among all age groups as a WASO of less than 20 minutes indicates good quality of sleep for all age groups. Furthermore, a SE of 85% or more and no more than one awakening exceeding five minutes are defined as indicators for good quality of sleep for all age groups (Ohayon et al., 2017). Further sleep characteristics include the subjective perception of sleep including components like the subjective sleep quality, calmness of sleep or ease of falling asleep which can be queried by self-reports, sleep logs or sleep questionnaires (Åkerstedt et al., 1997; Fino & Mazzetti, 2019). In summary, a definition and evaluation of key characteristics of good sleep require a combination of various subjective and objective sleep parameters assessed by adequate and complementary methods and instruments, which then can be interpreted with the use of National Sleep Foundation recommendations in consideration of individual variations.

All in good time – Circadian rhythm and chronotype

The aim of the chronobiology research field is to understand the biological rhythms of living organisms and how they are regulated by internal and external factors (Vitaterna et al., 2001). These biological rhythms exist at various levels, including molecular, cellular, organismal, and social aspects (Zaki et al., 2020). This research area has important implications for understanding human health and well-being. For instance, disruptions to circadian rhythms have been linked to a variety of health problems, including sleep disorders, metabolic disorders, and mental health issues (Abbott et al., 2020; Baron & Reid, 2014; Walker et al., 2020). Understanding the regulation of circadian rhythms and other biological rhythms may lead to improved treatments for these and other health issues.

The circadian rhythm is a 24-hour cycle that regulates various physiological processes in most organisms, including humans (Reilly et al., 1997; Teo et al., 2011). This rhythm is controlled by an internal biological clock which is located in the suprachiasmatic nucleus (SCN) of the hypothalamus (Gillette & Tischkau, 1999; Mouret et al., 1978). More precisely, it can be understood as a master clock that coordinates various physiological processes throughout the body to align with the 24-hour-day-night-cycle which is determined by a combination of endogenous and exogenous factors (Roenneberg, 2015; Roenneberg et al., 2003). For the successful interaction and entrainment between body and environment, the SCN receives signals from a variety of environmental cues, so-called *zeitgeber* (German term for giving time). The most dominant zeitgeber tends to be the natural dark-light-cycle, respectively, the solar clock (Czeisler et al., 1986). Further external cues represent changes in temperature, social activities, or meal timing. Understanding the role of zeitgebers is important for managing disruptions to the circadian rhythm.

One of the most important physiological processes regulated by the circadian rhythm is the sleep-wake cycle. The SCN plays a critical role in coordinating the timing and duration of sleep, as well as the timing of various stages of sleep, R sleep and NREM sleep (Beersma & Gordijn, 2007; Dijk & Czeisler, 1995). Also, the circadian rhythm influences further physiological processes, including metabolism, immune function, and hormone secretion (Serin & Acar Tek, 2019; Vitaterna et al., 2001). Thus, the timing of melatonin release, the main sleep-regulating hormone, is tightly controlled by the circadian rhythm (Cajochen et al., 2003; Zisapel, 2018). Similarly, the circadian rhythm also plays an important role in regulating the timing of glucose metabolism and insulin secretion (Johnston, 2014; Laposky et al., 2008).

Since almost all physiological and behavioural human functions follow a rhythmic pattern, irregularities, and abnormalities in consequence of unfavourable behaviour (e.g., shift work, jet lag) or illness may lead to disruptions to the circadian rhythm (Vitaterna et al., 2001). These disruptions can have significant health implications and have been linked to a variety of health problems, including sleep disorders, metabolic disorders, and mental health issues (Baron & Reid, 2014; Potter et al., 2016). Accordingly, individuals who work night shifts or have irregular sleep patterns may experience disruptions to their circadian rhythm, which can increase the risk of obesity, diabetes, and depression (Lee et al., 2023; Zuraikat et al., 2020).

One of the biggest manipulations influencing circadian rhythms is demonstrated by artificial light exposure, as it disrupts the natural pattern of light and darkness which mainly regulates the sleep-wake cycle (Kumar et al., 2019). Most affected by artificial lighting are individuals living in modern societies, especially in the evening hours when the circadian system is more sensitive to light exposure (Blume et al., 2019; Potter et al., 2016). Also, in comparison to natural light, it differs in timing, duration, and intensity (Tähkämö et al., 2019). Thus, a higher light exposure can delay circadian timing and lead to the suppression of melatonin production, since this hormonal process is regulated by the circadian rhythmic and, in turn, by exposure to darkness (Cho et al., 2015). Melatonin also plays a role in regulating immune function and has been shown to have anti-inflammatory effects (Reiter et al., 2000). Thus, a decreased melatonin secretion may illustrate a serious health risk. In accordance with this, Straif et al. (2007) reported an association between night shift work and light exposure during night time with an increased cancer risk, while McMullan et al. (2013) additionally mentioned a higher risk for developing type 2 diabetes. The use of blue-light emitting technologies, such as smartphones, tablets, and TV devices, may also cause delayed sleep onset latency and other sleep disruptions (Chang et al., 2015; Wahl et al., 2019). At the same time, the natural dark-light-cycle loses its influence as zeitgeber.

Depending on the circadian rhythm, the chronotype refers to an individual's inherent tendency for the preferred sleep timing and activity patterns. The extreme distributions are often described as *larks* (morning persons), who prefer to wake up early and go to bed early, and *owls* (evening persons), who prefer to stay up late and wake up late (Horne & Östberg, 1976). People with an intermediate chronotype tend to have a sleep-wake cycle that falls somewhere in the middle of the continuum, neither strongly favouring early mornings nor late nights. Also, intermediate types represent the largest group in the population (Kerkhof, 1985).

The chronotype is influenced by a combination of genetic and environmental factors and can significantly impact daily activity patterns as well as health and well-being (Walsh et al., 2021). Therefore, people with a morning chronotype may be at lower risk for obesity and metabolic disorders, as they tend to have better eating habits and to be more physically active (Partonen, 2015). Conversely, it is suggested that evening chronotypes may be more susceptible to sleep disorders like insomnia, as well as mental health issues like anxiety and depression (Kivelä et al., 2018; Taylor & Hasler, 2018; Walsh et al., 2022). This may be related to the fact that evening chronotypes have a delayed release of melatonin (Morera-Fumero et al., 2013). Additionally, evening chronotypes may be more likely to engage in unhealthy behaviours like low activity level, smoking, drinking, and poor diet, which can contribute to an increased risk of physical health problems such as obesity or metabolic disorders (Kivelä et al., 2018; Partonen, 2015). A further explanation for late chronotype being more vulnerable for misalignments of the circadian rhythm may be that the preferred sleep-wake-behaviour of evening types can be at odds with modern society schedules, such as early school start times or nine-to-five work schedules (Mota et al., 2016; Yuan et al., 2019). This misalignment between the individual's internal clock and the demands of the external world can lead to a condition known as *social jet lag*, which has been linked to a range of mental and physical health problems (Wittmann et al., 2006). The term *jet lag* is typically used to describe the temporary sleep disturbances and other symptoms that can occur when a person travels across different time zones. Social jet lag, on the other hand, is a more chronic condition that can arise from the misalignment between an individual's internal clock and the demands of their work or social schedule, even when there is no travel involved (Roenneberg et al., 2019). Social jet lag occurs when an individual's sleep patterns are disrupted by changes in social or work schedules, leading to a misalignment between the individual's internal clock and the demands of the external environment. This can result in a range of negative health outcomes, including an increased risk of obesity, diabetes, cardiovascular disease, and depression (Levandovski et al., 2011; Martínez-Lozano et al., 2020).

Sleep over the lifespan

Even if sleep represents a life-long reoccurring cycle, it differs and changes over the lifespan. Sleep patterns in infants are markedly different from those in adults. Thus, it is important to understand the development of sleep characteristics over the human lifespan, as this knowledge can be used to develop interventions and treatments for sleep disorders and to promote healthy sleep habits (Ohayon et al., 2004). The most reported sleep characteristic in research is sleep duration (Galland et al., 2012). The number of night awakenings, daytime naps, and the distribution of sleep phases are also sleep variables which are considered to investigate sleep behaviour over the lifespan. Further research is needed to fully understand the complex processes involved in the development of sleep characteristics, and to identify effective interventions for improving sleep quality and duration throughout the lifespan. While for new-borns (0–3 months), a ratio of 41% of time spent in R sleep to total sleep time is considered appropriate, a R activity of 21–30% indicates adequate and good quality of sleep among adults aged 26 to 64 (Ohayon et al., 2017). Concerning N1 sleep, 5% or less is postulated to indicate good sleep quality across many age categories from children at the age of six years and older to adults maximally aged 64 years. For the second NREM stage an equal sleep quality indicator applies to all age categories, as N2 sleep exceeding an amount of over 81% is considered an indicator of inappropriate sleep quality and does not indicate good quality of sleep accordingly.

Regarding stage N3, there are differing indicators for good quality of sleep among the age groups for children and teenagers aged six to 17 years, an amount of 20–25% of deep sleep is considered as an appropriate indicator of good sleep quality whereas for adults 16–20% of deep sleep are defined as the proper range for indicating good quality of sleep (Ohayon et al., 2017). For new-borns aged up to three months, 14 to 17 hours of sleep are recommended to ensure overall health, for school-aged children in the age range of six to 13 years, the advice is to sleep for nine to eleven hours considering well-being, components of health, as well as academic performance. For young adults aged 18 to 25 years and adults aged 26 to 64 years, the recommendation is to ensure a sleep duration of seven to nine hours regarding well-being, health, and components of health (Hirshkowitz et al., 2015).

Infants (0–2 years) sleep for around 14 hours a day, which includes both night-time and daytime sleep (Galland et al., 2012). Certainly, infants have the longest sleep duration with 14 to 15 hours during the first two months, which decreases to an average of twelve hours in the first two years of life. However, sleep is not consolidated at this stage, and infants may wake up frequently during the night (Weinraub et al., 2012). This fragmentation of sleep is due to the immature development of the circadian rhythm and the absence of a consolidated sleep-wake cycle (Davis et al., 2004). As children grow, they spend less time sleeping during the day, and their night-time sleep becomes more consolidated. By the age of six months, infants have established a more regular sleep pattern and typically sleep for nine to twelve hours a night, with daytime naps still occurring. By the age of two years, most children have consolidated their daytime sleep into a single nap and sleep for around eleven to 13 hours at night (Galland et al., 2012; Weinraub et al., 2012). For preschool-aged children (3–5 years) total average daily sleep duration of ten hours is reported (Galland et al., 2012; Ohayon et al., 2004). Furthermore, SWS as well as R latency are decreasing in children over time. The average sleep duration decreases with increasing age, as six-year-old children demonstrate an average total sleep time of still ten to eleven hours, while twelve-year-old individuals only have an average sleep duration of nine hours (Galland et al., 2012). Ohayon et al. (2004) suggest that the decrease in sleep duration in children older than five years to adolescents is associated more with environmental factors than with biological changes.

Since sleep is essential for healthy growth and development in children, sleep deprivation can have a wide range of consequences, both physical and cognitive (Leproult & Van Cauter, 2010; Maski & Kothare, 2013). Sleep deprivation refers to the condition of not getting enough sleep, either in terms of total or partial sleep deprivation and could also manifest in different ways, such as in R sleep deprivation (Dinges & Kribbs, 1991). Children who are not getting enough sleep may have problems with attention, memory, and learning. This could result in heavy consequences for paying attention in school, learning new concepts, and retaining information. Also, children who suffer from sleep deprivation potentially show behavioural problems such as hyperactivity, impulsivity, and irritability (Armstrong et al., 2014). They also tend to have more mood swings and show aggressive behaviour (O'Brien, 2009). On a physical level, delayed growth and development can be caused by insufficient sleep. This can lead to problems with height, weight, and other developmental milestones. Also, sleep deprivation in children causes a higher risk for obesity, diabetes, and cardiovascular diseases (Morrissey et al., 2020).

During adolescence (10–19 years), there are significant changes in sleep patterns, with a shift towards later sleep times and a decrease in the total amount of sleep (Carskadon et al., 1998; Fischer et al., 2017). This shift is caused by changes in the circadian rhythm, with a delay in the onset of the sleep phase because of a combination of biological and social factors, such as increased use of blue-light emitting electronic devices (Schweizer et al., 2017; Tarokh et al., 2019). Furthermore, several North American studies reported that adolescents show difficulties adjusting to early school start times (Ohayon et al., 2004). Roberts et al. (2009) indicated that the average adolescent requires around nine hours of sleep each night, but many do not get enough sleep, with some getting as little as six hours. This kind of sleep deprivation can have a significant impact on physical and mental health, including increased daytime sleepiness as well as a higher risk for obesity, diabetes, depression, and anxiety (Duraccio et al., 2019; Tarokh et al., 2019).

In adulthood (>19 years), sleep patterns become more stable, with a consistent amount of sleep required each night. Adults typically require seven to nine hours of sleep each night, with individual variations in the amount of sleep needed (Hirshkowitz et al., 2015; Ohayon et al., 2017). In increasing adult age, there is a gradual reduction in the amount of deep sleep and an increase in lighter sleep stages (Ohayon et al., 2004). This shift is caused by changes in the structure of sleep and changes in the circadian rhythm, which can result in earlier sleep onset and earlier wake times. There are also changes in the quality of sleep, with a higher prevalence of sleep disorders such as insomnia and sleep apnoea (McArdle et al., 2020). These sleep disorders can have significant impacts on physical and mental health, including an increased risk of cardiovascular disease and depression (Khalil et al., 2020; Nutt et al., 2008).

In older adulthood (>65 years) significant changes in sleep patterns occur, including a reduction in the total amount of sleep, a decrease in the quality of sleep, and an increase in the prevalence of sleep disorders (Gulia & Kumar, 2018; Haimov, 2001). Older adults typically require less sleep than younger adults, with most requiring around seven hours of sleep each night (Cooke & Ancoli-Israel, 2011). However, many older adults experience difficulties falling asleep, tend to wake up frequently during the night, and experience daytime fatigue (Rodriguez et al., 2015). These changes in sleep patterns are due to a combination of biological, environmental, and lifestyle factors, including changes in the circadian rhythm, a reduction in the production of hormones such as melatonin, and the increased prevalence of medical conditions such as sleep apnoea and chronic pain (Ferretti et al., 2018; Gulia & Kumar, 2018; Haimov, 2001).

Life stressors and occupational duties – A challenge for healthy sleep

In addition to the factor of age having a major impact on sleep and sleep needs, there are several other external factors affecting human sleep. The close link between stress and sleep is nowadays well assessed and is a field of growing societal and research interest (Martire et al., 2020). The relationship between sleep and stress is thereby assumed to be bidirectional as stressors were shown to influence sleep and wake phases and, on the other hand, sleep disturbances and sleep disorders can also affect stress responses and biological processes (Martire et al., 2020). In other words, an activated stress system could induce arousal and inhibit sleep as well as sleep loss could cause inhibited stress system responses (Chrousos, 2009). The focus of this section is on the influence of external and stress-inducing factors on sleep, whereby the extent of the impact depends on the characteristics of the stressor, the exposition duration, and variations between individuals (Martire et al., 2020). Stressors can thereby be defined as adverse external or internal, emotional, or physical stimuli challenging homeostasis (Chrousos, 2009). Furthermore, they can be understood as external events of actuality and moderate intensity whereby the focus is often set on persons' perceptions of and response to the relevant factors (Charles et al., 2021).

Regarding daily life stressors, empirical evidence points to a connection between work-related stress and impairments and disturbances of sleep. Moreover, psychosocial factors at work such as perception of control, social support and work schedules may affect prospective sleep problems (Linton et al., 2015). Furthermore, the effect of time pressure and effort-reward imbalance as two exemplary work stressors on sleep was shown to be mediated by ruminative thoughts implicating a significant effect of cognitions and thoughts about work-related stressors on the ability to recover (Berset et al., 2011). In addition, emotional stress due to shift work and being concerned about work in the morning can affect sleep architecture in terms of prolonged sleep latencies, reduced deep sleep and increased R sleep amounts (Kim & Dimsdale, 2007). Furthermore, shorter sleep durations and time spent in R sleep were found on nights before working days in comparison to free days in young workers (Söderström et al., 2004). Thus, work-related stressors have a high potential for negative impacts on sleep and recovery patterns.

Despite the well-known significance of sleep for memory and learning processes as well as for academic performance, impaired quality of sleep and sleep deprivation are often reported in students (Ahrberg et al., 2012; Curcio et al., 2006; Lund et al., 2010; Sing & Wong, 2010; Wolfson & Carskadon, 2003). Sleep deprivation, in turn, constitutes a stressor that has negative effects on cognitive and physical processes such as impaired retention and learning, increased oxidative stress, and heightened inflammatory reactions (McEwen, 2006). A recent review identified different determinants of sleep quality in college students including lifestyle factors, as well as factors of physical, social, and mental health (Wang & Bíró, 2021). Regarding behaviour patterns and lifestyle aspects, caffeine consumption, stress, and an irregularity of sleep-wake patterns can diminish the quality of sleep. Moreover, the understanding of sleep and the effects of nutrition were reported to determine sleep quality. Further reported potential contributing factors to disturbed sleep comprise fatigue and pain. The importance of mental health concerning sleep and sleep quality should hereby be emphasised as mental health issues including, inter alia, anxiety, depression, and stress are associated with impaired sleep and sleep quality in students (Wang & Bíró, 2021).

A study on American undergraduate students showed significant medium correlations between self-rated stress measures and subjectively perceived sleep quality and daytime sleepiness queried by standardised questionnaires indicating that sleep completes the relation between stress and health (Benham, 2010). School demands and academic stress can constitute a serious stress factor and cause for sleep impairments in terms of reduced sleep quality and sleep duration in adolescents (Van Schalkwijk et al., 2015). A moderating and buffering effect on the impact of academic stress on sleep was found for social support (Van Schalkwijk et al., 2015). Furthermore, a recent study on Chinese adolescents stated a hindering effect of academic stress on sleep quality which was found to be moderated by negative affect. Negative affect in turn was reported to be moderated by relationships with peers (Deng et al., 2023).

Physical activity and exercise constitute further influencing factors on sleep. Acute exercise' effects on sleep parameters are generally rather small but include possible enhancements of deep sleep, total sleep duration, SOL, SE, and WASO as well as reduced R sleep (Kredlow et al., 2015). Accordingly, acute exercise could contribute to less disturbed and interrupted sleep. Moreover, regular exercise was found to potentially benefit overall sleep quality, sleep duration as well as SE and SOL (Kredlow et al., 2015). Competitive and professional sports in turn also constitute potential risk factors for disturbed and reduced sleep. Sleep disturbances are reported in 50–78% of elite athletes, while seriously impaired sleep is reported for 22–26% (Walsh et al., 2021). Inadequate sleep in terms of inter alia average sleep durations of less than seven hours or prolonged SOL is said to be due to environmental conditions in sports potentially hindering sleep such as competition schedules and additional demands of training in addition to academic, work, and social demands (Fox et al., 2020; Walsh et al., 2021).

Another sleep-impairing factor and potential stressor of increasing and growing importance is the use of electronic media and smartphones (Heidari & Kellmann, this volume, Chapter 7; Hysing et al., 2015; Schweizer et al., 2017). Adolescents in possession of a smartphone were found to have a higher probability of sleep quantity reductions and deviations from recommended sleep durations (Schweizer et al., 2017). Furthermore, a relation was found between the use of electronic media prior to sleeping while lying in bed and reduced sleep quantity and an increase in sleep problems (Exelmans & Van den Bulck, 2016; Lemola et al., 2015). The sleep-hindering effects of media can thereby mainly be explained by game- and social media–induced arousal and possibly also by melatonin suppression processes through blue screen light potentially impeding sleep onset (Schweizer et al., 2017). For individuals showing problematic smartphone use, defined as excessively high smartphone use or addiction to smartphones in daily life with symptoms of dependence such as lowered self-control ability or priority of smartphone usage over other activities being present, an elevated risk of impaired and low sleep quality was stated (Yang et al., 2020).

On the psychological level, inter alia dysfunctional convictions about sleep and temporarily disturbed sleep due to stress constitute predisposing factors for clinically disturbed sleep i.e., insomnia (Yang et al., 2014). Furthermore, psychosocial stressors were shown to be related to a higher probability of reduced sleep quantity and quality in African Americans (Johnson et al., 2016). Recent research further demonstrated an association between daily stressors or stressful life events and the quality of sleep with a contributary role of rumination as a mechanism and manifestation of reappraising stressful events. This effect is moderated by the extent of resilience which can be favouring or diminishing sleep quality (Li et al., 2019). Behavioural factors associated with sleep are comprised by weight gain and obesity which are assumed to affect sleep (duration) on one hand and on the other hand to be influenced by sleep through contributing behavioural changes (Shochat, 2012). Further important lifestyle-related factors regarding inadequate and disturbed sleep are behaviours considered as causing risk to health such as consumption of caffeine in the evening, consumption and use of alcohol, nicotine, marihuana, and other drugs but also sitting for too long and having low levels of physical activity (Shochat, 2012).

To summarise, in addition to stress related to work and academic demands as crucial influencing factors for disturbed and reduced sleep, health and behavioural factors such as physical activity, electronic media use, cognitions about sleep as well as the consumption of alcohol, nicotine, and drugs can potentially affect sleep and sleep behaviour.

Conclusion and recommendations for practise

To manage stress and adequately react to stressors, it is recommended to secure and maintain adequate sleep and rest, establish regular sleep-wake patterns, do aerobic training, and to identify and address potential stressors (Jackson, 2013). Moreover, exercise can be summarised and considered as a suitable means of promoting sleep and stress management in healthy persons in general (Kredlow et al., 2015). Weight reduction and aerobic training were also shown to potentially decrease symptoms of sleep-related breathing disorders including obstructive sleep apnoea in overweight children and individuals (Shochat, 2012). Furthermore, exercise and physical activity are assumed to be beneficial for sleep quality in breast cancer and female heart patients, women after menopause as well as in older adult populations (Shochat, 2012).

In general, the relation between sleep and exercise is considered as reciprocal and complex, whereby regular training and moderately intense physical activity is recommended as an effective tool for treating and preventing sleeping disorders such as insomnia (Brand et al., 2009; Chennaoui et al., 2015). Moreover, beneficial effects of regular physical activity and exercise on academic stress and sleep quality during the COVID-19 pandemic have been demonstrated by a recent study (Yuan et al., 2022). The authors refer to the suggestions of light or medium intensity training when exercising in the evening, avoiding training during the last hour before bedtime and further recommend offering a range of sports courses and sports opportunities for colleges to increase the regularity of physical training and mitigate the effects of academic stress (Yuan et al., 2022). Regarding the potential effect of late-night exercise on sleep, it is important to note that some studies (Youngstedt et al., 1999) did not show any effects of late-night exercise on sleep, thus the recommendations concerning exercise in the evening hours should not be taken as a valid and universal advice but as a general recommendation. Regarding academic stress, adverse effects of stressors on health parameters including sleep and well-being could potentially also be diminished by physical activity and exercise during exam phases (Wunsch et al., 2017).

For promoting healthy sleep among students and among the general public, information on nutrition favourable to sleep (e.g., light- and high-carbohydrate dinners potentially aiding sleep onset) should be considered (Wang & Bíró, 2021). Furthermore, education on adequate nap and sleep behaviour and mental health promoting measures and interventions including information on stress and the relation between stress, sleep, and health seem to be of high importance to students (Wang & Bíró, 2021). One potential approach to provide sleep hygiene education for young adults might thereby be constituted by text messaging on sleep hygiene and health behaviour through an increase in self-efficacy (Gipson et al., 2019). Moreover, the authors of a study on academic stress in Chinese adolescents concluded and recommended a need to establish an academic environment which allows them to establish and maintain relationships that may in turn also promote sleep quality and academic performance (Deng et al., 2023).

Concerning work-related stress, employer-initiated interventions targeted to individual workplace conditions provide a possibility for sleep improvements in employees (Redeker et al., 2019). Besides sleep education pointing to the relevance of adequate sleep and sleep behaviour for shift and day work, programmes supporting adequate health and sleep behaviour including relaxation strategies, dietary instructions and exercise and physical activity recommendations could contribute to the improvement of sleep in working people (Redeker et al., 2019). According to a recent review, employers are recommended to provide environmental support through inter alia offering sleep education for all employees, establishing systems for risk management, modifications of environmental conditions such as light, or ensuring enough time to sleep by teleworking and respecting time offs (Redeker et al., 2019).

To address lifestyle-related factors, public health and cognitive behavioural therapy interventions could provide helpful measures targeting sleep-related behaviour in adolescents and children (Shochat, 2012). Sleep education should provide information on adequate sleep durations for the relevant age group and recommendations for sleep hygiene (Walsh et al., 2021). Sleep hygiene recommendations inter alia include a sleep-promoting environment (dark, cold, silent), comfortable clothes and bedclothes, no consumption of alcohol and no nicotine consumption, no more caffeine in the evening, light meals before bedtime, avoidance of smartphones and electronic devices 30 minutes before bedtime, a relaxing and low-stimulus bedtime routine in the evening and regular sleep and wake times with no large shifts (Caia et al., 2022; Irish et al., 2015; Walsh et al., 2021). Furthermore, regular exercise and stress management strategies comprise important sleep education components (Irish et al., 2015). Regarding media use, not only the duration of electronic media seems to play a crucial role, but also the choice of content. A replacement of heavy and brutal media content with prosocial, pedagogical content appropriate to children's age was shown to promote sleep in children of the age of three to five years and can thus provide a useful measure to establish and maintain healthy sleep in children (Garrison & Christakis, 2012). Moreover, regarding athletes' sleep, there are several recommendations that could also be transferred to other working populations and students including sleep education, sleep screenings to assess and identify potential sleep problems and disturbances, napping for a maximum of 30 minutes in the time frame between 1:00 and 4:00 pm as well as accumulating sleep before important events to soften adverse effects of reduced or disturbed sleep during special occasions and challenges (Walsh et al., 2021).

Regarding all the sleep hygiene recommendations and sleep management interventions outlined, several key aspects should be kept in mind. Most recommendations are assumed to be helpful for the general healthy public, individual differences should however always be considered, and sleep management interventions thus should always be tailored to individual needs and circumstances (Irish et al., 2015). Furthermore, lacking sleep hygiene and unfavourable sleep behaviour might be resulting from underlying sleep disturbances and sleeping disorders which should be treated in a different way. Another aspect worth considering is a change in behaviour in favour of sleep hygiene which might cause further behavioural changes, for example, reduction of caffeine intake could result in consequences such as reduced training frequency which could, in turn, influence sleep quality (Irish et al., 2015).

References

Abbott, S. M., Malkani, R. G., & Zee, P. C. (2020). Circadian disruption and human health: A bidirectional relationship. *The European Journal of Neuroscience*, *51*(1), 567–583.

Ahrberg, K., Dresler, M., Niedermaier, S., Steiger, A., & Genzel, L. (2012). The interaction between sleep quality and academic performance. *Journal of Psychiatric Research*, *46*(12), 1618–1622.

Åkerstedt, T., Hume, K. E. N., Minors, D., & Waterhouse, J. I. M. (1997). Good sleep – Its timing and physiological sleep characteristics. *Journal of Sleep Research*, *6*(4), 221–229.

Armstrong, J. M., Ruttle, P. L., Klein, M. H., Essex, M. J., & Benca, R. M. (2014). Associations of child insomnia, sleep movement, and their persistence with mental health symptoms in childhood and adolescence. *Sleep*, *37*(5), 901–909.

Baron, K. G., & Reid, K. J. (2014). Circadian misalignment and health. *International Review of Psychiatry, 26*(2), 139–154.

Beersma, D. G. M., & Gordijn, M. C. M. (2007). Circadian control of the sleep-wake cycle. *Physiology & Behavior, 90*(2–3), 190–195.

Benham, G. (2010). Sleep: An important factor in stress-health models. *Stress and Health, 26*(3), 204–214.

Berry, R. B., Brooks, R., Gamaldo, C. E., Harding, S. M., Marcus, C., & Vaughn, B. V. (2012). *The AASM manual for the scoring of sleep and associated events: Rules, terminology and technical specifications* (Vol. 2). American Academy of Sleep Medicine.

Berryhill, S., Morton, C. J., Dean, A., Berryhill, A., Provencio-Dean, N., Patel, S. I., Estep, L., Combs, D., Mashaqi, S., Gerald, L. B., Krishnan, J. A., & Parthasarathy, S. (2020). Effect of wearables on sleep in healthy individuals: A randomized crossover trial and validation study. *Journal of Clinical Sleep Medicine, 16*(5), 775–783.

Berset, M., Elfering, A., Lüthy, S., Lüthi, S., & Semmer, N. K. (2011). Work stressors and impaired sleep: Rumination as a mediator. *Stress and Health, 27*(2), e71–e82. https://doi.org/10.1002/smi.1337

Blume, C., Garbazza, C., & Spitschan, M. (2019). Effects of light on human circadian rhythms, sleep and mood. *Somnologie, 23*(3), 147–156.

Brand, S., Beck, J., Gerber, M., Hatzinger, M., & Holsboer-Trachsler, E. (2009). 'Football is good for your sleep': Favorable sleep patterns and psychological functioning of adolescent male intense football players compared to controls. *Journal of Health Psychology, 14*(8), 1144–1155.

Caia, J., Kelly, V. G., Driller, M. W., & Halson, S. L. (2022). The role of sleep in the performance of elite athletes. In M. Kellmann & J. Beckmann (Eds.), *Recovery and well-being in sport and exercise* (pp. 131–151). Routledge.

Cajochen, C., Kräuchi, K., & Wirz-Justice, A. (2003). Role of melatonin in the regulation of human circadian rhythms and sleep. *Journal of Neuroendocrinology, 15*(4), 432–437.

Carskadon, M. A., Wolfson, A. R., Acebo, C., Tzischinsky, O., & Seifer, R. (1998). Adolescent sleep patterns, circadian timing, and sleepiness at a transition to early school days. *Sleep, 21*(8), 871–881.

Carskadon, M. A., & Dement, W. C. (2011). Monitoring and staging human sleep. In M. H. Kryger, T. Roth, & W. C. Dement (Eds.), *Principles and practice of sleep medicine* (pp. 16–26). Elsevier.

Chang, A.-M., Aeschbach, D., Duffy, J. F., & Czeisler, C. A. (2015). Evening use of light-emitting eReaders negatively affects sleep, circadian timing, and next-morning alertness. *Proceedings of the National Academy of Sciences of the United States of America, 112*(4), 1232–1237.

Charles, S. T., Mogle, J., Chai, H. W., & Almeida, D. M. (2021). The mixed benefits of a stressor-free life. *Emotion, 21*(5), 962–971.

Chennaoui, M., Arnal, P. J., Sauvet, F., & Léger, D. (2015). Sleep and exercise: A reciprocal issue? *Sleep Medicine Reviews, 20*, 59–72.

Cho, Y., Ryu, S.-H., Lee, B. R., Kim, K. H., Lee, E., & Choi, J. (2015). Effects of artificial light at night on human health: A literature review of observational and experimental studies applied to exposure assessment. *Chronobiology International, 32*(9), 1294–1310.

Chokroverty, S. (2010). Overview of sleep & sleep disorders. *Indian Journal of Medical Research, 131*(2), 126–140.

Chrousos, G. (2009). Stress and disorders of the stress system. *Nature Reviews Endocrinology, 5*, 374–381.

Cook, J. D., & Charest, J. (2023). Sleep and performance in professional athletes. *Current Sleep Medicine Reports, 9*, 56–81.

Cooke, J. R., & Ancoli-Israel, S. (2011). Normal and abnormal sleep in the elderly. *Handbook of Clinical Neurology, 98*, 653–665.

Curcio, G., Ferrara, M., & De Gennaro, L. (2006). Sleep loss, learning capacity and academic performance. *Sleep Medicine Reviews, 10*(5), 323–337.

Czeisler, C. A., Allan, J. S., Strogatz, S. H., Ronda, J. M., Sánchez, R., Ríos, C. D., Freitag, W. O., Richardson, G. S., & Kronauer, R. E. (1986). Bright light resets the human circadian pacemaker independent of the timing of the sleep-wake cycle. *Science, 233*(4764), 667–671.

Davis, K. F., Parker, K. P., & Montgomery, G. L. (2004). Sleep in infants and young children: Part one: Normal sleep. *Journal of Pediatric Health Care, 18*(2), 65–71.

Deng, J., Zhang, L., Cao, G., & Yin, H. (2023). Effects of adolescent academic stress on sleep quality: Mediating effect of negative affect and moderating role of peer relationships. *Current Psychology, 42*, 4381–4390.

Dijk, D.-J., & Czeisler, C. A. (1995). Contribution of the circadian pacemaker and the sleep homeostat to sleep propensity, sleep structure, electroencephalographic slow waves, and sleep spindle activity in humans. *The Journal of Neuroscience, 15*(5), 3526–3538.

Dinges, D. F., & Kribbs, N. B. (1991). Performing while sleepy: Effects of experimentally-induced sleepiness. In T. H. Monk (Ed.), *Sleep, sleepiness and performance* (pp. 97–128). Wiley & Sons.

Duraccio, K. M., Krietsch, K. N., Chardon, M. L., Van Dyk, T. R., & Beebe, D. W. (2019). Poor sleep and adolescent obesity risk: A narrative review of potential mechanisms. *Adolescent Health, Medicine and Therapeutics, 10*, 117–130.

Erlacher, D. (2019). *Sport und Schlaf* [Sport and sleep]. Springer.

Exelmans, L., & Van den Bulck, J. (2016). Bedtime mobile phone use and sleep in adults. *Social Science & Medicine, 148*, 93–101.

Fino, E., & Mazzetti, M. (2019). Monitoring healthy and disturbed sleep through smartphone applications: A review of experimental evidence. *Sleep and Breathing, 23*, 13–24.

Ferretti, F., Santos, D. T. D., Giuriatti, L., Gauer, A. P. M., & Teo, C. R. P. A. (2018). Sleep quality in the elderly with and without chronic pain. *Brazilian Journal of Pain, 1*(2), 141–146.

Fischer, D., Lombardi, D. A., Marucci-Wellman, H., & Roenneberg, T. (2017). Chronotypes in the US – Influence of age and sex. *PloS One, 12*(6), e0178782. https://doi.org/10.1371/journal.pone.0178782

Fox, J. L., Scanlan, A. T., Stanton, R., & Sargent, C. (2020). Insufficient sleep in young athletes? Causes, consequences, and potential treatments. *Sports Medicine, 50*(3), 461–470.

Fullagar, H. H. K., Skorski, S., Duffield, R., Hammes, D., Coutts, A. J., & Meyer, T. (2015). Sleep and athletic performance: The effects of sleep loss on exercise performance, and physiological and cognitive responses to exercise. *Sports Medicine, 45*(2), 161–186.

Galland, B. C., Taylor, B. J., Elder, D. E., & Herbison, P. (2012). Normal sleep patterns in infants and children: A systematic review of observational studies. *Sleep Medicine Reviews, 16*(3), 213–222.

Garrison, M. M., & Christakis, D. A. (2012). The impact of a healthy media use intervention on sleep in preschool children. *Pediatrics, 130*(3), 492–499.

Gillette, M. U., & Tischkau, S. A. (1999). Suprachiasmatic nucleus: The brain's circadian clock. *Recent Progress in Hormone Research*, *54*, 33–58.

Gipson, C. S., Chilton, J. M., Dickerson, S. S., Alfred, D., & Haas, B. K. (2019). Effects of a sleep hygiene text message intervention on sleep in college students. *Journal of American College Health*, *67*(1), 32–41.

Gulia, K. K., & Kumar, V. M. (2018). Sleep disorders in the elderly: A growing challenge. *Psychogeriatrics*, *18*(3), 155–165.

Haimov, I. (2001). Melatonin rhythm abnormalities and sleep disorders in the elderly. *CNS Spectrums*, *6*(6), 502–506.

Hirshkowitz, M., Whiton, K., Albert, S. M., Alessi, C., Bruni, O., DonCarlos, L., Hazen, N., Herman, J., Katz, E. S., Kheirandish-Gozal, L., Neubauer, D. N., O'Donnell, A. E., Ohayon, M., Peever, J., Rawding, R., Sachdeva, R. C., Setters, B., Vitiello, M. V., Ware, J. C., & Adams Hillard, P. J. (2015). National Sleep Foundation's sleep time duration recommendations: Methodology and results summary. *Sleep Health*, *1*(1), 40–43.

Horne, J. A., & Östberg, O. (1976). A self-assessment questionnaire to determine morningness-eveningness in human circadian rhythms. *International Journal of Chronobiology*, *4*, 97–110.

Hysing, M., Pallesen, S., Stormark, K. M., Jakobsen, R., Lundervold, A. J., & Sivertsen, B. (2015). Sleep and use of electronic devices in adolescence: Results from a large population-based study. *BMJ Open*, *5*(1), e006748. https://doi.org/ 10.1136/bmjopen-2014-006748

Irish, L. A., Kline, C. E., Gunn, H. E., Buysse, D. J., & Hall, M. H. (2015). The role of sleep hygiene in promoting public health: A review of empirical evidence. *Sleep Medicine Reviews*, *22*, 23–36.

Jackson, E. M. (2013). Stress relief: The role of exercise in stress management. *ACSM's Health & Fitness Journal*, *17*(3), 14–19.

Johnson, D. A., Lisabeth, L., Lewis, T. T., Sims, M., Hickson, D. A., Samdarshi, T., Taylor, H., & Roux, A. V. D. (2016). The contribution of psychosocial stressors to sleep among African Americans in the Jackson Heart Study. *Sleep*, *39*(7), 1411–1419.

Johnston, J. D. (2014). Physiological links between circadian rhythms, metabolism and nutrition. *Experimental Physiology*, *99*(9), 1133–1137.

Kellmann, M., Bertollo, M., Bosquet, L., Brink, M., Coutts, A. J., Duffield, R., Erlacher, D., Halson, S. L., Hecksteden, A., Heidari, J., Kallus, K. W., Meeusen, R., Mujika, I., Robazza, C., Skorski, S., Venter, R., & Beckmann, J. (2018). Recovery and performance in sport: Consensus statement. *International Journal of Sports Physiology and Performance*, *13*(2), 240–245.

Kerkhof, G. A. (1985). Inter-individual differences in the human circadian system: A review. *Biological Psychology*, *20*, 83–112.

Khalil, M., Power, N., Graham, E., Deschênes, S. S., & Schmitz, N. (2020). The association between sleep and diabetes outcomes – A systematic review. *Diabetes Research and Clinical Practice*, *161*, 108035. https://doi.org/10.1016/j.diabres.2020.108035

Kim, E. J., & Dimsdale, J. E. (2007). The effect of psychosocial stress on sleep: A review of polysomnographic evidence. *Behavioral Sleep Medicine*, *5*(4), 256–278.

Kivelä, L., Papadopoulos, M. R., & Antypa, N. (2018). Chronotype and psychiatric disorders. *Current Sleep Medicine Reports*, *4*(2), 94–103.

Kölling, S., Duffield, R., Erlacher, D., Venter, R., & Halson, S. L. (2019). Sleep-related issues for recovery and performance in athletes. *International Journal of Sports Physiology and Performance*, *14*(2), 144–148.

Kredlow, M. A., Capozzoli, M. C., Hearon, B. A., Calkins, A. W., & Otto, M. W. (2015). The effects of physical activity on sleep: A meta-analytic review. *Journal of Behavioral Medicine, 38*, 427–449.

Kumar, P., Ashawat, M. S., Pandit, V., & Sharma, D. K. (2019). Artificial light pollution at night: A risk for normal circadian rhythm and physiological functions in humans. *Current Environmental Engineering, 6*(2), 111–125.

Laposky, A. D., Bass, J., Kohsaka, A., & Turek, F. W. (2008). Sleep and circadian rhythms: Key components in the regulation of energy metabolism. *FEBS Letters, 582*(1), 142–151.

Lee, S., Lee, J., Jeon, S., Hwang, Y., Kim, J., & Kim, S. J. (2023). Sleep disturbances and depressive symptoms of shift workers: Effects of shift schedules. *Journal of Psychiatric Research, 161*, 371–376.

Lemola, S., Perkinson-Gloor, N., Brand, S., Dewald-Kaufmann, J. F., & Grob, A. (2015). Adolescents' electronic media use at night, sleep disturbance, and depressive symptoms in the smartphone age. *Journal of Youth and Adolescence, 44*(2), 405–418.

Leproult, R., & Van Cauter, E. (2010). Role of sleep and sleep loss in hormonal release and metabolism. *Endocrine Development, 17*, 11–21.

Levandovski, R., Dantas, G., Fernandes, L. C., Caumo, W., Torres, I., Roenneberg, T., Hidalgo, M. P. L., & Allebrandt, K. V. (2011). Depression scores associate with chronotype and social jetlag in a rural population. *Chronobiology International, 28*(9), 771–778.

Li, Y., Gu, S., Wang, Z., Li, H., Xu, X., Zhu, H., Deng, S., Xianjun, M., Feng, G., Wang, F., & Huang, J. H. (2019). Relationship between stressful life events and sleep quality: Rumination as a mediator and resilience as a moderator. *Frontiers in Psychiatry, 10*, 348. https://doi.org/10.3389/fpsyt.2019.00348

Linton, S. J., Kecklund, G., Franklin, K. A., Leissner, L. C., Sivertsen, B., Lindberg, E., Svensson, A. C., Hansson, S. O., Sundin, Ö., Hetta, J., & Hall, C. (2015). The effect of the work environment on future sleep disturbances: A systematic review. *Sleep Medicine Reviews, 23*, 10–19.

Lund, H. G., Reider, B. D., Whiting, A. B., & Prichard, J. R. (2010). Sleep patterns and predictors of disturbed sleep in a large population of college students. *Journal of Adolescent Health, 46*(2), 124–132.

Manfredini, R., Cappadona, R., Tiseo, R., Bagnaresi, I., & Fabbian, F. (2023). Light, circadian rhythms and health. In S. Capalongo, M. Botta, & A. Rebecchi (Eds.), *Therapeutic landscape design* (pp. 81–92). Springer.

Martínez-Lozano, N., Barraco, G. M., Rios, R., Ruiz, M. J., Tvarijonaviciute, A., Fardy, P., Madrid, J. A., & Garaulet, M. (2020). Evening types have social jet lag and metabolic alterations in school-age children. *Scientific Reports, 10*(1), 16747. https://doi.org/10.1038/s41598-020-73297-5

Martire, V. L., Caruso, D., Palagini, L., Zoccoli, G., & Bastianini, S. (2020). Stress & sleep: A relationship lasting a lifetime. *Neuroscience & Biobehavioral Reviews, 117*, 65–77.

Maski, K. P., & Kothare, S. V. (2013). Sleep deprivation and neurobehavioral functioning in children. *International Journal of Psychophysiology, 89*(2), 259–264.

McArdle, N., Ward, S. V., Bucks, R. S., Maddison, K., Smith, A., Huang, R.-C., Pennell, C. E., Hillman, D. R., & Eastwood, P. R. (2020). The prevalence of common sleep disorders in young adults: A descriptive population-based study. *Sleep, 43*(10). https://doi.org/10.1093/sleep/zsaa072

McEwen, B. S. (2006). Sleep deprivation as a neurobiologic and physiologic stressor: Allostasis and allostatic load. *Metabolism, 55*, S20–S23.

McMullan, C. J., Schernhammer, E. S., Rimm, E. B., Hu, F. B., & Forman, J. P. (2013). Melatonin secretion and the incidence of type 2 diabetes. *Journal of the American Medical Association*, *309*(13), 1388–1396.

Morera-Fumero, A. L., Abreu-González, P., Henry-Benítez, M., Díaz-Mesa, E., Yelmo-Cruz, S., & Gracia-Marco, R. (2013). Chronotype as modulator of morning serum melatonin levels. *Actas Españolas de Psiquiatría*, *41*(3), 149–153.

Morrissey, B., Taveras, E., Allender, S., & Strugnell, C. (2020). Sleep and obesity among children: A systematic review of multiple sleep dimensions. *Pediatric Obesity*, *15*(4), e12619. https://doi.org/10.1111/ijpo.12619

Mota, M. C., Waterhouse, J., De-Souza, D. A., Rossato, L. T., Silva, C. M., Araújo, M. B. J., Tufik, S., de Mello, M. T., & Crispim, C. A. (2016). Association between chronotype, food intake and physical activity in medical residents. *Chronobiology International*, *33*(6), 730–739.

Mouret, J., Coindet, J., Debilly, G., & Chouvet, G. (1978). Suprachiasmatic nuclei lesions in the rat: Alterations in sleep circadian rhythms. *Electroencephalography and Clinical Neurophysiology*, *45*(3), 402–408.

Nutt, D., Wilson, S., & Paterson, L. (2008). Sleep disorders as core symptoms of depression. *Dialogues in Clinical Neuroscience*, *10*(3), 329–336.

O'Brien, L. M. (2009). The neurocognitive effects of sleep disruption in children and adolescents. *Child and Adolescent Psychiatric Clinics of North America*, *18*(4), 813–823.

Ohayon, M. M., Wickwire, E. M., Hirshkowitz, M., Albert, S. M., Avidan, A., Daly, F. J., Dauvilliers, Y., Ferri, R., Fung, C., Gozal, D., Hazen, N., Krystal, A., Lichstein, K., Mallampalli, M., Plazzi, G., Rawding, R., Scheer, F. A., Somers, V., & Vitiello, M. V. (2017). National sleep foundation's sleep quality recommendations: First report. *Sleep Health*, *3*(1), 6–19.

Ohayon, M. M., Carskadon, M. A., Guilleminault, C., & Vitiello, M. V. (2004). Meta-analysis of quantitative sleep parameters from childhood to old age in healthy individuals: Developing normative sleep values across the human lifespan. *Sleep*, *27*(7), 1255–1273.

Partonen, T. (2015). Chronotype and health outcomes. *Current Sleep Medicine Reports*, *1*(4), 205–211.

Patel, A. K., Reddy, V., & Araujo, J. F. (2022). *Physiology, sleep stages*. StatPearls Publishing.

Peever, J., & Fuller, P. M. (2017). The biology of REM sleep. *Current Biology*, *27*(22), R1237–R1248.

Potter, G. D. M., Skene, D. J., Arendt, J., Cade, J. E., Grant, P. J., & Hardie, L. J. (2016). Circadian rhythm and sleep disruption: Causes, metabolic consequences, and countermeasures. *Endocrine Reviews*, *37*(6), 584–608.

Rasch, B., & Born, J. (2013). About sleep's role in memory. *Physiological Reviews*, *93*(2), 681–766.

Redeker, N. S., Caruso, C. C., Hashmi, S. D., Mullington, J. M., Grandner, M., & Morgenthaler, T. I. (2019). Workplace interventions to promote sleep health and an alert, healthy workforce. *Journal of Clinical Sleep Medicine*, *15*(4), 649–657.

Reilly, T., Aktionson, G., & Waterhouse, J. (1997). *Biological rhythms and exercise*. Oxford University Press.

Reiter, R. J., Calvo, J. R., Karbownik, M., Qi, W., & Tan, D. X. (2000). Melatonin and its relation to the immune system and inflammation. *Annals of the New York Academy of Sciences*, *917*, 376–386.

Roberts, R. E., Roberts, C. R., & Duong, H. T. (2009). Sleepless in adolescence: Prospective data on sleep deprivation, health and functioning. *Journal of Adolescence*, *32*(5), 1045–1057.

Rodriguez, J. C., Dzierzewski, J. M., & Alessi, C. A. (2015). Sleep problems in the elderly. *The Medical Clinics of North America*, *99*(2), 431–439.

Roenneberg, T. (2015). Having trouble typing? What on earth is chronotype? *Journal of Biological Rhythms*, *30*(6), 487–491.

Roenneberg, T., Daan, S., & Merrow, M. (2003). The art of entrainment. *Journal of Biological Rhythms*, *18*(3), 183–194.

Roenneberg, T., Pilz, L. K., Zerbini, G., & Winnebeck, E. C. (2019). Chronotype and social jetlag: A (self-) critical review. *Biology*, *8*(3), 54. https://doi.org/10.3390/biology8030054

Schweizer, A., Berchtold, A., Barrense-Dias, Y., Akre, C., & Suris, J.-C. (2017). Adolescents with a smartphone sleep less than their peers. *European Journal of Pediatrics*, *176*(1), 131–136.

Serin, Y., & Acar Tek, N. (2019). Effect of circadian rhythm on metabolic processes and the regulation of energy balance. *Annals of Nutrition & Metabolism*, *74*(4), 322–330.

Shochat, T. (2012). Impact of lifestyle and technology developments on sleep. *Nature and Science of Sleep*, *4*, 19–31.

Siegel, J. M. (2005). Clues to the functions of mammalian sleep. *Nature*, *437*, 1264–1271.

Siegel, J. M. (2008). Do all animals sleep? *Trends in Neurosciences*, *31*(4), 208–213.

Sing, C. Y., & Wong, W. S. (2010). Prevalence of insomnia and its psychosocial correlates among college students in Hong Kong. *Journal of American College Health*, *59*(3), 174–182.

Söderström, M., Ekstedt, M., Akerstedt, T., Nilsson, J., & Axelsson, J. (2004). Sleep and sleepiness in young individuals with high burnout scores. *Sleep*, *27*(7), 1369–1377.

Straif, K., Baan, R., Grosse, Y., Secretan, B., El Ghissassi, F., Bouvard, V., Altieri, A., Benbrahim-Tallaa, L., & Cogliano, V. (2007). Carcinogenicity of shift-work, painting, and fire-fighting. *Lancet Oncology*, *8*(12), 1065–1066.

Sullivan, S. S., Carskadon, M. A., Dement, W. C., & Jackson, C. L. (2021). Normal human sleep: An overview. In M. H. Kryger, T. Roth, & C. A. Goldstein (Eds.), *Principles and practice of sleep medicine* (7th ed., pp. 16–26). Elsevier.

Tähkämö, L., Partonen, T., & Pesonen, A.-K. (2019). Systematic review of light exposure impact on human circadian rhythm. *Chronobiology International*, *36*(2), 151–170.

Tarokh, L., Short, M., Crowley, S. J., Fontanellaz-Castiglione, C. E. G., & Carskadon, M. A. (2019). Sleep and circadian rhythms in adolescence. *Current Sleep Medicine Reports*, *5*(4), 181–192.

Taylor, B. J., & Hasler, B. P. (2018). Chronotype and mental health: Recent advances. *Current Psychiatry Reports*, *20*(8), 59. https://doi.org/10.1007/s11920-018-0925-8

Teo, W., Newton, M. J., & McGuigan, M. R. (2011). Circadian rhythms in exercise performance: Implications for hormonal and muscular adaptation. *Journal of Sports Science & Medicine*, *10*(4), 600–606.

Van Schalkwijk, F. J., Blessinga, A. N., Willemen, A. M., Van der Werf, Y. D., & Schuengel, C. (2015). Social support moderates the effects of stress on sleep in adolescents. *Journal of Sleep Research*, *24*(4), 407–413.

Vitaterna, M. H., Takahashi, J. S., & Turek, F. W. (2001). Overview of circadian rhythms. *Alcohol Research & Health*, *25*(2), 85–93.

Wahl, S., Engelhardt, M., Schaupp, P., Lappe, C., & Ivanov, I. V. (2019). The inner clock-blue light sets the human rhythm. *Journal of Biophotonics*, *12*(12), e201900102. https://doi.org/10.1002/jbio.201900102

Walker, W. H., Walton, J. C., DeVries, A. C., & Nelson, R. J. (2020). Circadian rhythm disruption and mental health. *Translational Psychiatry*, *10*(1), 28. https://doi.org/10.1038/s41398-020-0694-0

Walsh, N. P., Halson, S. L., Sargent, C., Roach, G. D., Nédélec, M., Gupta, L., Leeder, J., Fullagar, H. H., Coutts, A. J., Edwards, B. J., Pullinger, S. A., Robertson, C. M., Burniston, J. G., Lastella, M., Le Meur, Y., Hausswirth, C., Bender, A. M., Grandner, M. A., & Samuels, C. H. (2021). Sleep and the athlete: Narrative review and 2021 expert consensus recommendations. *British Journal of Sports Medicine*, *55*, 356–368.

Walsh, N., Repa, L. M., & Garland, S. N. (2022). Association between chronotype and mental health in Canadian university students. In A. D. Nesbitt (Ed.), *Oxford handbook of sleep medicine* (Vol. 41, pp. 242–243). Oxford University Press.

Wang, F., & Bíró, É. (2021). Determinants of sleep quality in college students: A literature review. *Explore*, *17*(2), 170–177.

Weinraub, M., Bender, R. H., Friedman, S. L., Susman, E. J., Knoke, B., Bradley, R., Houts, R., & Williams, J. (2012). Patterns of developmental change in infants' nighttime sleep awakenings from 6 through 36 months of age. *Developmental Psychology*, *48*(6), 1511–1528.

Wittmann, M., Dinich, J., Merrow, M., & Roenneberg, T. (2006). Social jetlag: Misalignment of biological and social time. *Chronobiology International*, *23*(1–2), 497–509.

Wolfson, A. R., & Carskadon, M. A. (2003). Understanding adolescent's sleep patterns and school performance: A critical appraisal. *Sleep Medicine Reviews*, 7(6), 491–506.

Wunsch, K., Kasten, N., & Fuchs, R. (2017). The effect of physical activity on sleep quality, well-being, and affect in academic stress periods. *Nature and Science of Sleep*, *9*, 117–126.

Yang, C. M., Hung, C. Y., & Lee, H. C. (2014). Stress-related sleep vulnerability and maladaptive sleep beliefs predict insomnia at long-term follow-up. *Journal of Clinical Sleep Medicine*, *10*(9), 997–1001.

Yang, J., Fu, X., Liao, X., & Li, Y. (2020). Association of problematic smartphone use with poor sleep quality, depression, and anxiety: A systematic review and meta-analysis. *Psychiatry Research*, *284*, 112686. https://doi.org/10.1016/j.psychres.2019.112686

Yuan, M. Z., Chen, C. C., Chen, I. S., Yang, C. C., & Hsu, C. H. (2022). Research on the impact of regular exercise behavior of college students on academic stress and sleep quality during the COVID-19 pandemic. *Healthcare*, *10*(12), 2534. https://doi.org/10.3390/healthcare10122534

Youngstedt, S. D., Kripke, D. F., & Elliott, J. A. (1999). Is sleep disturbed by various late-night exercise? *Medicine and Science in Sports and Exercise*, *31*(6), 864–869.

Zaki, N. F. W., Spence, D. W., Subramanian, P., Bharti, V. K., Karthikeyan, R., BaHammam, A. S., & Pandi-Perumal, S. R. (2020). Basic chronobiology: What do sleep physicians need to know? *Sleep Science*, *13*(4), 256–266.

Zisapel, N. (2018). New perspectives on the role of melatonin in human sleep, circadian rhythms and their regulation. *British Journal of Pharmacology*, *175*(16), 3190–3199.

Zuraikat, F. M., Makarem, N., Redline, S., Aggarwal, B., Jelic, S., & St-Onge, M.-P. (2020). Sleep regularity and cardiometabolic health: Is variability in sleep patterns a risk factor for excess adiposity and glycaemic dysregulation? *Current Diabetic Reports*, *20*, 38. https://doi.org/10.1007/s11892-020-01324-w

Part IV

Organisational prevention approaches

11 Optimising fatigue agility and recovery within military settings

Enhancing capability, well-being, and performance

Raymond W. Matthews, Gerard J. Fogarty, Eugene Aidman, and Tom Patrick

Introduction

High-performing professionals experience considerable internal and external stress due to the nature of their roles across several high-performance organisations and industries. In sport, for example, coaches at the professional level are constantly experiencing the inherent pressures and stressors of their chosen career (Altfeld et al., 2018). The same can be said for those working in military environments, who must perform at the highest possible level to ensure they are capable of delivering, in full, their operational outcomes as required to achieve mission success. Military personnel often operate within challenging, multi-stressor environments that can compromise performance and recovery (Tait, Drain, Corrigan, et al., 2022).

Sustained military operations are conducted around the clock, with periods of high stress and fatigue (Krueger, 1989). In these environments, personnel's lives and the lives of their colleagues are at risk to a degree that is not common in civilian sustained operations (Kavanagh, 2005). Modern military platforms are becoming more complex with ever-increasing technological systems and greater informational flow, placing a greater burden on their operators to make superior decisions. Additionally, they must manage both draining high workload periods along with long monotonous intervals of low workload (Belenkey, 1997). This combination of high fatigue, high stress, and varying workload creates a distinctive challenge for the modern warfighter. It has been acknowledged that fatigue and stress account for up to 50% of casualties in war (Mareth & Brooker, 1985), making this a challenge that modern militaries ignore at their peril.

Matthews, R. W., Fogarty, G. J., Aidman, E., & Patrick, T. (2024). Optimising fatigue agility and recovery within military settings: Enhancing capability, well-being, and performance. In M. Kellmann & J. Beckmann (Eds.), *Fostering Recovery and Well-being in a Healthy Lifestyle: Psychological, Somatic, and Organizational Prevention Approaches* (pp. 165–181). Routledge.

DOI: 10.4324/9781003250654-15

The authors of this chapter have considerable experience working in, and supporting, the development of programs and initiatives that can proactively target stress and fatigue in military environments towards ensuring the following:

1)   that unit readiness is optimised through the application of appropriate training and processes based on recovery optimisation and fatigue mitigation evidence;
2)   that the environments within the units are conducive to promoting optimal performance through the active valuing and promotion of personal recovery and well-being efforts; and
3)   that members understand how to autonomously develop and maintain the physical and mental performance requirements of their respective occupational roles.

Stress, sleep, recovery, and burnout

The biological definition of stress encompasses a response to a demand that will increase the chances of successfully handling a threatening situation (Selye, 1956). It was first considered in terms of a concept of the 'fight-or-flight' response (Cannon, 1914), and later a model of stress and general adaptation syndrome, which is composed of stages of alarm, resistance, and exhortation (Selye, 1956). The ability of the body to increase or decrease its state of activation to meet external challenges is described by the term allostasis (McEwen & Wingfield, 2003). Through this process, the long-term effect of stress moves the body's set state of activation to a high level. This results in an allostatic load, which is the long-term cost to the body of a stressful event (Peters et al., 2017). This cost can take the form of altered brain architecture and systemic pathophysiology resulting in stress diseases such as cardiovascular diseases, insomnia, and clinical burnout syndrome (McEwen & Wingfield, 2003).

The goal of recovery is to relieve and attenuate stress, moderate the effects of stress, and decrease the allostatic load. Kellmann and Kallus (2001) described its complexities, which can include psychological, physiological, and social dimensions to recovery. At its most basic level, however, all animals use the physiological state of 'sleep' for recovery (Matthews et al., 2023). Our homeostatic drive for sleep increases not only with wakefulness but with stress, which results in symptoms of fatigue, and is alleviated by sleep (Kullik & Kiel, this volume, Chapter 10; Martire et al., 2020).

When considering a relatively well-slept athlete or businessman, it is easy to overlook the recovery aspect of sleep and place the focus on action-orientated, pro-active recovery strategies. In fact, for most people, a healthy homeostatic sleep drive will keep the sleep-wake system functioning within reasonably tight parameters without issue. For individuals who work outside of the natural endogenous diurnal rhythm of activity (i.e., shift workers), sleep becomes the primary moderator of stress responses and recovery effectiveness. High-intensity operational environments are frequently also prolonged by their nature and push individuals to the physiological extremes of wakefulness and stress. Within this context, recovery is dependent upon sleep.

A significant workforce issue in high-tempo operational settings is that long-term failures to recover adequately can lead to burnout (Åkerstedt et al., 2011). The links between stress, sleep, recovery, and burnout are interconnected in multiple ways. If sleep is removed or limited in the stress/recovery equation, poor outcomes are inevitable. As Åkerstedt, a preeminent researcher in stress, sleep, and recovery, succinctly wrote; "Sleep impairment seems to be a prerequisite for developing burnout" (Åkerstedt et al., 2011, p. 814).

Workload and stress in military environments

In addition to innate biological processes, task factors and external factors such as workload impact fatigue, reducing cognitive performance. One common definition of workload considers the tempo of the task, time on task, complexity, and expenditure of effort to meet demands (Popkin, 1999). There is debate, however, surrounding how workload is conceptualised and operationalised (Winter, 2014). A common conceptualisation is that when workload is too high, alertness decreases due to an inability to cope with demands (Warm et al., 2008). However, both underload (during periods of low tempo boring work) and overload (during periods of very high tempo and stressful work) have been identified as potential causes of fatigue (Hancock & Verwey, 1997), and the optimal level of task demand may change over time. Therefore, in some circumstances having too little work to do may be just as fatiguing and cognitively demanding as having too much work to do. Chronically low levels of cognitive load (low tempo) produce low arousal, making it difficult to maintain alertness and attention, thereby producing the subjective experience of fatigue (Hancock & Desmond, 2001). Increases in task demands produce an increase in arousal, which can be energising and increase alertness, decreasing fatigue. However, as task demands approach and then exceed an individual's capacity limit, the individual will need to compensate by applying extra effort (Hancock & Desmond, 2001). For example, the individual may have to reallocate resources among tasks, change their strategies or goals, and/or regulate their emotional reactions. Compensatory effort drains energy reserves and produces cognitive fatigue.

The interaction effects among these factors are complex, and there are various factors that impact workload and influence the maintenance of alertness. Undertaking tasks for long periods is common in sustained operations. A military operator may be required to attend to a screen in a control room for a prolonged period or drive a vehicle for many hours. Research has shown that extended time on a task during the day can increase sleepiness and reduce alertness (Van Dongen et al., 2011). It has been postulated from animal models that this could be due to areas of the brain 'falling asleep' when overworked, even while the whole organism is functionally awake (Rector et al., 2005). These brain changes could lead to performance instability while an individual is otherwise functionally awake and why with longer time on task operators might miss signals and make errors (Van Dongen et al., 2011).

The effect of different workload and task factors on fatigue levels has been observed in military operations. A comparison study was undertaken onboard the USS *America* between Operation Desert Shield and Operation Desert Storm. Higher levels of fatigue were observed in pilots during Operation Desert Storm, and this was directly attributed to mission duration (time on task), workload task differences (between the aircraft type involved), as well as mission time of day (DeJohn et al., 1992; Shappell & Neri, 1993). In a separate study of this operation, other aircrew (flying C141's) reported that this combination of fatiguing factors resulted in them being fatigued to the point that they were unable to function (Neville et al., 1994). These field studies demonstrate that in a military operational environment factors such as time on task and workload are extremely important.

The challenges of operational sleeping

The military context not only brings high stress and workload but also many varied and context-specific challenges for sleep. For example, movement conditions such as rocking side-to-side or head-to-toe on a ship will have a large impact on the recovery value of sleep obtained (Matthews et al., 2021). Side-to-side rocking not only leads to shorter sleep time, reduced sleep efficiency, and waking more frequently from sleep, it also significantly decreases rapid eye movement sleep. This particular sleep change may have the effect of impairing memory, learning, emotional regulation, and stress recovery. Similarly, sleeping in a chair in an aircraft can lead to compromised sleep. As well as noise and vibration, a significant variable is the recline angle of the chair (Roach et al., 2018). An 'economy class chair' (with the equivalent back angle of 20-degrees to the vertical), has been shown to decrease total sleep time by 30% but also removes 80% of the rapid eye movement sleep (compared to a flat 90-degrees to the vertical first-class chair). Even a business class equivalent reclined chair (with a back angle of 40-degrees to the vertical) will decrease rapid eye movement sleep by 40%. These two examples along with other sleeping conditions that are hot, cold, loud, bright, or even dangerous, show that sleeping in operational environments comes with significant challenges that disrupt sleep, the recovery value of that sleep, and the functionality for that sleep to be used for stress recovery.

There are many examples of high sleep propensity and performance impairment in military operations. For example, a US study of 78 F/A-18 and F-14 Navy and Marine aviators reported that their job performance was compromised by fatigue to the degree that a third disclosed having fallen asleep in their cockpits (Williams et al., 1998). Reporters during Operation Iraqi Freedom also described US tank, Bradley Fighting Vehicle, and Humvee drivers falling asleep while driving (Miller et al., 2018). Soldiers on foot had to repeatedly wake the drivers to keep to convoys moving. Sleep deprivation has contributed to cases of friendly fire, with an example documented during the 100-hour ground war of

Operation Desert Storm (Belenky et al., 1996). These examples show that for performance optimisation to be achieved within continuous operations, effective recovery is needed, and the foundation of that recovery is sleep.

An applied model to address chronic stress in military settings

Military members will face multi-dimensional physical and mental stressors resulting from training, operational delivery, as well as during and post-deployment. When recovery is not achieved sufficiently, a negative balance will occur in an individual's recovery-stress states, which can lead to impaired performance and compromised well-being (Kellmann et al., 2018). Importantly, the accumulation of mental fatigue can lead to performance impairment if a sufficient degree of mental recovery has not taken place (Loch et al., 2022).

In addition, military settings require high degrees of performance readiness and the link between recovery and well-being optimisation will be demonstrated as part of an emerging *Cognitive Fitness Model* (Aidman, 2020) to ensure all within the environment can deliver fully against their occupational roles when required and for the duration needed to achieve the outcome that is desired.

The *Cognitive Fitness Framework* (CF2; Figure 11.1) model is based on a 'Cognitive Gym' concept, that name conveying a sense that cognitive skills can be developed in the same way as physical skills, by repeatedly executing drills that are designed to improve performance on specific cognitive abilities. The overarching themes informing CF2 stem from the findings of a multinational research program (Albertella et al., 2022) aimed at discovering those cognitive processes particularly relevant in high-risk situations where maximum performance is required to succeed.

A notable feature of the CF2 model is that it aligns with an operational cycle where the notion of readiness can be applied to the different stages that inform an individuals' degree of psychological/operational readiness. In the first part of the cycle, cognitive primaries such as attention, impulse control, and co-action are seen as underpinning cognitive capacity. These skills can be acquired through what the CF2 model refers to as 'Foundational Training'. Some of them are acquired during initial military training.

Cognitive readiness. Moving in a clockwise direction around the CF2 model, the competencies regarding 'Advanced Training' include stress management, arousal regulation, adaptability, teamwork, situation awareness, and decision making. Within this phase, cognitive readiness has been achieved when individuals feel comfortable across the cognitive operational performance areas. Whilst they are all internal processes, affected by the external elements mentioned by Murphy and Fogarty (2009), they are largely under the volitional control of the individual.

It is worth noting that the training of these cognitive skill areas is best achieved through scenarios that mimic real-life situations as this will improve the transference of learning within the actual operational setting. Much can be accomplished

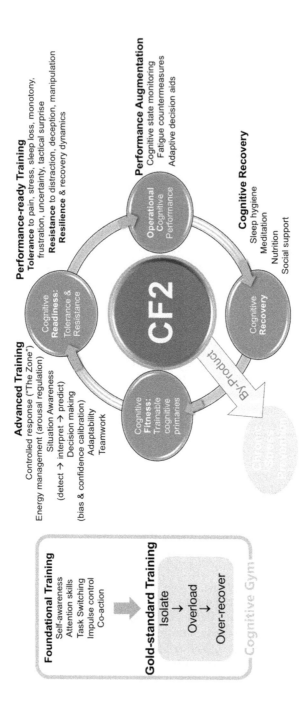

Figure 11.1 The cognitive fitness cycle.
Adapted with permission from Aidman (2020).

by individuals working on their own provided that the exercises they are completing develop the cognitive skills that drive performance in their real-world settings. For example, stress can be mitigated through the use of various breathing drills that have been shown to lead to improved mood and reduced state of anxiety (Balban et al., 2023). Drills of this nature have ample historical evidence of being embraced across several occupational areas (e.g., pilot pathway, special forces in Army, Navy, and Air Force). In addition, these skills are taught through a formal Performance Enhancement Program as part of the pilot pathway within the Royal Australian Air Force.

Operational cognitive performance. The 'Performance-Ready training' phase describes an advanced state of physical and cognitive readiness. It considers what psychological readiness might mean in an operational context. In addition to all the foundational and advanced cognitive skills, there is now a demand for tolerances and resistances. The tolerances are for pain, sleep loss, monotony, frustration, fear, and uncertainty. The resistances are for elements such as distraction (versus task focus), deception (versus situation awareness), and manipulation (versus mission-focus). Some of these tolerances and resistances spill over into the physical domain where they draw upon strengths developed through exercise and lifestyle habits that optimise sleep and recovery stores.

Performance augmentation. The 'Performance Augmentation' phase refers to the operational aids, many of them technical, that help to boost performance or to maintain high levels of performance. Examples include tools like decision aids and fatigue countermeasures. The underlying notion here is that there is a stage of readiness that refers to the will to maintain high levels of performance in the face of an almost overwhelming desire to quit.

Cognitive recovery. This phase completes the cycle. While the body will need to recover using ingrained restorative practices such as healthy eating, hydration, and sleep hygiene, it is also imperative that enough attention be given to achieving a sufficient level of cognitive recovery given the cognitive load that may have accumulated (Loch et al., 2022). External factors as mentioned by Murphy and Fogarty (2009) are also particularly important: Social support, unit cohesion, and leadership. At the end of the cognitive fitness cycle, the individual factors that help to rebuild cognitive fitness, in addition to those already mentioned, will include a period of restoration before re-engaging the foundational skills leading back to a state of readiness for renewed operational delivery.

Evidence for the usefulness of the CF2 model in civilian and military populations

A combination of CF2-informed interventions was incorporated in a study by Taylor (2021) which utilised The Resilient Mind Program (RMP), aimed at developing cognitive fitness through a blended methodology, with three hours of face-to-face delivery augmented with a four-week program via a mobile application. Taylor reported that the RMP produced improvements in mental well-being and resilience and a reduction in burnout for 800 workers in a range of businesses in the Australian corporate sector.

Taylor et al. (2021) extended the RMP evaluation in a block-randomised study with Navy aviators. Seventy-eight members of a Royal Australian Navy Fleet Air Arm Squadron completed the four-week RMP, with half the participants combining it with self-paced 'Functional Imagery' practice. The RMP intervention, which is based on a combination of goal-setting and imagery techniques, was found to be effective in reducing burnout symptoms while improving self-reported mental well-being and resilience. Similar training programs are being developed and evaluated for training defence operators' situation awareness (Black et al., 2020), decision making (Immink et al., 2020), and stress management skills (Kluge et al., 2021).

Managing fatigue and improving decision making

Many fatigue mitigation strategies have been considered for use in sustained operations. These can broadly be considered as structural, behavioural, and technological countermeasures. In civilian industrial settings, structural countermeasures such as scheduling or rostering have been useful in mitigating periods of high fatigue by limiting long prior wakefulness, short sleep, and biological performance troughs (Darwent et al., 2015). While these structural methods have applications in military contexts, the nature of sustained operations will require operators to continue to operate beyond the limits of their schedules (U.S. Department of Defense, 2021). For this reason, structural countermeasures are limited in military sustained operations.

Behavioural countermeasures, such as napping, or caffeine use, have been shown to be advantageous to combat the effects of fatigue. However, again in military operational settings there can be limits to their use (Johnson et al., 2014). Caffeine is highly effective in increasing alertness but its impact on higher cognitive functions is less well known. Additionally, the effect of caffeine is temporary – it cannot replace sleep and recovery. Continuous high consumption of caffeine can reduce its effectiveness and there are physiological symptoms such as elevated heart rate (Goldfarb et al., 2014; Shah et al., 2019). Napping is another popular behavioural countermeasure. It is not always possible in military operational environments where there is a risk of sleep inertia upon waking. Sleep inertia is the feeling of confusion and grogginess on waking that is the result of the brain transitioning from sleep to wake (Hilditch & McHill, 2019). Many studies have shown impaired performance and decision making on waking due to the effects of sleep inertia (Hilditch et al., 2016).

While these structural and behavioural countermeasures are used in military environments, they can be problematic. Where technological countermeasures are concerned, however, there are new tools that show promise. Artificial intelligence (AI) has been utilised to help manage decision making and information flow and display in many industries such as health care, manufacturing, education, finance, social networking, and streaming services (Baker, 2015; Israni & Verghese, 2019;

Jordan & Mitchell, 2015; Shortliffe & Sepúlveda, 2018). In medicine, AI has been utilised in medical diagnostic and predictive analysis (Park & Han, 2018), which has been shown to improve workflow and reduce medical errors (Topol, 2019). These approaches could be used in military control room environments to support situational awareness and inform decision making both on and off the platform. Attempts have been made to develop systems, such as those with adaptable capabilities to alter the flow of information and provide decision-making assistance when operators performance efficacy is reduced. However, it should be noted that even the most competent operator supported by AI and other technology may fail in complex environments due to fatigue, boredom, anxiety, stress, and environmental factors. We need humans in the loop and optimising their performance will still matter.

Optimisation of rest–activity cycles

Rest-activity cycles can affect health and performance at both the physiological and neurobehavioural levels (Calogiuri et al., 2013). In sport, a complete cycle often consists of the days leading up to an event, the hours covering the event, and the hours or days it takes to recover. For a military operation, the cycle might be considered over several months of preparation, several months of operation, and several months of recovery. Both example time scales for recovery ignore all the rest-activity cycles that take place on finer and broader time scales.

Observations of biological rhythms date back to the 1700s with pioneering work by de Mairan. This early work demonstrated that the daily rhythm of plant leaves was not a result of sunlight but was derived from an internal biological mechanism (Dement, 2000). Later, using bunkers and caves as research laboratories, the human circadian rhythms were mapped and explored (Aschoff, 1960; Aschoff & Wever, 1976; Kleitman, 1961). This work continues in modern laboratories and extreme environments such as space shuttles and submarines (Dijk et al., 2001; Mallis & DeRoshia, 2005; Matthews et al., 2021, 2023; Marando et al., 2022). The primary characteristic of this cycle is its 24-hour oscillation, its continued pattern in an environment devoid of time cues, and consistency under altered sleep-wake behaviour (Kleitman 1961; Matthews, Ferguson, Zhou, Kosmadopoulos, et al., 2012; Matthews, Ferguson, Zhou, Sargent, et al., 2012; Vitaterna et al., 2001). Other, shorter, rest-activity cycles were first published in in the 1960's and 70's (Friedman & Fisher, 1967; Kleitman, 1961; Orr et al., 1976; Sterman & Hoppenbrouwers, 1971). Observations were made that basic human behaviour such as eating, drinking, human performance, and sleep followed approximately 90-min 'ultradian cycles'. Of particular note was the demonstration that these rhythms existed as a general activity pattern of the brain observed in both wake and sleep (Kleitman, 1961; Othmer et al., 1969).

Infradian rhythms, which follow four longer periods of weekly (circaseptan cycle), monthly (circatrigintan cycle), seasonal, and yearly cycles (circannual cycle) were also explored and documented in humans and animals (Aschoff, 1981; Swaab et al., 1996). The scientific community now understands the important roles that all these rhythms play in human and animal functioning. Humans have the ability to exert unprecedented control over their rest-activity cycles, often with poor outcomes (Matthews et al., 2013, 2023). Despite this research starting in the 1960s and 1970s, with the modern application of this work we are only beginning to acknowledge that by optimising rest and recovery on each of these scales we are able to optimise our performance and functioning.

In humans, the fundamental rhythm in our rest-active cycle is our 24-hour (circadian) rhythm. This rhythm provides us with our sleep/wake rest-active cycle which forms the basis of our physiological and psychological recovery. Both the shorter 90-min ultradian cycle and longer weekly infradian cycle can also be optimised to 'take up the slack' of our daily cycle. For example, it is now commonplace for people to sleep less than their need during the week (six to seven hours per night) and then recover their sleep debt during the weekend. It is also common practice for shift workers to nap at 45-, 90-, 120- or 360-min periods within a 24-hour day to supplement a disrupted circadian cycle. In both cases, infradian or ultradian rest-activity cycles are being used to recover and optimise performance. On longer time scales, our weekly, monthly, seasonally, and yearly infradian rhythms guide our longer rest and recovery periods of days off and holiday breaks. Ignoring our weekly or monthly days off for recovery will mean seasonal or yearly cycles become more important, and vice versa.

There are examples showing that good short-time-scale peri-operation recovery can mean that post-operational recovery is not necessary. An example of this was demonstrated on a civilian maritime ferry service, where high-intensity summer operations led to high-risks 'double sailing' (Thomas et al., 2019). What was normally an overnight operation became consecutive day and night sailings, through a stretch of Australian waters that was notoriously rough and known for extreme wave height. These operations meant the crew lost their usual recovery time between sailings and had an increased workload. However, more frequent short recovery (which also included napping), resulted in more sleep obtained, no increase in fatigue, and sustained performance, irrespective of the increased work and loss of pre and post sailing recovery (Thomas et al., 2019). It should be noted that all the sailors in this study had more than ten years of experience and were practised in optimising their peri-operation recovery. In addition, they worked for a company that trusted them to prioritise rest and defer non-safety-related ancillary tasks during high high-intensity periods.

Conclusion and recommendations for practice

The utilisation of various cognitive enhancement skills and strategies that include the optimisation of recovery and well-being as foundation skills has received considerable attention in various high-performance environments (Guo et al., 2019;

Jha et al., 2010). High-performing organisations must pay particular attention to their ability to foster and facilitate recovery and cognitive performance competencies in their workforce and to ensure that the leaders within the environment both understand and appreciate the efficacy of doing so (see also Kuntz, this volume, Chapter 12).

This contemporary approach to fostering a workforce that has a high degree of mental health, is prepared to perform on demand, and is resilient allowing for operational delivery to be optimised while ensuring that each member has the agency to take care of themselves during their careers and once their careers are over.

Human performance optimisation in military settings

Efforts to enhance the psychosocial health are of critical importance for Defence Force members, their families, and the healthcare system as a whole (Vanhove et al., 2018). Human Performance Optimisation (HPO) programs and initiatives within military environments endeavour to address the physical, mental, and socio-cultural factors that enhance operational performance while ensuring sufficient recovery and well-being are achieved.

Of particular importance is the need to ensure that those undergoing initial training in military and civilian environments have the skills and strategies that will enable them to deliver optimal performance on demand. Part of this skill set should be the ability personal responsibility for managing and mitigating stress, fatigue, and distraction through the application of personal well-being and recovery habits that were formed early on in their careers.

Sleep recommendations for optimising capability in operational environments

1) Prioritise sleep where possible during the operation to ensure there is 'sustainment sleep'. This consists of short sleeps or naps totaling to five to seven hours of sleep each 24-hour period. Continuous operations, or long periods of high tempo can only be accomplished if some sleep is achieved. This sleep is to slow the growth of cumulative fatigue and restrict fatigue and stress from growing exponentially. The presence of even some sleep will also help alleviate the symptoms of stress and fatigue.

2) Rest activity cycles need to be considered so recovery is factored into multiple time scales, including 90-min, daily, weekly, monthly, quarterly, and yearly.

3) When stress causes impaired sleep, rely on pro-active stress recovery behaviours (such as Mindfulness-Based-Stress-Reduction) to decrease stress and allow the homeostatic sleep drive to function.

4) As soon as possible, and as frequently as possible, receive naturally induced 'recovery sleep'. This would be uninterrupted time in bed of eight to 14 hours in duration, for at least two periods.

Mindfulness training on stress and recovery

As part of the HPO curriculum within military environments, Mindfulness-Based-Stress-Reduction (MBSR) training should be offered as part of Initial Military Training and as part of a pre-deployment protocol. For example, Chen et al. (2022) found that MBSR training significantly reduced the perceived stress levels within a military cadet population. Jha et al. (2017) demonstrated that Marines who received mindfulness meditation training showed faster recovery from combat training that those who did not receive mindfulness training.

Monitoring stress, fatigue, and recovery

Performance monitoring is common practice within high performance environments (Coutts et al., 2022). Civilian populations entering IMT environments are considered a high physical and psychological risk. Ensuring a balance exists between the training demands and recovery during basic military training is of critical importance to optimise the progression of recruits (Tait, Drain, Bulmer, et al., 2022). Ongoing monitoring with a suite of easily administered measures can assist with the early detection of training maladaptation in recruits and assist both the recruits and the unit with enhanced self-awareness of current well-being, recovery, and performance readiness states.

Military training units can benefit from the implementation of a monitoring system as follows:

1) Optimisation of trainee progression through early detection of training maladaptation and/or compromised well-being and recovery.
2) Facilitation of self-awareness and self-knowledge associated with human performance optimisation skills and competencies aligned with stress, fatigue and well-being optimisation.
3) Improved physical conditioning and mental performance from entry to graduation and enhanced preparation for initial employment training.

References

Aidman, E. (2020). Cognitive fitness framework: Towards assessing, training and augmenting individual-difference factors underpinning high-performance cognition. *Frontiers in Neuroscience, 13*, 466. https://doi.org/10.3389/fnhum.2019.00466

Åkerstedt, T., Perski, A., & Kecklund, G. (2011). Sleep, stress, and burnout. In M. H. Kryger, T. Roth, & W. C. Dement (Eds.), *Principles and practice of sleep medicine* (5th ed., pp. 814–821). Saunders.

Albertella, L., Kirkham, R., Adler, A. B., Crampton, J., Drummond, S. P. A., Fogarty, G. J., Gross J. J., Zaichkowsky, L., Andersen, J. P., Bartone, P. T., Boga, D., Bond, J., Brunyé, T. T., Campbell, M. J., Ciobanu, L. G., Clark, S. R., Crane, M. F., Dietrich, A., Doty, T. J., & Yücel, M. (2022). Building a transdisciplinary expert consensus on the cognitive drivers of performance under pressure: An international multi-panel Delphi study. *Frontiers in Psychology, 13*, 1017675. https://doi.org/10.3389/fpsyg.2022.1017675

Altfeld, S., Schaffran, P., Kleinert, J., & Kellmann, M. (2018). Minimising the risk of coach burnout: From research to practice. *International Sport Coaching Journal, 5*(1), 71–78.

Aschoff, J. (1960). Exogenous and endogenous components in circadian rhythms. *Cold Spring Harbor Symposia on Quantitative Biology, 25*(11), 11–28.

Aschoff, J. (1981). A survey on biological rhythms. In J. Aschoff (Eds.), *Biological rhythms* (pp. 3–10). Springer.

Aschoff, J., & Wever, R. (1976). Human circadian rhythms: A multioscillatory system. *Federation Proceedings, 35*(12), 2326–2332.

Baker, M. (2015). Data science: Industry allure. *Nature, 520*(7546), 253–255.

Balban, M. Y., Neri, E., Kogan, M. M., Weed, L., Nouriani, B., Booil, J., Holl, G., Zeitzer, J. M., Spiegel, D., & Huberman, A. D. (2023). Brief structured respiration practices enhance mood and reduce physiological arousal. *Cell Reports Medicine, 4*, 100895. https://doi.org/10.1016/j.xcrm.2022.100895

Belenky, G., Marcy, S. C., & Martin, J. A. (1996). Debriefings and battle reconstructions following combat. In J. A. Martin, L. Sparacino, & G. Belenky (Eds.), *The Gulf War and mental health: A comprehensive guide* (pp. 105–115). Praeger.

Black, S., Whitney, S., Bender, A., Lipp, O., Loft, S., & Visser, T. (2020, December 7–9). *The effect of mobile app-based multitasking training on situation awareness and performance in Army personnel* [Paper presentation]. Defence Human Sciences Symposium 2020, Adelaide, South Australia.

Calogiuri, G., Weydahl, A., & Carandente, F. (2013). Methodological issues for studying the rest–activity cycle and sleep disturbances: A chronobiological approach using actigraphy data. *Biological Research for Nursing, 15*(1), 5–12.

Cannon, W. B. (1914). The emergency function of the adrenal medulla in pain and the major emotions. *American Journal of Physiology, 33*, 356–372.

Chen, Y.-H., Chiu, F.-C., Lin, Y.-N., & Chang, Y.-L. (2022). The effectiveness of mindfulness-based-stress-reduction for military cadets on perceived stress. *Psychological Reports, 125*(4), 1915–1936.

Coutts, A. J., Crowcroft, S., & Kempton, T. (2022). Developing athlete monitoring systems: Theoretical basis and practical applications. In M. Kellmann & J. Beckmann (Eds.), *Recovery and well-being in sport and exercise* (pp. 17–31). Routledge.

Darwent, D., Dawson, D., Paterson, J. L., Roach, G. D., & Ferguson, S. A. (2015). Managing fatigue: It really is about sleep. *Accident Analysis & Prevention, 82*, 20–26.

DeJohn, C. A., Shappell, S. A., & Neri, D. F. (1992). *Subjective fatigue in A-6, F-14, and F/A-18 aircrews during Operations Desert Shield and Storm.* Navel Aerospace Medical Research Laboratory.

Dement, W. C. (2000). History of sleep physiology and medicine. In M. K. Kryer, T. Roth, & W. C. Dement (Eds.), *Principles and practice of sleep medicine* (3rd ed., pp. 1–12). Saunders.

Dijk, D. J., Neri, D. F., Wyatt, J. K., Ronda, J. M., Riel, E., Ritz-De Cecco, A., Hughes, R. J., Elliott, A. R., Prisk, G. K., West, J. B., & Czeisler, C. A. (2001). Sleep, performance, circadian rhythms, and light-dark cycles during two space shuttle flights. *American Journal of Physiology-Regulatory, Integrative and Comparative Physiology, 281*(5), R1647–R1664.

Friedman, S., & Fisher, C. (1967). On the presence of a rhythmic, diurnal, oral instinctual drive cycle in man. *Journal of the American Psychoanalytic Association, 15*(2), 317–351.

Goldfarb, M., Tellier, C., & Thanassoulis, G. (2014). Review of published cases of adverse cardiovascular events after ingestion of energy drinks. *The American Journal of Cardiology, 113*(1), 168–172.

Guo, D., Sun, L., Yu, X., Lie, T., Wu, L., Sun, Z., Zhang, F., Zhou, Y., Shen, M., & Lie, W. (2019). Mindfulness-based stress reduction improves the general health and stress of Chinese military recruits: A pilot study. *Psychiatry Research, 281,* 112571. https://doi.org/10.1016/j.psychres.2019.112571

Hancock, P. A., & Desmond, P. A. (2001). *Stress, workload, and fatigue.* Lawrence Erlbaum Associates Publishers.

Hancock, P. A., & Verwey, W. B. (1997). Fatigue, workload and adaptive driver systems. *Accident Analysis & Prevention, 29*(4), 495–506.

Hilditch, C. J., Dorrian, J., & Banks, S. (2016). Time to wake up: Reactive countermeasures to sleep inertia. *Industrial Health, 54*(6), 528–541.

Hilditch, C. J., & McHill, A. W. (2019). Sleep inertia: Current insights. *Nature and Science of Sleep, 11,* 155–165.

Immink, M. A., Chatburn, A., Baumeister, J., Pomeroy, D., Schlesewsky, M., & Bornkessel-Schlesewsky, I. (2020, December 7–9). *Multi-modal cognitive training with an immersive virtual reality marksmanship task and mindfulness mediation* [Paper presentation]. *Defence Human Sciences Symposium 2020,* Adelaide, South Australia.

Israni, S. T., & Verghese, A. (2019). Humanizing artificial intelligence. *Journal of the American Medical Association, 321*(1), 29–30.

Jha, A. P., Morrison, A. B., Parker, S. C., & Stanley, E. A. (2017). Practice is protective: Mindfulness training promotes cognitive resilience in high-stress cohorts. *Mindfulness, 8*(1), 46–58.

Jha, A. P., Stanley, E. A., Kiyonaga, A., Wong, L., & Gelfand, L. (2010). Examining the protective effects of mindfulness training on working memory capacity and affective experience. *Emotion, 10*(1), 54–64.

Johnson, L. A., Foster, D., & McDowell, J. C. (2014). Energy drinks: Review of performance benefits, health concerns, and use by military personnel. *Military Medicine, 179*(4), 375–380.

Jordan, M. I., & Mitchell, T. M. (2015). Machine learning: Trends, perspectives, and prospects. *Science, 349*(6245), 255–260.

Kavanagh, J. (2005). *Stress and performance: A review of the literature and its applicability to the military.* Rand.

Kellmann, M., Bertollo, M., Bosquet, L., Brink, M., Coutts, A. J., Duffield, R., Erlacher, D., Halson, S. L., Hecksteden, A., Heidari, J., Kallus, K. W., Meeusen, R., Mujika, I., Robazza, C., Skorski, S., Venter, R., & Beckmann, J. (2018). Recovery and performance in sport: Consensus statement. *International Journal of Sports Physiology and Performance, 13*(2), 240–245.

Kellmann, M., & Kallus, K. W. (2001). *Recovery-Stress Questionnaire for Athletes: User manual.* Human Kinetics.

Kleitman, N. (1961). The nature of dreaming. In G. E. W. Wolstenholme & M. O'Connor (Eds.), *The nature of sleep* (pp. 349–364). Churchill.

Kluge, M. G., Maltby, S., Walker, N., Bennett, N., Aidman, E., Nalivaiko, E., & Walker, F. R. (2021). Development of a modular stress management platform (Performance Edge VR) and a pilot efficacy trial of a bio-feedback enhanced training module for controlled breathing. *PLoS One, 16*(2), e0245068. https://doi.org/10.1371/journal.pone.0245068

Krueger, G. P. (1989). Sustained work, fatigue, sleep loss and performance: A review of the issues. *Work & Stress, 3*(2), 129–141.

Loch, F., Jakowski, S., Hof zum Berge, A., & Kellmann, M. (2022). Mental fatigue and the concept of mental recovery in sport. In M. Kellmann & J. Beckmann (Eds.), *Recovery and well-being in sport and exercise* (pp. 187–200). Routledge.

Mallis, M. M., & DeRoshia, C. W. (2005). Circadian rhythms, sleep, and performance in space. *Aviation, Space, and Environmental Medicine, 76*(6), B94–B107.

Marando, I., Lushington, K., Matthews, R., & Banks, S. (2022). The sleep, performance, and physiological health consequences of watchkeeping schedules: A scoping review. *Sleep Advances: A Journal of the Sleep Research Society, 3*(Suppl. 1), A53–A54. https://doi.org/10.1093/sleepadvances/zpac029.143

Mareth, T. R., & Brooker, A. E. (1985). Combat stress reaction: A concept in evolution. *Military Medicine, 150*(4), 186–190.

Martire, V. L., Caruso, D., Palagini, L., Zoccoli, G., & Bastianini, S. (2020). Stress & sleep: A relationship lasting a lifetime. *Neuroscience & Biobehavioral Reviews, 117*, 65–77.

Matthews, R. W., Ferguson, S. A., Zhou, X., Kosmadopoulos, A., Kennaway, D. J., & Roach, G. D. (2012). Simulated driving under the influence of extended wake, time of day and sleep restriction. *Accident Analysis & Prevention, 45*, 55–61.

Matthews, R. W., Ferguson, S. A., Zhou, X., Sargent, C., Darwent, D., Kennaway, D. J., & Roach, G. D. (2012). Time-of-day mediates the influences of extended wake and sleep restriction on simulated driving. *Chronobiology International, 29*(5), 572–579.

Matthews, R. M., Ferguson, S. A., & Banks, S. (2013). Partial and sleep-stage-selective deprivation. In C. A. Kushida (Ed.), *Encyclopedia of sleep* (pp. 162–168). Academic Press.

Matthews, R., Fraysse, F., Daniell, N., Schumacher, P., & Banks, S. (2021). Rockabye sailor: Investigating the impact of simulated motion on sleep and cognitive performance. *Sleep Advances: A Journal of the Sleep Research Society, 2*(Suppl. 1), A15–A16. https://doi.org/10.1093/sleepadvances/zpab014.033

Matthews, R. W., Guzzetti, J., & Banks, S. (2023). Partial and sleep-stage-selective deprivation. In C. A. Kushida (Ed.), *Encyclopedia of sleep and circadian rhythms* (2nd ed., pp. 162–168). Academic Press.

McEwen, B. S., & Wingfield, J. C. (2003). The concept of allostasis in biology and biomedicine. *Hormones and Behavior, 43*(1), 2–15.

Miller, N. L., Matsangas, P., & Shattuck, L. G. (2018). Fatigue and its effect on performance in military environments. In J. Szalma & P. A. Hancock (Eds.), *Performance under stress* (pp. 247–266). CRC Press.

Murphy, P. J., & Fogarty, G. J. (2009). Good to go? The human dimensions of mission readiness. In P. J. Murphy (Ed.), *Focus on human performance in land operations* (Vol. 1, pp. 46–55). Australian Department of Defence, Department of Psychology.

Neville, K. J., Bisson, R. U., French, J., Boll, P. A., & Storm, W. F. (1994). Subjective fatigue of C-141 aircrews during Operation Desert Storm. *Human Factors, 36*(2), 339–349.

Othmer, E., Hayden, M. P., & Segelbaum, R. (1969). Encephalic cycles during sleep and wakefulness in humans: A 24-hour pattern. *Science, 164*, 447–449.

Orr, W. C., Hoffman, H. J., & Hegge, F. W. (1976). The assessment of time-dependent changes in human performance. *Chronobiologia, 3*(4), 293–305.

Park, S. H., & Han, K. (2018). Methodologic guide for evaluating clinical performance and effect of artificial intelligence technology for medical diagnosis and prediction. *Radiology, 286*(3), 800–809.

Peters, A., McEwen, B. S., & Friston, K. (2017). Uncertainty and stress: Why it causes diseases and how it is mastered by the brain. *Progress in Neurobiology, 156*, 164–188.

Popkin, S. M. (1999). An examination and comparison of workload and subjective measures collected from railroad dispatchers. *Proceedings of the Human Factors and Ergonomics Society Annual Meeting, 43*(18), 997–1001.

Rector, M. R., Topchiy, I. A., Carter, K. M., & Rojas, M. J. (2005). Local functional state differences between rat cortical columns. *Brain Research, 1047*(1), 45–55.

Roach, G. D., Matthews, R., Naweed, A., Kontou, T. G., & Sargent, C. (2018). Flat-out napping: The quantity and quality of sleep obtained in a seat during the daytime increase as the angle of recline of the seat increases. *Chronobiology International, 35*(6), 872–883.

Selye, H. (1956). *The stress of life*. McGraw-Hill.

Shah, S. A., Szeto, A. H., Farewell, R., Shek, A., Fan, D., Quach, K. N., Bhattacharyya, M., Elmiari, J., Chan, W., O'Dell, K., Nguyen, N., McGaughey, T. J., Nasir, J. M., & Kaul, S. (2019). Impact of high volume energy drink consumption on electrocardiographic and blood pressure parameters: A randomized trial. *Journal of the American Heart Association, 8*(11), e011318. https://doi.org/10.1161/JAHA.118.011318

Shappell, S. A., & Neri, D. F. (1993). Effect of combat on aircrew subjective readiness during Operations Desert Shield and Desert Storm. *The International Journal of Aviation Psychology, 3*(3), 231–252.

Shortliffe, E. H., & Sepúlveda, M. J. (2018). Clinical decision support in the era of artificial intelligence. *Journal of the American Medical Association, 320*(21), 2199–2200.

Sterman, M. B., & Hoppenbrouwers, T. (1971). The development of sleep-waking and rest-activity patterns from fetus to adult in man. In M. B. Sterman, D. J. McGinty, & A. Adinolfi (Eds.), *Brain development and behavior* (pp. 203–227). Academic Press.

Swaab, D. F., Van Someren, E. J. W., Zhou, J. N., & Hofman, M. A. (1996). Biological rhythms in the human life cycle and their relationship to functional changes in the suprachiasmatic nucleus. In R. M. Buijs, A. Kalsbeek, H. J. Romijn, C. M. A. Pennartz, & M. Mirmiran (Eds.), *Progress in brain research* (Vol. 111, pp. 349–368). Elsevier.

Topol, E. J. (2019). High-performance medicine: The convergence of human and artificial intelligence. *Nature Medicine, 25*(1), 44–56.

Tait, J. L., Drain, J. R., Bulmer, S., Gastin, P. B., & Main, L. C. (2022). Factors predicting training delays and attrition of recruits during basic military training. *International Journal of Environmental Research and Public Health, 19*(12), 7271. https://doi.org/10.3390/ijerph19127271

Tait, J. L., Drain, J. R., Corrigan, S. L., Drake, J. M., & Main, L. C. (2022). Impact of military training stress on hormone response and recovery. *PloS One, 17*(3), e0265121. https://doi.org/10.1371/journal.pone.0265121

Taylor, P. (2021). Physical and cognitive fitness training in the workplace: Validating a multimodal intervention in Australian corporate settings. *International Journal of Sport and Exercise Psychology, 19*, S14–S15.

Taylor, P., Heathcote, A., & Aidman, E. (2021). Effects of multimodal physical and cognitive fitness training on subjective well-being, burnout and resilience in a military cohort. *Journal of Science and Medicine in Sport, 24*, S35–S36.

Thomas, M. J., Paterson, J. L., Jay, S. M., Matthews, R. W., & Ferguson, S. A. (2019). More than hours of work: Fatigue management during high-intensity maritime operations. *Chronobiology International, 36*(1), 143–149.

U.S. Department of Defense. (2021). *Study on effects of sleep deprivation on readiness of members of the Armed Forces*. Retrieved July 01, 2023 from https://www.google.com/url?sa=t&rct=j&q=&esrc=s&source=web&cd=&ved=2ahUKEwijkcb3pPL_AhWStqQKHQJ_CNYQFnoECA4QAQ&url=https%3A%2F%2Fwww.health.mil%2FReference-Center%2FReports%2F2021%2F02%2F26%2FStudy-on-Effects-of-Sleep-Deprivation-on-Readiness-of-Members-of-the-Armed-Forces-Final-Report&usg=AOvVaw2YLGllJGkWG21eEnD8orDf&opi=89978449

Van Dongen, H., Belenky, G., & Krueger, J. M. (2011). Investigating the temporal dynamics and underlying mechanisms of cognitive fatigue. In P. L. Ackerman (Ed.), *Cognitive fatigue: Multidisciplinary perspectives on current research and future applications* (pp. 127–147). American Psychological Association.

Vanhove, A. J., Brutus, T., & Sowden, K. A. (2018). Psychosocial health prevention programs in military organizations: A quantitative review of the evaluative rigor evidence. In P. D. Harms & P. L. Perrewé (Eds.), *Occupational stress and well-being in military contexts* (pp. 129–156). Emerald Publishing.

Vitaterna, M. H., Takahashi, J. S., & Turek, F. W. (2001). Overview of circadian rhythms. *Alcohol Research & Health, 25*(2), 85–93.

Warm, J. S., Matthews, G., & Finomore, V. S. (2008). Vigilance, workload, and stress. In J. L. Szalma, P. A. A. Hancock, D. Harris, E. Salas, & N. A. Stanton (Eds.), *Performance under stress* (pp. 115–141). CRC Press LLC.

Williams, D., Streeter, J., & Kelly, T. (1998). *Fatigue in naval tactical aviators.* Naval Health Research Centre.

Winter, J. C. (2014). Controversy in human factors constructs and the explosive use of the NASA-TLX: A measurement perspective. *Cognition, Technology & Work, 16*(3), 289–297.

12 Building recovery into organisations to foster resilience

Joana C. Kuntz

Introduction

Over the past two decades, a surge of scholarly research has demonstrated how physical and psychological recovery from work offset the impact of job stressors on health and performance, and sustain well-being (Beckmann & Kellmann, 2004; Bennett et al., 2018; Sonnentag et al., 2022; Steed et al., 2021). The literature is rich in examples of recovery activities people carry out within and outside the workplace (Chan et al., 2022; de Bloom et al., 2018; Kim et al., 2018) and the recovery experiences derived from those activities, which reflect physical and psychological states associated with energy restoration and stress reduction (Newman et al., 2014; Sonnentag & Fritz, 2007). Growing evidence shows that recovery experiences produce desirable outcomes including restored energy levels, improved sleep quality, and increased engagement, creativity, helping behaviours, and performance (Karabinski et al., 2021; Verbeek et al., 2019; Weinberger et al., 2018). Nevertheless, scholars and practitioners have noted the need to deepen our understanding of the biopsychosocial mechanisms that underpin our capacity to recover from work, and of the ways organisations optimally support recovery experiences (Sonnentag et al., 2022; Steed et al., 2021; ten Brummelhuis & Trougakos, 2014). This chapter discusses how overlaying resilience and work recovery research reveals intrapersonal mechanisms of recovery and how organisations can leverage the mutually enhancing resilience-recovery processes.

Work recovery overview

Work recovery is defined as the "unwinding and restoration processes during which a person's strain level that has increased as a reaction to a stressor or any other demand returns to its prestressor level" (Sonnentag et al., 2017, p. 366).

Kuntz, J. C. (2024). Building recovery into organisations to foster resilience. In M. Kellmann & J. Beckmann (Eds.), *Fostering Recovery and Well-being in a Healthy Lifestyle: Psychological, Somatic, and Organizational Prevention Approaches* (pp. 182–198). Routledge.

DOI: 10.4324/9781003250654-16

Opportunities for work recovery are essential to restoring functioning following the depletion of energy and other personal resources caused by physical, cognitive, or social job demands. The recovery process relies on activities carried out outside of work (e.g., holidays, sleep, family time), in a place of work (e.g., socialisation, microbreaks, task switching), or during work hours in remote work situations (e.g., voluntary breaks, nature walks). Given that boundaryless work is increasingly pervasive in contemporary societies and that recovery activities carried out within and outside the organisation have complementary effects on worker well-being and performance, the restorative experiences that ensue from both 'recovery at work' and 'recovery from work' should be considered in tandem (Chan et al., 2022; de Bloom et al., 2018; Kim et al., 2018; Smith et al., 2022). Recovery experiences characterise the subjective experiences of energy and affect repair that mediate the relationship between recovery activities and well-being outcomes (Sonnentag & Geurts, 2009). When people select recovery activities because they fit with their needs and preferences, the strength of the relationship between recovery activities, recovery experiences, and well-being is greater (Bennett et al., 2018; de Bloom et al., 2017, 2018; Rost et al., 2021). It is therefore essential to understand the individual and contextual factors that account for the linkages among the selection of recovery activities, recovery experiences, and recovery outcomes.

Recovery experiences

The first taxonomy of recovery experiences comprised psychological detachment from work, control, mastery, and relaxation (Sonnentag & Fritz, 2007). Newman et al. (2014) later extended this four-dimension taxonomy to include experiences of meaning and affiliation.

Psychological detachment (Balk, this volume, Chapter 4) is arguably the most widely studied recovery experience and it describes a process of mental disengagement where thoughts and feelings about work are temporarily set aside as people carry out recovery activities in their own time (Sonnentag & Fritz, 2015). While psychological detachment from work is a well-established means to recover, researchers have recently stated that not all instances of thinking about work equate to the sort of negative rumination that depletes well-being. For example, problem-solving pondering (i.e., reflecting on ways to improve performance and address job challenges) and positive work reflection (i.e., reflecting on the positive features of one's job; Weigelt et al., 2019; Zijlstra et al., 2014) can happen outside of work and lead to recovered states through control and mastery experiences. It follows that certain individual factors may explain why people differ in their tendency to ruminate about work or to rely on positive work-related thinking, and in their capacity to psychologically detach from work.

Control reflects a sense of agency over the selection and timing of both work and recovery activities (Ouyang et al., 2019; Sonnentag et al., 2017, 2022), and has been identified as a protective factor against energy depletion (Trougakos et al., 2014). Experiences of control can take place during work hours and, as exemplified, also outside of work through voluntary reflection about the positive aspects of the job and ways to render it more fulfilling. Further to control, mastery experiences occur when workers engage in recovery activities tied to learning and growth (Sonnentag et al., 2017). The restorative effects of mastery experiences such as overcoming job challenges, developing competencies, and, outside work, pursuing meaningful hobbies, sustain engagement and well-being. As with psychological detachment and control, the need for mastery experiences and extent of their impact on recovered states differs among individuals.

Relaxation experiences decrease sympathetic activation and are essential to restoring functioning and well-being at times of high stress (e.g., peak performance; Sonnentag et al., 2022). Akin to other recovery experiences, relaxation can occur within and outside the workplace, and achieved through activities such as meditation, technology breaks, and socialisation. The positive impact of these activities on relaxation experiences and recovered states has been tied to personal resources such as resilience and regulatory capacity (Baethge et al., 2020; Trougakos et al., 2014).

Lastly, meaning experiences pertain to subjective positive experiences that arise from purposeful or impactful activities, including volunteering, work projects that have a positive impact on the community, and participating in sports events; whereas affiliation experiences reflect a sense of social connection and support derived from social activities within and outside work (Bosch et al., 2018; Newman et al., 2014; Virtanen et al., 2021).

Recovery frameworks

One of the main challenges for organisations is to identify how work demands deplete energy, positive affect, cognitive function, and motivation, and under what conditions recovery activities restore functioning and well-being (Bakker & de Vries, 2021; Sonnentag et al., 2022). These phenomena have been explored through the lens of stress, motivation, and affect-regulation theories.

The *Effort-Recovery Model* (ERM; Meijman & Mulder, 1998) and *Conservation of Resources Theory* (COR; Hobfoll, 1989) are ubiquitous in the literature and have been extensively relied upon to explain recovery processes from a demands and resources perspective (Ragsdale & Beehr, 2016; Steed et al., 2021). The ERM provides a physiological account of how stress impacts human functioning. It contends that work demands require effort expenditure, including energies devoted to self-regulation, and that strain responses to effort expenditure (e.g., fatigue) will worsen in the absence of respite from these demands (Meijman & Mulder, 1998). COR theory postulates that people are motivated to safeguard existing resources and to generate new ones (Hobfoll et al., 2018). The theory elucidates how recovery activities and experiences restore personal resources that are depleted by work demands and contribute to further resource development (Blanco-Donoso et al., 2017; Kim et al., 2018). An integrative perspective of these theories suggests that a reservoir of personal resources such as energy and regulatory capacity protects against the impact of work demands, guides the selection of recovery activities, and supports recovery experiences (Beckmann & Kellmann, 2004). In turn, when organisations provide opportunities for recovery, they ensure that workers continue to develop their personal resources (Niks et al., 2016).

Further to the contributions of ERM and COR theory to our understanding of how recovery influences stress and resource management, *Self-Determination Theory* (SDT) elucidates the motivational underpinnings of recovery. SDT describes how the satisfaction of basic psychological needs (BPN) at work – autonomy, competence, and relatedness – promotes engagement and well-being by restoring personal and social resources. In practice, the positive motivational and emotional states associated with BPN satisfaction at work are linked to the production of hormones that regulate stress responses, and direct attention to new resource acquisition (van Hooff et al., 2018). In doing so, SDT emphasises the role of organisations in satisfying BPN to foster recovery experiences (Deci & Ryan, 2008; Trougakos et al., 2014).

Lastly, affect- and regulation-based theories underscore the importance of recovery in offsetting the deleterious effect of emotional job demands on worker energy and well-being (Chong et al., 2020; Virtanen et al., 2021). The theories suggest common recovery mechanisms, the importance of attending to the interplay of workers and their organisational environment, and the role of individual differences linked to regulatory capacity in enabling or disrupting recovery. For instance, *Ego-Depletion Theory* (EDT) posits that most work behaviours involve regulatory capacity (personal resource), that the energy expended on self-regulation throughout the workday must be replenished through recovery activities and experiences, and that individuals differ with regards to their capacity for self-regulation (Muraven & Baumeister, 2000; Trougakos et al., 2014). Regarding the latter, scholars note that emotional stability is a trait associated with lower need for recovery, and that this trait underpins the necessary regulatory capacity to ensure psychological detachment and relaxation experiences (Fostervold & Watten, 2022; Jalonen et al., 2015; Sonnentag & Fritz, 2007).

The stress, motivation, and affect-regulation theories outlined have advanced recovery research by explaining the effect of job demands-resources imbalances on well-being and performance, worker motivation to select specific recovery activities, and the contextual factors that determine whether recovery experiences will ensue from recovery activities. However, scholars have recently called for further research that uncovers the psychological factors and mechanisms interacting with organisational factors to influence recovery processes and trajectories (Cham et al., 2021; Chan et al., 2022; Sonnentag et al., 2021, 2022).

Integrating resilience with work recovery

In the organisational research, contemporary definitions of resilience draw on and integrate psychological, transformational, and ecological perspectives. From a psychological perspective, resilience is described as a personal resource that influences the ability to self-regulate, restore functioning, and show positive adaptation following exposure to adversity (Bonanno, 2004; Hartmann et al., 2020). This resource has been ascribed to individual differences such as personality traits and resilience biomarkers. Regarding the latter, the Neuropeptide Y gene has been linked with resilience due to its role in regulating cortisol, which improves stress reactivity and coping among gene carriers by supporting emotional regulation and cognitive functioning following exposure to adverse events (Crane et al., 2019; Gan et al., 2019; Lau et al., 2021).

The transformational view of resilience builds on the notion that resilience results from a constellation of psychophysiological factors and is both demonstrated through and further developed by ongoing learning and adaptive processes that assist recovery from stress (Hartmann et al., 2020; Kuntz, 2021). Relatedly, the ecological perspective underscores the critical role of the environment (e.g., organisations, family) in promoting or weakening resilience. Hence, the capacity to cope with stressors, learn, and show positive adaptation is contingent on the availability of contextual resources, including social support (Kuntz, Connell, & Näswall, 2017; Southwick et al., 2014).

The resilience scholarship is grounded on similar stress models, motivational mechanisms, and affect-regulation precepts to the ones that guide contemporary work recovery research, which suggests opportunities to overlay insights from the resilience research onto work recovery models in order to advance the literature. For instance, scholars have relied on resilience biomarkers (e.g., cortisol levels) as indicators of recovery experiences and states (Kubo et al., 2021), and noted the impact of social and job resources on the autonomic regulation that signals recovery (Baethge et al., 2020). Yet, a cursory examination of the resilience and recovery literatures exposes conceptual entanglements and missed opportunities for integration. For instance, while the recovery literature frames resilience either as a personal resource that facilitates recovery experiences (Baethge et al., 2020; Ragsdale & Beehr, 2016; Yang et al., 2020) or the upshot of recovery experiences (Jo & Lee, 2022), the resilience literature regards recovery as a facet of resilience (Maltby & Hall, 2022), or the stage within a resilience trajectory that precedes adaptation (IJntema et al., 2023). In addition, although much of the recovery research has relied on regulation- and motivation-based theories to uncover energy management mechanisms at work, explain the selection of recovery activities, and identify the impact of job resources and demands imbalances on worker outcomes (Niks et al., 2016; Trougakos et al., 2014; van Hooff et al., 2018; Virtanen et al., 2021), scholars have recently called for the identification of specific personal resources that contribute to positive recovery trajectories and strengthen the relationship between recovery processes and well-being outcomes (Chan et al., 2022; Sonnentag et al., 2022).

The resilience literature may contribute to addressing these gaps by putting forth resilience as a personal resource that is inextricable from regulatory capacity and essential to work recovery (Fisher et al., 2019; Hartmann et al., 2020). Resilience has been linked to a decreased likelihood of experiencing job demands as significant stressors and to an improved capacity to identify and leverage job resources (Kuntz, Connell, & Näswall, 2017). Consequently, it may also enable workers to direct energy to and select effective recovery activities. Though limited, the research that intersects resilience and recovery in occupational settings offers preliminary evidence to establish its role as a foundational recovery resource (IJntema et al., 2023; Ragsdale & Beehr, 2016). Further, the research suggests that resilience is sustained and enhanced in workplaces that promote recovery and create the conditions to maximise recovery experiences (Malinen et al., 2019).

Resilience as a personal resource for recovery

Individuals are labelled as resilient when they demonstrate low stress reactance, the ability to quickly rebound from and cope with adverse events, and a propensity to identify specific stressors, including workplace stressors, as challenges that contribute to personal growth and development rather than as hindrances (Bonanno, 2004; Connor & Davidson, 2003; Crane et al., 2019). In essence, individuals with higher levels of resilience show greater tolerance to stress exposure through their ability to self-regulate. They also tend to reflect on the nature and severity of a stressor to regulate affective states, require less time to recover, and enjoy better experiences of recovery (Blanco-Donoso et al., 2017; IJntema et al., 2023; Troy et al., 2023). This conclusion is consistent with recent insights that link individual differences with recovery, positing that "individuals with a strong sense of psychosomatic or psychological well-being may be better able to engage in the recovery process" (Steed et al., 2021, p. 892). It also positions resilience as a personal resource that contributes to disentangling the 'recovery paradox'. According to the recovery paradox, when workers experience fatigue and negative emotions following effort expenditure at work, they often decide to limit further energy expenditure. However, this includes energy that could be allocated to recovery activities aimed at offsetting fatigue and negative states (Cham et al., 2021; van Hooff et al., 2018). Higher levels of resilience may disentangle the paradox by ensuring that workers have the regulatory capacity to prioritise recovery over additional effort expenditure at work and guides the decision to invest extra effort in recovery activities. Hence, resilience may represent an important personal resource in the recovery process through its association with greater stress tolerance and capacity to effectively allocate energies to recovery.

Further to its influence on regulatory processes essential to stress and energy management, resilience has also been associated with the ability to identify and capitalise on resources available in the organisation (Kuntz, Connell, & Näswall, 2017; Kuntz, Malinen, & Näswall, 2017), and to assess when and how to utilise resources to offset demands and stressors (Diotaiuti et al., 2021; Fletcher & Sarkar, 2013). The same way workers with greater regulatory capacity are better able to select effective approaches to cope with stressors (Bakker & de Vries, 2021), resilient workers will arguably select the recovery activities with greater potential to reduce the negative impact of job demands (i.e., activities that will elicit recovery experiences).

Resilience as a dynamic capability in recovery

Much of the recovery research has only indirectly drawn on psychological resilience principles and scholarship (Zijlstra et al., 2014), and the connections between resilience and recovery at work have been mainly explored from the perspective of physiological phenomena caused by stress exposure (Baethge et al., 2020; Schilbach et al., 2021). This research has provided useful insights that inform work recovery research by positioning resilience as an essential personal resource that interacts with job demands and resources to explain recovery trajectories, and that is also susceptible to the availability of recovery opportunities in the environment (Ragsdale & Beehr, 2016).

Healthy organisations represent ecosystems that provide recovery opportunities and other resources to lessen the detrimental effects of perceived job demands on physical, cognitive, and emotional functioning. Although the capacity to restore functioning or to bounce back is greater among workers with higher baseline resilience, healthy organisations promote resilience development by exposing workers to sporadic situations that elevate cortisol levels and prompt adaptive stress responses, while ensuring that the necessary resources and recovery opportunities are present (Baethge et al., 2020; Schilbach et al., 2021). This is beneficial all around, as recovered workers are more likely to develop further job resources (e.g., social support; Steed et al., 2021), along with resilience capability that improves organisational functioning. Conversely, in unhealthy organisations, where prolonged stress exposure or activation are not adequately managed through the provision of recovery opportunities, workers show impaired physical and psychological functioning, and decreased ability to cope with stress over time. In these organisations, depleted functioning can be a sign of diminished resilience capability due to lack of recovery.

This reciprocal resilience-recovery dynamic highlights the importance of an enabling organisational ecosystem where workers are encouraged to engage in activities that elicit recovery experiences. It also illustrates how resilience facilitates recovery by ensuring that workers possess the regulatory capacity to manage stress and energy expenditure at work – quickly restoring energy, positive affect, and focus – and to select recovery activities that achieve desired recovery experiences and end states. In turn, the availability of recovery opportunities and the quality of recovery experiences builds resilience capability over time.

To recap, resilience as a personal resource promotes work recovery by ensuring that workers: a) have greater tolerance to everyday stressors that deplete energy, b) select the suite of recovery activities that best sustain their well-being and functioning, and c) effectively allocate time and energy to these activities. Resilience as a dynamic capability interacts with enabling environments to ensure adaptation, and is associated with recovery through a mutually enhancing process supported by the organisation.

Developing organisations for resilience and recovery

The psychological resilience and work recovery nexus have been primarily examined in the context of recovery from injury or illness, and crisis recovery. A deeper examination of the regulatory and motivational underpinnings of resilience and recovery, namely their commonalities and complementarity, suggests that resilience is an essential personal resource that both supports work recovery, and is influenced by recovery processes. Recent meta-analytical evidence underscores the effect of personal resources on recovery (Steed et al., 2021), corroborating the centrality of individual factors to recovery processes and outcomes. The research also underscores the merits of developing an enabling organisational context that leverages the diversity of personal resources, motivations, and capabilities that characterise the workforce (Parker et al., 2021), and of steering clear of overly prescriptive approaches to recovery activities assumed to embody 'best practice'. For example, although organisational scholars have advocated for the inclusion of resilience as a key selection criterion due to its strong relationship with desirable worker behaviours, this practice is not always defensible (Nolzen, 2018). Instead, the literature offers a plethora of ways organisations can facilitate resilience development (Hartmann et al., 2020; Kuntz, Malinen, & Näswall, 2017). This includes helping workers reframe stressors to support stress management, providing them with discretion to manage job demands, setting clear expectations around job roles and performance, signaling resource availability, and creating an environment rich in technical, developmental, and social resources (Fisher et al., 2019; Kuntz, 2021; Kuntz, Malinen, & Näswall, 2017).

Shaping views of work and organisation to promote recovery

Many of the resilience-building approaches proposed in the literature would address the concerns and propositions outlined in the recovery research, as they underscore the mutually enhancing mechanisms of recovery and resilience and illustrate the centrality of leadership and organisation to positive adaptation and well-being (IJntema et al., 2023). For instance, resilience scholars advocate the development of resilience and stress management literacy, which invites workers to reflect on stressors, job demands, and resource availability as a means to reduce stress and leverage resources (Kuntz, 2021). Given recent evidence suggesting that worker perceptions of their role and organisation influence recovery processes (Perko et al., 2017), organisations can promote recovery through the development of stress literacy, namely reframing stressors and stress experiences. Alongside support from leaders, helping workers distinguish between hindrance stressors (i.e., job demands that decrease energy and cause distress) and challenge stressors (i.e., job demands that sustain engagement and eustress; Bennett et al., 2018; Conlin et al., 2020), may contribute to stress reduction by allowing workers to reduce hindrance demands, and to pursue fulfilling tasks that elicit control and mastery experiences. Relatedly, evidence linking exposure to job challenges with resilience development (Schilbach et al., 2021) supports the reciprocal resilience-recovery dynamic whereby the control and mastery recovery experiences that arise from challenging demands foster resilience. This increased resilience will subsequently bolster workers' ability to cope with further job demands and to engage in effective recovery.

The benefits of shaping worker perceptions of their roles and the organisation can also be realised by guiding positive reflection about work, specifically around its purpose-oriented features (Clauss et al., 2018; Newman et al., 2014). When organisations invite workers to identify how their jobs promote personal and professional growth, sustain the development of meaningful connections, and have a significant impact on the community, this positive reflection has a restorative effect on energy and affect through mastery, affiliation, and meaning experiences.

Recent research also emphasises the importance of recovery self-efficacy to processes of energy restoration at work. Organisations that clearly communicate the connection between recovery activities, replenished energy levels, and restored emotional states, reinforce workers' belief in their ability to offset the negative impact of job demands through recovery activities, and to select the activities that best suit their individual characteristics and contextual demands (Sonnentag & Fritz, 2007; Steed et al., 2021; Yang et al., 2020).

Designing work and organisations for recovery

Autonomy. The regulatory processes that underpin energy management at work, and by extension recovery experiences, rely on the extent to which people are free to decide when to take breaks from work (Ragsdale & Beehr, 2016), what they do with free time at-work (i.e., selection of recovery activities; Trougakos et al., 2014), and how to manage their job tasks (Steed et al., 2021). The provision of autonomy sustains worker motivation by satisfying this basic psychological need (Deci & Ryan, 2008; van Hooff et al., 2018) and supports recovery through an increased sense of agency and control over the environment (Ouyang et al., 2019; Parker et al., 2021; Sonnentag et al., 2022). Further, autonomy paves the way for other effective recovery experiences such as mastery (e.g., electing to engage in challenging projects), relaxation (e.g., withdrawing from or pausing activities that produce negative affective states), and meaning (e.g., selecting job tasks or recovery activities that align with a sense of purpose; Chan et al., 2022; Newman et al., 2014; Sonnentag et al., 2022; Virtanen et al., 2021).

Based on insights from the resilience literature, autonomy-enabling organisations contribute to the ongoing development of resilience as a personal resource (Kuntz, Malinen, & Näswall, 2017). In turn, the regulatory capacity that characterises resilient workers enables them to detect when they need to recover at work and which activities will result in restored functioning. For example, taking microbreaks or switching tasks represent minor yet significant instances of respite that allow individuals to redirect their attention when faced with cognitively or emotionally taxing duties, and to replenish energy (Kim et al., 2018; Troy et al., 2023). The freedom to decide when to recover and which activities to select is necessary to elicit recovery experiences such as control (Beckmann, 2002; Parker et al., 2021; Sonnentag et al., 2022).

Further to the role of autonomy and resilience in the effective timing and selection of recovery activities, having agency to decide when to participate in or withdraw from job tasks also allows workers to reframe their organisation as an accommodating environment within which stress management is both possible and encouraged (Kim et al., 2018; Kuntz, 2021). This is important as workers have unique experiences of the restorative effects of recovery activities; while for some physical exercise or socialisation promote recovery, for others these activities may be perceived as energy depleting (Rost et al., 2021; Trougakos et al., 2014). By explicitly endorsing autonomous decision making around recovery activities and broader job tasks, organisations are simultaneously contributing to effective recovery and to resilience development, setting up an environment where workers remain adaptable through the exploration of new ways of working that help manage emerging demands to sustain energy and engagement. To this end, organisations may provide information about types of recovery activities and job crafting suitable to their unique functional requirements and structure (Kim et al., 2018). In addition, workers might benefit from workshops where they are invited to share energy management and emotion regulation strategies that work for them (Yang et al., 2020), and learn about resilience and the shared role of people and organisations in building resilience capability.

Agency over one's recovery and work management is also vital given the increasing prevalence of non-traditional jobs and complex organisational contexts, including remote work, leaderless organisations, radical change, and global uncertainty. Organisations stand to gain by renegotiating boundaries with workers and providing training that supports effective work recovery across new and emerging occupational environments (Sonnentag et al., 2022; Weigelt et al., 2019).

Social support. In the recovery research, social support from peers and supervisors has been associated with replenished energy, decreased physiological activation (Fostervold & Watten, 2022; Fu et al., 2023; Schilbach et al., 2021; Volmer et al., 2023), and identified as a protective factor linked to resilience (Baethge et al., 2020). The resilience literature has similarly extolled the importance of social support (Degbey & Einola, 2020; Malinen et al., 2019; Näswall et al., 2019), and described how organisations can set up a resilience-promoting environment. In essence, resilience-promoting organisations ensure that workers have opportunities for and are encouraged to seek support and feedback from managers and peers, to engage in meaningful social interactions, and to extend and strengthen personal and professional networks. Organisations that intentionally capitalise on social support create favourable conditions for worker recovery. By investing in feedback elicitation and provision skills, specifying the value of social connections to well-being, designing co-located and remote work for successful collaboration, and implementing research-informed diversity and inclusion strategies, organisations develop resilience capability and support effective worker recovery through increased opportunities for mastery, affiliation, and meaning experiences.

On the flipside of social support, the research shows that incivility perpetrated by organisational members or external stakeholders has been linked to poor recovery outcomes (Demsky et al., 2019). While trait resilience attenuates the detrimental effect of incivility on recovery (Yang et al., 2020) and recovery experiences such as relaxation and psychological detachment from work buffer against the impact of negative affective states caused by incivility, the depletion of cognitive and emotional resources that ensues from exposure to incivility poses a threat to resilience. Together, these findings suggest that opportunities to recover from work, coupled with the regulatory capacity to psychologically detach from work and relax, mitigate the negative impact of incivility on recovery and well-being outcomes. Nevertheless, leaders should strive to safeguard a psychologically safe environment. By setting clear standards of constructive communication and promoting worker voice, leaders will reduce the frequency of negative exchanges and the detrimental effects of low agency on resilience and other personal resources linked to recovery (Edmondson, 2019; Yulita et al., 2022).

Balancing at-work and off-work recovery. A holistic approach to organisational recovery relies on the assumption that effective recovery requires a balance between, and integration of, at-work and off-work recovery activities (Chan et al., 2022; Ginoux et al., 2021; Smith et al., 2022). This approach ensures that workers restore energy and psychological functioning through experiences of control, mastery, and relaxation, and by engaging in psychological detachment from work. A holistic view of recovery intersects with an ecological perspective of resilience development, which underscores the significance of a broad resource ecosystem and deems factors outside the work sphere (e.g., family support) as vital to building resilience capability as those available from work (e.g., leader support). Resilience development is therefore contingent on the extent to which the organisation provides opportunities to draw on resources from work and non-work domains to manage demands (Kuntz, Malinen, & Näswall, 2017). Likewise, contemporary recovery research demonstrates how organisations foster recovery experiences by endorsing both at-work and off-work recovery activities (for recent reviews, see Chan et al., 2022; Karabinski et al., 2021; Smith et al., 2022; Steed et al., 2021). Importantly, organisations have a critical role in considering the exigencies of peak performance times specific to their sector (e.g., end of financial year, pre-holiday periods), and support staff to manage stress and sustain resilience by implementing recovery interventions consistent with anticipated stress levels (Kellmann & Heidari, 2020).

Conclusion and recommendations for practice

The selection of effective recovery activities, timely engagement in recovery, and strength of association between recovery activities and recovery experiences are predicated on the interplay of resilience (personal resource) with an autonomy-enabling and supportive organisational environment. Viewed through a resilience lens, organising for recovery serves not only as a protective approach that improves workers' ability to cope with everyday stressors, but also as a preparedness tactic that equips workers and organisations to successfully navigate stress through periods of high job demand, uncertainty, and crises. Organisations can create environments that concurrently promote work recovery and resilience development by considering the following:

1. ***Recovery is personal*:** Workers vary in their preference for recovery activities and in the extent to which these activities result in stress reduction, energy restoration, and resilience development. What's more, individual preferences for and the effectiveness of specific recovery activities vary from day-to-day and over time. While this may suggest that fostering recovery requires organisations to identify each worker's unique needs and have a tailored approach to recovery, this would represent a taxing and unreasonable proposition for many workplaces. Instead, organisations can clearly communicate the importance of recovery activities and experiences to worker performance, well-being, and resilience (e.g., through training and leadership communications), delineate the parameters of what constitute acceptable at-work recovery activities within their unique context (e.g., microbreaks, task-switching, relaxation techniques, socialisation, exercise), and allow workers the discretion to select the activities that best fit their needs to ensure recovered states and resilience development.
2. ***Lead for recovery*:** Leaders are pivotal in building recovery into organisations through communication, support, and other leadership functions. First, they should clearly communicate the importance of recovery and the availability of at-work recovery activities in one-on-one conversations and team debriefs. These communications serve to reiterate the impact of stress on human functioning, underscore that recovery activities are not 'one size fits all', and to guide workers through the options available to maximise effective outcomes. Second, leaders should role model recovery by also engaging in these activities at work. Role modelling signals that recovery is an endorsed organisational practice and normalises recovery activities during the workday. Relatedly, leaders' espousal of and openness to discuss work recovery and its benefits contributes to the development of a psychologically safe environment where employees feel empowered not only to carry out recovery activities, but also to explore, propose, and modify these activities to offset new or heightened work demands and develop personal resources.
3. ***Organise for recovery*:** Further to the provision of training that covers the importance of work recovery to stress management, performance, and well-being, and of clear communication around the range of recovery activities that are commensurate with the organisation's characteristics and occupational requirements, including activities tailored to reduce stress

through periods of high demand, workplaces can set up practices and structures to support recovery. In some organisations, this may entail setting boundaries around email accessibility outside business hours, thereby managing technostress (e.g., techno-invasion or the pressure to be constantly connected to work) which impedes psychological detachment and relaxation experiences. In others, recovery may be supported by job design options that permit greater flexibility around scheduling and breaks, promote frequent informal interactions and group recovery activities that leverage the restorative effects of social support, or allow workers to engage in job crafting and regular upskilling that elicits mastery, control, and other recovery experiences.

References

Baethge, A., Vahle-Hinz, T., & Rigotti, T. (2020). Coworker support and its relationship to allostasis during a workday: A diary study on trajectories of heart rate variability during work. *Journal of Applied Psychology, 105*(5), 506–526.

Bakker, A., & de Vries, J. (2021). Job demands-resources theory and self-regulation: New explanations and remedies for job burnout. *Anxiety, Stress, and Coping, 34*(1), 1–21.

Beckmann, J. (2002). Interaction of volition and recovery. In M. Kellmann (Ed.), *Enhancing recovery: Preventing underperformance in athletes* (pp. 269–282). Human Kinetics.

Beckmann, J., & Kellmann, M. (2004). Self-regulation and recovery: Approaching an understanding of the process of recovery from stress. *Psychological Reports, 95*(3), 1135–1153.

Bennett, A., Bakker, A., & Field, J. (2018). Recovery from work-related effort: A meta-analysis. *Journal of Organizational Behavior, 39*(3), 262–275.

Blanco-Donoso, L. M., Garrosa, E., Demerouti, E., & Moreno-Jiménez, B. (2017). Job resources and recovery experiences to face difficulties in emotion regulation at work: A diary study among nurses. *International Journal of Stress Management, 24*(2), 107–134.

Bonanno, G. A. (2004). Loss, trauma, and human resilience: Have we underestimated the human capacity to thrive after extremely aversive events? *The American Psychologist, 59*(1), 20–28.

Bosch, C., Sonnentag, S., & Pinck, A. S. (2018). What makes for a good break? A diary study on recovery experiences during lunch break. *Journal of Occupational and Organizational Psychology, 91*(1), 134–157.

Cham, B. S., Boeing, A. A., Wilson, M. D., Griffin, M. A., & Jorritsma, K. (2021). Endurance in extreme work environments. *Organizational Psychology Review, 11*(4), 343–364.

Chan, P. H. H., Howard, J., Eva, N., & Tse, H. H. M. (2022). A systematic review of at-work recovery and a framework for future research. *Journal of Vocational Behavior, 137*, 103747. https://doi.org/10.1016/j.jvb.2022.103747

Chong, S., Kim, Y., Lee, H., Johnson, R., & Lin, S. (2020). Mind your own break! The interactive effect of workday respite activities and mindfulness on employee outcomes via affective linkages. *Organizational Behavior and Human Decision Processes, 159*, 64–77.

Clauss, E., Hoppe, A., O'Shea, D., González Morales, M. G., Steidle, A., & Michel, A. (2018). Promoting personal resources and reducing exhaustion through positive work reflection among caregivers. *Journal of Occupational Health Psychology, 23*(1), 127–140.

Conlin, A., Hu, X., & Barber, L. K. (2020). Comparing relaxation versus mastery microbreak activity: A within-task recovery perspective. *Psychological Reports*, *124*(1), 248–265.

Connor, K. M., & Davidson, J. R. T. (2003). Development of a new resilience scale: The Connor-Davidson resilience scale (CD-RISC). *Depression and Anxiety*, *18*(2), 76–82.

Crane, M. F., Searle, B. J., Kangas, M., & Nwiran, Y. (2019). How resilience is strengthened by exposure to stressors: The systematic self-reflection model of resilience strengthening. *Anxiety, Stress, and Coping*, *32*(1), 1–17.

de Bloom, J., Rantanen, J., Tement, S., & Kinnunen, U. (2018). Longitudinal leisure activity profiles and their associations with recovery experiences and job performance. *Leisure Sciences*, *40*(3), 151–173.

de Bloom, J., Sianoja, M., Korpela, K., Tuomisto, M., Lilja, A., Geurts, S., & Kinnunen, U. (2017). Effects of park walks and relaxation exercises during lunch breaks on recovery from job stress: Two randomized controlled trials. *Journal of Environmental Psychology*, *51*, 14–30.

Deci, E. L., & Ryan, R. M. (2008). Self-determination theory: A macrotheory of human motivation, development, and health. *Psychologie Canadienne*, *49*(3), 182–185.

Degbey, W. Y., & Einola, K. (2020). Resilience in virtual teams: Developing the capacity to bounce back. *Applied Psychology*, *69*(4), 1301–1337.

Demsky, C. A., Fritz, C., Hammer, L. B., & Black, A. E. (2019). Workplace incivility and employee sleep: The role of rumination and recovery experiences. *Journal of Occupational Health Psychology*, *24*(2), 228–240.

Diotaiuti, P., Corrado, S., Mancone, S., & Falese, L. (2021). Resilience in the endurance runner: The role of self-regulatory modes and basic psychological needs. *Frontiers in Psychology*, *11*, 558287. https://doi.org/10.3389/fpsyg.2020.558287

Edmondson, A. (2019). The role of psychological safety. *Leader to Leader*, *92*, 13–19.

Fisher, D. M., Ragsdale, J. M., & Fisher, E. C. (2019). The importance of definitional and temporal issues in the study of resilience. *Applied Psychology*, *68*(4), 583–620.

Fletcher, D., & Sarkar, M. (2013). Psychological resilience: A review and critique of definitions, concepts, and theory. *European Psychologist*, *18*(1), 12–23.

Fostervold, K. I., & Watten, R. G. (2022). Put your feet up: The impact of personality traits, job pressure, and social support on the need for recovery after work. *Current Psychology*. https://doi.org/10.1007/s12144-022-02950-1

Fu, X., Du, B., Chen, Q., Norbäck, D., Lindgren, T., Janson, C., & Runeson-Broberg, R. (2023). Self-rated health (SRH), recovery from work, fatigue, and insomnia among commercial pilots concerning occupational and non-occupational factors. *Frontiers in Public Health*, *10*, 1050776. https://doi.org/10.3389/fpubh.2022.1050776

Gan, Y., Chen, Y., Han, X., Yu, N. X., & Wang, L. (2019). Neuropeptide Y gene × environment interaction predicts resilience and positive future focus. *Applied Psychology: Health and Wellbeing*, *11*(3), 438–458.

Ginoux, C., Isoard-Gautheur, S., & Sarrazin, P. (2021). "What did you do this weekend?" Relationships between weekend activities, recovery experiences, and changes in work-related well-being. *Applied Psychology: Health and Well-Being*, *13*(4), 798–816.

Hartmann, S., Weiss, M., Newman, A., & Hoegl, M. (2020). Resilience in the workplace: A multilevel review and synthesis. *Applied Psychology*, *69*(3), 913–959.

Hobfoll, S. E. (1989). Conservation of resources: A new attempt at conceptualizing stress. *The American Psychologist*, *44*(3), 513–524.

Hobfoll, S. E., Halbesleben, J., Neveu, J., & Westman, M. (2018). Conservation of resources in the organizational context: The reality of resources and their consequences. *Annual Review of Organizational Psychology and Organizational Behavior, 5*(1), 103–128.

IJntema, R. C., Schaufeli, W. B., & Burger, Y. D. (2023). Resilience mechanisms at work: The psychological immunity-psychological elasticity (PI-PE) model of psychological resilience. *Current Psychology, 42*, 4719–4731.

Jalonen, N., Kinnunen, M., Pulkkinen, L., & Kokko, K. (2015). Job skill discretion and emotion control strategies as antecedents of recovery from work. *European Journal of Work and Organizational Psychology, 24*(3), 389–401.

Jo, Y., & Lee, D. (2022). Activated at home but deactivated at work: How daily mobile work leads to next-day psychological withdrawal behavior. *Journal of Organizational Behavior, 43*(1), 1–16.

Karabinski, T., Haun, V. C., Nübold, A., Wendsche, J., & Wegge, J. (2021). Interventions for improving psychological detachment from work: A meta-analysis. *Journal of Occupational Health Psychology, 26*(3), 224–242.

Kellmann, M., & Heidari, J. (2020). Changes in the perception of stress and recovery in German secondary school teachers. *Teacher Development, 24*(2), 242–257.

Kim, S., Park, Y., & Headrick, L. (2018). Daily micro-breaks and job performance: General work engagement as a cross-level moderator. *Journal of Applied Psychology, 103*(7), 772–786.

Kubo, T., Sugawara, D., & Masuyama, A. (2021). The effect of ego-resiliency and COVID-19-related stress on mental health among the Japanese population. *Personality and Individual Differences, 175*, 110702. https://doi.org/10.1016/j.paid.2021.110702

Kuntz, J. C. (2021). Resilience in times of global pandemic: Steering recovery and thriving trajectories. *Applied Psychology, 70*(1), 188–215.

Kuntz, J. C., Connell, P., & Näswall, K. (2017). Workplace resources and employee resilience: The role of regulatory profiles. *Career Development International, 22*(4), 419–435.

Kuntz, J. C., Malinen, S., & Näswall, K. (2017). Employee resilience: Directions for resilience development. *Consulting Psychology Journal, 69*(3), 223–242.

Lau, W. K., Tai, A. P., Chan, J., Lau, B., & Geng, X. (2021). Integrative psycho-biophysiological markers in predicting psychological resilience. *Psychoneuroendocrinology, 129*, 105267. https://doi.org/10.1016/j.psyneuen.2021.105267

Malinen, S., Hatton, T., Näswall, K., & Kuntz, J. C. (2019). Strategies to enhance employee well-being and organisational performance in a postcrisis environment: A case study. *Journal of Contingencies and Crisis Management, 27*(1), 79–86.

Maltby, J., & Hall, S. S. (2022). Less is more: Discovering the latent factors of trait resilience. *Journal of Research in Personality, 97*, 104193. https://doi.org/10.1016/j.jrp.2022.104193

Meijman, T. F., & Mulder, G. (1998). Psychological aspects of workload. In P. J. D. Drenth, H. Thierry, & C. J. de Wolff (Eds.), *Handbook of work and organizational psychology. Work psychology* (pp. 5–33). Psychology Press.

Muraven, M., & Baumeister, R. F. (2000). Self-regulation and depletion of limited resources: Does self-control resemble a muscle? *Psychological Bulletin, 126*(2), 247–259.

Näswall, K., Malinen, S., Kuntz, J., & Hodliffe, M. (2019). Employee resilience: Development and validation of a measure. *Journal of Managerial Psychology, 34*(5), 353–367.

Newman, D. B., Tay, L., & Diener, E. (2014). Leisure and subjective well-being: A model of psychological mechanisms as mediating factors. *Journal of Happiness Studies, 15*(3), 555–578.

Niks, I., Gevers, J., de Jonge, J., & Houtman, I. (2016). The relation between off-job recovery and job resources: Person-level differences and day-level dynamics. *European Journal of Work and Organizational Psychology, 25*(2), 226–238.

Nolzen, N. (2018). The concept of psychological capital: A comprehensive review. *Management Review Quarterly, 68*(3), 237–277.

Ouyang, K., Cheng, B. H., Lam, W., & Parker, S. K. (2019). Enjoy your evening, be proactive tomorrow: How off-job experiences shape daily proactivity. *Journal of Applied Psychology, 104*(8), 1003–1019.

Parker, S. L., Dawson, N., Van den Broeck, A., Sonnentag, S., & Neal, A. (2021). Employee motivation profiles, energy levels, and approaches to sustaining energy: A two-wave latent-profile analysis. *Journal of Vocational Behavior, 131*, 103659. https://doi.org/10.1016/j.jvb.2021.103659

Perko, K., Kinnunen, U., & Feldt, T. (2017). Long-term profiles of work-related rumination associated with leadership, job demands, and exhaustion: A three-wave study. *Work and Stress, 31*(4), 395–420.

Ragsdale, J. M., & Beehr, T. A. (2016). A rigorous test of a model of employees' resource recovery mechanisms during a weekend. *Journal of Organizational Behavior, 37*(6), 911–932.

Rost, E. A., Glasgow, T. E., & Calderwood, C. (2021). Active today, replenished tomorrow? How daily physical activity diminishes next-morning depletion. *Applied Psychology: Health and Well-Being, 13*(1), 219–238.

Schilbach, M., Baethge, A., & Rigotti, T. (2021). Do challenge and hindrance job demands prepare employees to demonstrate resilience? *Journal of Occupational Health Psychology, 26*(3), 155–174.

Smith, T. A., Butts, M. M., Courtright, S. H., Duerden, M. D., & Widmer, M. A. (2022). Work-leisure blending: An integrative conceptual review and framework to guide future research. *Journal of Applied Psychology, 107*(4), 560–580.

Sonnentag, S., Cheng, B. H., & Parker, S. L. (2022). Recovery from work: Advancing the field toward the future. *Annual Review of Organizational Psychology and Organizational Behavior, 9*(1), 33–60.

Sonnentag, S., & Fritz, C. (2007). The Recovery Experience Questionnaire: Development and validation of a measure for assessing recuperation and unwinding from work. *Journal of Occupational Health Psychology, 12*(3), 204–221.

Sonnentag, S., & Fritz, C. (2015). Recovery from job stress: The stressor-detachment model as an integrative framework. *Journal of Organizational Behavior, 36*(S1), S72–S103.

Sonnentag, S., & Geurts, S. A. E. (2009). Methodological issues in recovery research. In S. Sonnentag, P. L. Perrewé, & D. C. Ganster (Eds.), *Current perspectives on job-stress recovery* (pp. 1–46). Emerald Group Publishing Limited.

Sonnentag, S., Stephan, U., Wendsche, J., de Bloom, J., Syrek, C., & Vahle-Hinz, T. (2021). Recovery in occupational health psychology and human resource management research: An interview with Prof. Sabine Sonnentag and Prof. Ute Stephan. *German Journal of Human Resource Management, 35*(2), 274–281.

Sonnentag, S., Venz, L., & Casper, A. (2017). Advances in recovery research: What have we learned? What should be done next? *Journal of Occupational Health Psychology, 22*(3), 365–380.

Southwick, S. M., Bonanno, G. A., Masten, A. S., Panter-Brick, C., & Yehuda, R. (2014). Resilience definitions, theory, and challenges: Interdisciplinary perspectives. *European Journal of Psychotraumatology, 5*, 25338. https://doi.org/10.3402/ejpt.v5.25338

Steed, L. B., Swider, B. W., Keem, S., & Liu, J. T. (2021). Leaving work at work: A meta-analysis on employee recovery from work. *Journal of Management*, *47*(4), 867–897.

ten Brummelhuis, L. L., & Trougakos, J. P. (2014). The recovery potential of intrinsically versus extrinsically motivated off-job activities. *Journal of Occupational and Organizational Psychology*, *87*(1), 177–199.

Trougakos, J. P., Hideg, I., Cheng, B. H., & Beal, D. J. (2014). Lunch breaks unpacked: The role of autonomy as a moderator of recovery during lunch. *Academy of Management Journal*, *57*(2), 405–421.

Troy, A. S., Willroth, E. C., Shallcross, A. J., Giuliani, N. R., Gross, J. J., & Mauss, I. B. (2023). Psychological resilience: An affect-regulation framework. *Annual Review of Psychology*, *74*, 1810–1830.

van Hooff, M. L., Flaxman, P. E., Söderberg, M., Stride, C. B., & Geurts, S. A. (2018). Basic psychological need satisfaction, recovery state, and recovery timing. *Human Performance*, *31*(2), 125–143.

Verbeek, J., Ruotsalainen, J., Laitinen, J., Korkiakangas, E., Lusa, S., Mänttäri, S., & Oksanen, T. (2019). Interventions to enhance recovery in healthy workers: A scoping review. *Occupational Medicine*, *69*(1), 54–63.

Virtanen, A., Van Laethem, M., de Bloom, J., & Kinnunen, U. (2021). Dramatic breaks: Break recovery experiences as mediators between job demands and affect in the afternoon and evening. *Stress and Health*, *37*(4), 801–818.

Volmer, J., Schulte, E., & Fritz, C. (2023). Facilitating employee recovery from work: The role of leader-member-exchange. *Occupational Health Science*, *7*, 297–319.

Weigelt, O., Syrek, C. J., Schmitt, A., & Urbach, T. (2019). Finding peace of mind when there still is so much left undone: A diary study on how job stress, competence need satisfaction, and proactive work behavior contribute to work-related rumination during the weekend. *Journal of Occupational Health Psychology*, *24*(3), 373–386.

Weinberger, E., Wach, D., Stephan, U., & Wegge, J. (2018). Having a creative day: Understanding entrepreneurs' daily idea generation through a recovery lens. *Journal of Business Venturing*, *33*(1), 1–19.

Yang, F., Lu, M., & Huang, X. (2020). Customer mistreatment and employee well-being: A daily diary study of recovery mechanisms for frontline restaurant employees in a hotel. *International Journal of Hospitality Management*, *91*, 102665. https://doi.org/10.1016/j.ijhm.2020.102665

Yulita Idris, M., & Abdullah, S. (2022). Psychosocial safety climate improves psychological detachment and relaxation during off-job recovery time to reduce emotional exhaustion: A multilevel shortitudinal study. *Scandinavian Journal of Psychology*, *63*(1), 19–31.

Zijlstra, F. R. H., Cropley, M., & Rydstedt, L. W. (2014). From recovery to regulation: An attempt to reconceptualize "recovery from work". *Stress and Health*, *30*(3), 244–252.

13 Death due to overwork

Problems and solutions

Tomohide Kubo, Xinxin Liu, and Tomoaki Matsuo

Introduction

The Japanese word, *Karoshi* has been internationally recognised since it was listed in the *Oxford English Dictionary* in 2002 (North & Morioka, 2016). Generally, *Karoshi* is defined as a fatal incidence and an associated work disability due to cardiovascular or cerebrovascular attacks, which could occur due to aggravated hypertensive or arteriosclerotic diseases, triggered by a heavy workload (Uehata, 1991). Meanwhile, according to Act Promoting Measures to Prevent Death and Injury from Overwork (Ministry of Justice Japan, 2014) in Japan, *Karoshi* is legally defined as a) 'death and injury from overwork' means death due to cerebrovascular disease or heart disease that is brought by an overload of work, b) death by suicide due to a mental disorder that is brought by an intense psychological burden at work, or c) cerebrovascular disease, heart disease, or a mental disorder brought on by such work-related causes. Thus, *Karoshi* officially includes survival cases, but this chapter focuses on death cases due to overwork.

Karoshi still occur in Japan because approximately 200 *Karoshi* cases are compensated annually (Ministry of Health Labour and Welfare Japan, 2022). This problem has spread throughout other countries, especially in Asia, during the last decade (Cheng et al., 2012; Kim et al., 2019; Lin et al., 2017). Besides, the World Health Organization (WHO) and International Labour Organization (ILO) recently reported that exposure to long working hours (≥55 hours/week) is common and causes a large attributable burden of ischaemic heart disease and stroke. Based on a previous report, the estimated 745,194 deaths (705,786–784,601) from ischaemic heart disease and stroke combined were attributable to this exposure worldwide (Pega et al., 2021). Thus, the problem regarding long working hours and *Karoshi* is serious not only in Japan but also in other parts of the world. Moreover, coronavirus disease (COVID-19) changed the working

Kubo, T., Liu, X., & Matsuo, T. (2024). Death due to overwork: Problems and solutions. In M. Kellmann & J. Beckmann (Eds.), *Fostering Recovery and Well-being in a Healthy Lifestyle: Psychological, Somatic, and Organizational Prevention Approaches* (pp. 199–217). Routledge.

DOI: 10.4324/9781003250654-17

style, such as the establishment of remote/mobile working, which made the boundary between work and private life blurry. Given the worldwide changes in working style, more serious consequences from 'invisible' overwork are expected to surface in the future. For instance, boundaryless work could have the potential risks of sleep disturbance linked to health problems (Barber & Jenkins, 2014; Vieten et al., 2022).

National criteria for recognising and compensating Karoshi cases in Japan

The following three viewpoints regarding work overload are stipulated to compensate whether a claimed case should be applicable as *Karoshi* (Park et al., 2012) in Japan. The length of working hours is the most critical viewpoint. Particularly, working >80 hours of overtime a month is defined as the *Karoshi* line, which is closely related to the occurrence of *Karoshi*.

1) **Short-term work overload**
   A worker has taken on a clearly excessive workload, imposing a very significant physical or mental burden (compared with that of normal work) within approximately one week prior to disease appearance.
2) **Long-term work overload**
   A worker has engaged in long-term excessive heavy work. A stronger correlation can be assumed between an individual's work and disease appearance, if a worker has experienced working overtime more than approximately 100 hours during the one month prior to disease appearance, or by working overtime of approximately 80 hours per month during a period of two to six months prior to the appearance of such disease.
3) **Abnormal event**
   An abnormal event includes a) extreme tension, excitement, fear, or wonder or, b) an accidental or unpredictable incident, which urgently places a worker under a physical burden, or c) a rapid and significant change in the working environment.

Park et al. (2012) reported that only three countries in the world have national criteria for recognising and compensating *Karoshi* cases. In addition to the Japanese criteria (Ministry of Health Labour and Welfare Japan, 2001), similar criteria were established in Taiwan in 2004 (Occupational Safety and Health Administration, 2021) and in the Republic of Korea in 2013 (Republic of Korea, 2021). Basically, those criteria stipulate that *Karoshi* could be caused by overwork, after excluding personal and other workplace risk factors. Moreover, the Japanese criteria were recently updated in 2021 (Ministry of Health Labour and Welfare Japan, 2021). Notably, the viewpoint of daily rest period between working days (i.e., work-interval system), stipulated by the European Union's (EU) Working Time Directive (EUR-Lex, 2003), was added in the new criteria.

Risky occupations for Karoshi cases

It would be informative to understand what kind of occupations have potential risks of *Karoshi* in Japan. As shown in Figure 13.1, the number of compensated *Karoshi* cases varied among occupations (Takahashi, 2019). Transport and postal activities showed the largest number of compensation cases. To control for the number of employees working in the given industry, the incidence rate (IR), which is the number of compensated cases per 1 million employees in each occupation, was calculated. Consequently, Figure 13.1 shows that the highest IR was observed in fisheries, but the number was only 14 compensated cases. The second highest IR was transport and postal activities, thereby suggesting that they are thought to be most risky occupations. Besides, the study reports that the highest generation was 50s, followed by 40s. Overall, *Karoshi* cases are more present in males than in females.

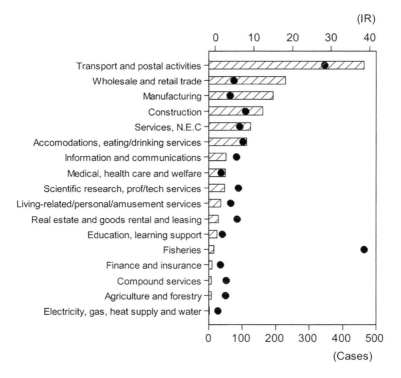

Figure 13.1 Number of compensated cases (▨) and incidence rates (IRs, ●) for over-work-related cerebrovascular and cardiovascular diseases from January 2010 to March 2015.
Note: Services, NEC: Services, Not elsewhere classified.
Reprinted with permission from Takahashi, M. (2019). Sociomedical problems of overwork-related deaths and disorders in Japan. *Journal of Occupational Health*, *61*(4), 269–277.

Sakai and Sasaki (2018) focused on truck drivers who have one of the riskiest occupations in *Karoshi* cases and analysed the data of workers' compensation claims (including not-accepted claims) coupled with work shift schedules. Truck drivers who worked fixed and irregular schedules with an early morning start (i.e., pattern 6 and 7 in Figure 13.2) showed the highest percentage of cerebro-vascular and cardiovascular diseases in all work schedule patterns regardless of compensation situation. It should be noted that higher cases were observed in fixed and irregular schedules with an early morning start than long working hour schedules (i.e., pattern 1 and 2 in Figure 13.2). These findings suggest that early morning work could negatively affect health at work compared with long working hours. Namely, the management of time of day is also important to prevent overwork-related disease in addition to the management of length of working hours.

Furthermore, mental disorder is another aspect of adverse consequences resulting from long working hours. Yamauchi et al. (2018) examined the association between work-related adverse events and workers' compensation for mental disorders by using a Japanese database containing industrial accident compensation insurance claims for mental disorders (Yamauchi et al., 2018).

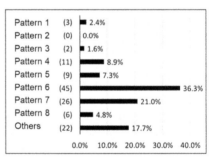

Figure 13.2 Work schedule patterns and cerebrovascular and cardiovascular diseases among truck drivers.
Reprinted with permission from Sakai, T., & Sasaki, T. (2018). 過労死等の実態解明と防止対策に関する総合的な労働安全衛生研究 [An analytical study for preventing and predicting Karoshi cases in transport and postal activities]. *Report of the industrial disease clinical research grants from the Ministry of Health, Labour and Welfare, Government of Japan* (pp. 102–132). https://www.jniosh.johas.go.jp/publication/houkoku/houkoku_overwork_2018.pdf

Among 1,362 cases, almost all cases with compensation for mental disorders were attributed to 'long working hours' (Figure 13.3). However, mental health disorders also occurred due to other work-related events, such as 'accidents/disasters' and 'interpersonal conflict'. Moreover, the trend was different considering gender and industries. Particularly, the occurrence of mental disorders among male employees was more closely related to 'long working hours'. In the future, therefore, preventive measures against mental disorders should be implemented considering gender- and industry-based differences.

Long working hours and mortality

Working long hours is equal to shortening private life, thereby deteriorating recovery. Although the definition of recovery is different among research areas, Kellmann et al. (2018) reported that recovery is regarded as a multifaceted (e.g., physiological, psychological) restorative process relative to time. Moreover, they pointed out that an imbalance of long-term fatigue and insufficient recovery initiates an unfavorable development, resulting in negative consequences. Considering the link between long working hours and insufficient recovery, it is natural that sleep plays an essential role in recovering from work-related fatigue. Namely, shortened sleep resulting from long working time or overtime would increase the likelihood of the occurrence of *Karoshi*.

As introduced earlier, the riskiest trigger of *Karoshi* is considered to be the long working hours in any country with the *Karoshi* criteria. In a previous systematic review, the relationship between long working hours and heart disease and stroke was examined by using data of 603,838 individuals derived from 25 studies (Kivimäki et al., 2015). Consequently, the dose-response relationship was more evident in stroke cases than in heart disease cases. The finding is consistent with the previously mentioned WHO and ILO collaborative study (Pega et al., 2021). The study showed that the population-attributable fractions for deaths were 3.7% (95% uncertainty range; 3.4–4.0) for ischaemic heart disease and 6.9% for stroke (95% uncertainty range; 6.4–7.5). Moreover, 8.9% of the global population was reportedly exposed to long working hours (≥55 hours per week). Hence, long working hours should be avoided in order to prevent health issues, although the adverse effects might be different by individual trait (e.g., gender, age, and physical strength), or work-related factors (e.g., time of day, options for regenerative breaks, and job-demand-control-balance).

Meanwhile, both studies mentioned above (Kivimäki et al., 2015; Pega et al., 2021) did not examine the effect of ≥80 working hours (i.e., *Karoshi* line) on health outcomes. Probably, that is the reason why available data regarding excessive long working hours are lacking in European countries and the US. Further studies are needed to better understand the mechanisms underlying the occurrence of *Karoshi*.

Additionally, the length of working hours is one of the biggest triggers of *Karoshi*, but the quality of workload, i.e., job stress, is also critical to understand its occurrence. To examine the association between job stress and mortality,

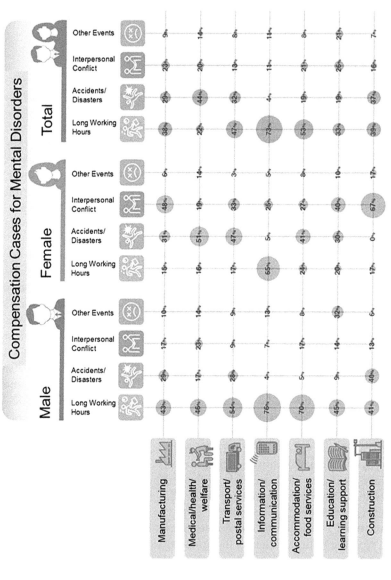

Figure 13.3 Percentage of compensated cases for mental disorders according to industry- and work-related events in males and females. Reprinted with permission from Yamauchi, T., Sasaki, T., Yoshikawa, T., Matsumoto, S., Takahashi, M., Suka, M., & Yanagisawa, H. (2018). Differences in work-related adverse events by sex and industry in cases involving compensation for mental disorders and suicide in Japan from 2010 to 2014. *Journal of Occupational and Environmental Medicine, 60*(4), e178–e182.

Kivimäki et al. (2018) conducted a meta-analysis using data of 102,663 individuals from seven cohort studies (initiated between 1985 and 2002 in Finland, France, Sweden, and the UK). As shown in Figure 13.4, in men with cardiometabolic disease, job stress could increase mortality risk, whereas no difference was found between women with and without the disease. Therefore, managing job stress is necessary to prevent the occurrence of *Karoshi*, especially among male employees with diseases such as diabetes, stroke, and myocardial infarction.

The level of job stress could be expected to be higher with longer working hours, although individual differences could mediate the linkage between long working hours and job stress (Kallus & Gaisbachgrabner, 2018; Kuntz, this volume, Chapter 12). However, currently, the *Karoshi* criteria do not consider the effect of job stress because it is difficult to detect the casual link between job stress and the occurrence of *Karoshi* by using the data of the national investigation report.

Accordingly, an appropriate measure to evaluate the stress levels among employees is required in the future. For instance, the use of annual health check-ups including stress measurements may be effective to investigate whether a claim is a compensated *Karoshi* case.

Age-related vulnerability for long working hours

Long working hours is the most potent risk factor for the occurrence of *Karoshi*. However, little is known about how individual differences, such as age, gender, and physical strength, could be related to the occurrence of *Karoshi*. Among the individual differences, the aging effect should be given more attention as *Karoshi* commonly occurs in the elderly working population. To fill the gap, Liu et al. (2019) conducted an experimental study investigating the association between long working hours and hemodynamic functions among workers in their 30s, 40s, and 50s (Liu et al., 2019). Under the simulated 12-hour working condition, all age groups significantly showed increased systolic blood pressure with longer working hours (Figure 13.5).

Notably, the tendency was more obvious in those in their 50s as compared with the other groups, especially in the latter half of working hours. Based on the findings of previous studies (Boehme et al., 2017; Finegold et al., 2013), aging could contribute to the occurrence of stroke and heart disease, but the findings of Liu et al. (2019) provide novel insights into the effect of aging on hemodynamic functions in terms of time-on-task. However, such age-related vulnerability for long working hours is not currently considered in the *Karoshi* criteria. Considering vulnerability is important when establishing the criteria of *Karoshi* in the future.

Preventive solutions against the occurrence of Karoshi

Some preventive solutions at the organisational and individual levels are discussed in this section. As a regulatory-based solution, the work-interval system,

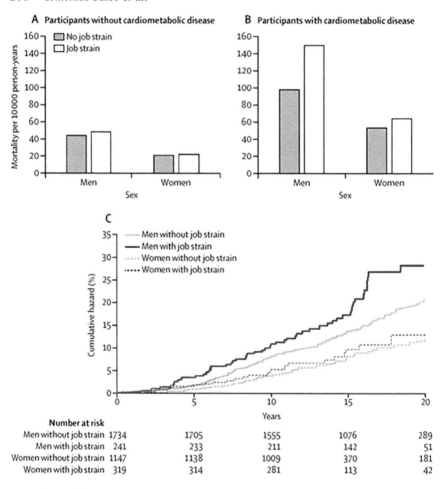

Figure 13.4 Job strain and age-adjusted mortality.
          Note: Job strain and mortality in participants without (A) and with cardio-
          metabolic disease (B) at baseline, and cumulative hazard in participants with
          cardiometabolic disease at baseline (C).
          Reprinted with permission from Kivimäki, M., Pentti, J., Ferrie, J. E.,
          Batty, G. D., Nyberg, S. T., Jokela, M., Virtanen, M., Alfredsson, L.,
          Dragano, N., Fransson, E. I., Goldberg, M., Knutsson, A., Koskenvuo, M.,
          Koskinen, A., Kouvonen, A., Luukkonen, R., Oksanen, T., Rugulies, R.,
          Siegrist, J., ... IPD-Work Consortium. (2018). Work stress and risk of death
          in men and women with and without cardiometabolic disease: A multico-
          hort study. *Lancet Diabetes Endocrinology, 6*(9), 705–713.

the right to disconnect from work, and fatigue risk management are quite
important (Balk, this volume, Chapter 4; Kuntz, this volume, Chapter 12).
Additionally, self-care solutions requiring individual effort are discussed, such as
cardiorespiratory fitness, leisure activities, and self-monitoring wearable tools.

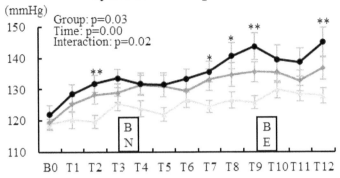

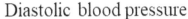

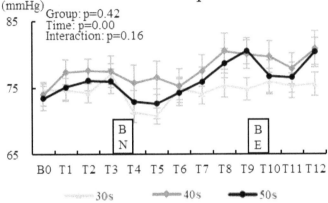

Figure 13.5 Blood pressure responses under simulated long working hours. Forty-seven males participate in and were divided into three age groups: 30s (33.9 ± 2.7 years old, *n* = 16), 40s (45.5 ± 2.9 years old, *n* = 15), and 50s (54.1 ± 2.7 years old, *n* = 16).
Note: Values are shown in terms of mean and SE. ★50s > 30s, *p* < .05; ★★50s > 30s, *p* < .01. BN: break at noon, BE: break in the evening.
Reprinted with permission from Liu, X., Ikeda, H., Oyama, F., & Takahashi, M. (2019). Haemodynamic responses to simulated long working hours in different age groups. *Occupational and Environmental Medicine*, 76(10), 754–757.

Organisational level

The biggest cause of occupational fatigue is the way employees work, namely working conditions. However, it is difficult for individuals to change working conditions. Hence, the primary prevention solution should be conducted by an organisational-level approach, such as changing the working rule.

Work-interval system

Much interest has been paid to the EU's working time directive, which stipulates recovery periods as "11 consecutive hour rest-intervals between working days (so-called work–interval system)" (Ministry of Health Labour and Welfare Japan, 2019, w. p.) to prevent *Karoshi* problems in Japan. Regarding fatigue recovery, the EU's regulation would be more effective in preventing overwork than Japan's regulation because ensuring off-job time is very important to ensure recovery from work-induced fatigue. However, to the best of our knowledge, evidence regarding the association between working conditions and appropriate recovery time is lacking even in EU countries. Especially, little is known about the effects of quick return (eleven-hour interval between working days) and health-related outcomes among daytime workers. To fill the gap, our research team has conducted some studies examining the association between recovery period and fatigue among daytime workers (Ikeda, Kubo, Izawa, et al., 2022; Ikeda et al., 2017, 2018; Kubo et al., 2018; Tsuchiya et al., 2017). Consequently, our findings suggested the links between insufficient weekday off-job time and higher blood pressure (Ikeda et al., 2017), poor mental health (Tsuchiya et al., 2017), and deteriorated sleep quantity and quality (Ikeda et al., 2018; Kubo et al., 2018). Moreover, our latest findings showed that the combination of quick returns and shorter sleep duration was related to low work productivity (i.e., presenteeism; Ikeda, Kubo, Izawa, et al., 2022). Hence, the above-mentioned work-interval system to ensure off-job time for employees would be one of the effective measures to prevent *Karoshi*.

The right to disconnect from work

Meanwhile, the boundaries between work and private life are becoming blurry with the advancement of information communication technology (ICT). Given that working remotely has become widespread worldwide due to the COVID-19 pandemic, boundaryless work could negatively affect the worker's health. Job-related communications outside official working hours would be a potential risk for health issues (Arlinghaus & Nachreiner, 2014). Notably, France has introduced the right to disconnect from work since 2017, which forbids employers from taking adverse employment action against workers who do not reply to work-related emails during off-job time. A similar law has been considered in other areas (e.g., Belgium, Germany, and New York City). Probably, such work rule-based strategy could be necessary to protect the employees' private life, although the work-interval system has already been introduced in EU countries. Kubo, Izawa, et al. (2021) examined how work-related emailing after work and off-job duration are associated with health outcomes using data from a one-month observational study. The findings suggested that deteriorated self-reported outcomes and sleep quality were more likely to occur in those with a higher frequency of work-related emailing even though off-job time was a longer condition (Figure 13.6).

It is likely that employees who often email outside working hours could have difficulty in psychologically detaching from work (Balk, this volume, Chapter 4), thereby experiencing deterioration in sleep quality and carry-over fatigue. To sum up, our finding provides empirical evidence to support the benefits of

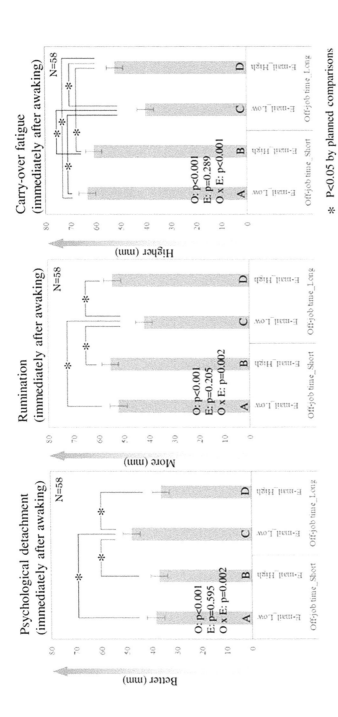

Figure 13.6 Self-reported parameters (visual analogue scale [VAS] measured psychological detachment from work, rumination, and carry-over fatigue) associated with the frequency of work-related emailing after work hours and amount of off-job time.

Note: The data regarding the VAS-measured work emailing frequency were divided into two levels (email frequency [high, low]) according to the median (median email frequency = 38 mm). Off-job time was divided into two levels (off-job time [short = less than 15h, long = 15h or more]) based on whether employees worked overtime.

Reprinted with permission from Kubo, T., Izawa, S., Ikeda, H., Tsuchiya, M., Miki, K., & Takahashi, M. (2021). Work e-mail after hours and off-job duration and their association with psychological detachment, actigraphic sleep, and saliva cortisol: A 1-month observational study for information technology employees. *Journal of Occupational Health, 63*(1), e12300. https://doi.org/10.1002/1348-9585.12300

introducing the concepts of 'the right to disconnect' and 'the work-interval system' to protect the workers' recovery opportunities by ensuring optimal sleep (Ikeda, Kubo, Sasaki, et al., 2022; Kubo et al., 2018; Kubo, Izawa, et al., 2021; Kuntz, this volume, Chapter 12).

Fatigue risk management system

To ensure safety, the International Civil Aviation Organization has recommended a Fatigue Risk Management System (FRMS) defined as "a data-driven means of continuously monitoring and managing fatigue-related safety risks, based upon scientific principles and knowledge as well as operational experience that aims to ensure relevant personnel are performing at adequate levels of alertness" (International Air Transport Association, 2011, p. 1). A traditional regulatory approach to managing crewmember fatigue has been to prescribe limits on maximum daily, monthly, and yearly flight, and duty hours, and to require minimum breaks within and between duty periods. However, prescriptive flight and duty time limits represent a somewhat simplistic view of safety – being inside the limits is safe while being outside the limits is unsafe – and they represent a single defensive strategy. Meanwhile, an FRMS employs multi-layered defensive strategies to manage fatigue-related risks regardless of their source. It includes data-driven, ongoing adaptive processes that can identify fatigue hazards and then develop, implement, and evaluate controls and mitigation strategies. Also, much attention has been paid to the FRMS as an effective solution to protect safety at work (Sprajcer et al., 2022). At the moment, the FRMS focuses on safety risks linking to a fatigue-related error and is adopted for flight crews or drivers. However, fatigue is also well known as a health risk. Hence, its applicability could be fully considered in other occupations to prevent the development of health risks.

Individual level

In principle, the preventive solution should be conducted by an organisational level approach. However, the regulatory-based solution, such as changing working conditions or establishing a new work rule, need a lot of time. Besides, new working issues, which cannot cope with the current regulatory system, have been increased by COVID-19 (e.g., gig work, remote work, etc.). Therefore, individual-based preventive solutions to counter new working issues are also critical in 'new normal' working life.

Cardiorespiratory fitness

The abovementioned organisational strategies are important to prevent *Karoshi*; however, individual strategies would be also effective. Particularly, a lower level of cardiorespiratory fitness is reported to be closely related to increased health issues and mortality (Kodama et al., 2009). Some effective measures to enhance cardiorespiratory fitness were developed in previous research. For instance, high-intensity interval training (HIIT) described as "brief intervals of vigorous activity interspersed with periods of low activity or rest" (Cassidy et al., 2017, p. 8) is well known in this area. Of the available empirical findings, an eleven-week randomised controlled trial showed that HIIT coupled with caloric restriction could be effective in increasing cardiorespiratory fitness (So & Matsuo, 2020). However, it would be challenging to evaluate cardiorespiratory fitness in normal settings because the gold standard measurement is maximal oxygen consumption, which is costly and requires a considerable amount of measurement time. Our research team then developed the Modified Worker's Living Activity-time Questionnaire (m-WLAQ; Matsuo et al., 2020) to easily predict cardiorespiratory fitness. The predicted VO_{2max} assessed by m-WLAQ significantly correlated with VO_{2max} assessed by the treadmill exercise test ($r = .77$, $p < .01$). Age, sex, and body fat-related values accounted for 43–51% of the variance in the objectively-measured VO_{2max}. The accounted variance increased 11–16% by adding the score of m-WLAQ to those factors. The test–retest reliability analyses showed that the intraclass correlation coefficient (ICC) was .87 (.82–.91) suggesting high reliability. Given that self-care and organisational management for cardiorespiratory fitness require an easy assessment, the m-WLAQ is a practical tool to promote health at work.

Leisure activity

Recovery often occurs outside official working hours. Since work and private life are the head and tail of a coin, work influences private life and vice versa. Considering *Karoshi* prevention, the primary strategy is to manage the working condition, but ensuring a recuperative opportunity during off-duty is also critical. Mentally detaching from work during off-job time (i.e., psychological detachment from work) is well known to contribute to recovery from work (Sonnentag et al., 2014). Previous research showed that individuals with higher levels of active leisure activities (e.g., exercise, creative, and social activity) reported significantly better recovery outcomes, as compared with their counterparts (Winwood et al., 2007). Accordingly, active and fulfilling off-job behaviours could be effective in promoting recovery from work. Moreover, much attention has been paid to the concept of leisure crafting, defined as "the proactive pursuit of leisure activities targeted at goal setting, human connection, learning and personal development" (Petrou & Bakker, 2016, p. 508). With ICT development, the boundaries between work and private life have been blurred. Particularly, the COVID-19 pandemic accelerated boundaryless work worldwide. Thus, employees should obtain more recovery opportunities and skills with psychological detachment from work to protect themselves.

Self-monitoring wearable tool

Much interest has been paid to digital health care since the Apple watch was sold from 2015. Notably, since 2021, the Apple watch can detect possible episodes of atrial fibrillation. According to Perez et al.'s (2019) study, of the 419,297 participants, only 0.52% received an irregular pulse notification from their Apple watch. However, 84% (95% CI, 76–92) of their subsequent notifications were confirmed to be atrial fibrillation (Perez et al., 2019). Hence, the use of a digital health care tool would be very useful to protect worker's health. Moreover, it is expected that such digital health care management will be more widespread and be required in the future (Brüßler et al., this volume, Chapter 3). Meanwhile, little is known about the early signs of *Karoshi*. Thus, Kubo, Matsumoto, et al. (2021) analyzed 1,564 documents from all areas of Japan, which were compensated for *Karoshi* from January 2010 to March 2015. Of these, 190 documents listed the prodromes of *Karoshi*, which were used to develop the Excessive Fatigue Symptom Inventory (EFSI; Kubo, Matsumoto, et al., 2021). As shown in Figure 13.7, these prodromes were classified into 26 excessive fatigue symptoms.

Then, Kubo, Matsumoto, et al. (2021) distributed a survey with EFSI to 5,410 truck drivers to investigate the association between EFSI score and history of cerebrovascular and cardiovascular diseases. Among the collected 1,992 samples, multiple logistic regression analysis showed that the occurrences of cerebrovascular and cardiovascular diseases were significantly higher in the middle [adjusted odd ratios = 3.56 (1.28–9.94)] and high-score groups [3.55 (1.24–10.21)] than in the low-score group. Therefore, the findings suggest that the EFSI is effective in evaluating a worker's potential risk for *Karoshi*.

Conclusion and recommendations for practice

Karoshi is a problem observed not only in Asia but also in other parts of the world. This chapter summarised the definitions and causes of *Karoshi* as well as its preventive and management strategies based on previous studies. The length of working hours is regarded as the most important factor in recognising *Karoshi* cases, although there are some differences among countries. The Japanese criteria stipulates that its onset is more closely related to 100 hours of overtime work in a month or an average of 80 hours of overtime work per month for up to six months. Hence, a primary strategy for handling the *Karoshi* problem should be managing working hours so as not to exceed the upper limit of working hours. On the other hand, the boundaries between work and private life will become increasingly unclear in the future due to the advancement in ICT. Accordingly, it would be more difficult to detect and manage the length of working hours in the future workplace than in the current workplace. Of course, the primary preventive strategies should be recommendable for an organisational approach, such as introducing the work-interval system, the right to disconnect from work, and the fatigue risk management system. However, more individual care may also be required to prevent overwork-related diseases in new working styles

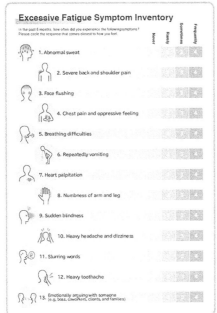

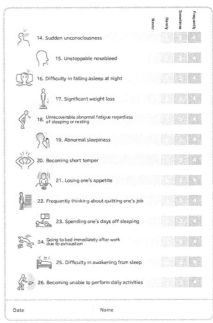

Figure 13.7 Twenty-six excessive fatigue symptoms listed in the Excessive Fatigue Symptom Inventory.

Note: Those symptoms were extracted from an information of investigators report which were accepted to compensate *Karoshi* cases from January 2010 through March 2015. Of 1,564 investigation reports, 190 documents listed the Karoshi prodromes, which were used to develop the Excessive Fatigue Symptom Inventory (EFSI). A labour standards inspector recorded those prodromes based on a medical certificate or an interview from the victim's family. We condensed a sentence into a short word regarding excessive fatigue symptoms, and thereby 162 words were derived from 190 documents. After that, we categorised the prodromes by similar symptoms with the K–J method. Consequently, those prodromes were classified into 26 excessive fatigue symptoms.

Reprinted with permission from Kubo, T., Matsumoto, S., Sasaki, T., Ikeda, H., Izawa, S., Takahashi, M., Koda, S., Sasaki, T., & Sakai, K. (2021). Shorter sleep duration is associated with potential risks for overwork-related death among Japanese truck drivers: Use of the Karoshi prodromes from worker's compensation cases. *International Archives of Occupational Environmental Health*, *94*(5), 991–1001.

(e.g., increasing individual cardiorespiratory fitness, obtaining skills to spend leisure time for effective recovery, and using wearable tools). The importance of psychological detachment from work could expand as boundaryless work between work and private life spreads globally. Therefore, ensuring recovery opportunities and skills coupled with psychological detachment from work is essential to protect all workers' health in the future.

References

Arlinghaus, A., & Nachreiner, F. (2014). Health effects of supplemental work from home in the European Union. *Chronobiology International, 31*(10), 1100–1107.

Barber, L. K., & Jenkins, J. S. (2014). Creating technological boundaries to protect bedtime: Examining work-home boundary management, psychological detachment and sleep. *Stress Health, 30*(3), 259–264.

Boehme, A. K., Esenwa, C., & Elkind, M. S. V. (2017). Stroke risk factors, genetics, and prevention. *Circulation Research, 120*(3), 472–495.

Cassidy, S., Thoma, C., Houghton, D., & Trenell, M. I. (2017). High-intensity interval training: A review of its impact on glucose control and cardiometabolic health. *Diabetologia, 60*(1), 7–23.

Cheng, Y., Park, J., Kim, Y., & Kawakami, N. (2012). The recognition of occupational diseases attributed to heavy workloads: Experiences in Japan, Korea, and Taiwan. *International Archives of Occupational and Environmental Health, 85*(7), 791–799.

EUR-Lex. (2003). Directive 2003/88/EC of the European parliament and of the council of 4 November 2003 concerning certain aspects of the organisation of working time. *Official Journal of the European Union, L299*, 9–19.

Finegold, J. A., Asaria, P., & Francis, D. P. (2013). Mortality from ischaemic heart disease by country, region, and age: Statistics from World Health Organisation and United Nations. *International Journal of Cardiology, 168*(2), 934–945.

Ikeda, H., Kubo, T., Izawa, S., Nakamura-Taira, N., Yoshikawa, T., & Akamatsu, R. (2022). The joint association of daily rest periods and sleep duration with worker health and productivity: A cross-sectional web survey of Japanese daytime workers. *International Journal of Environmental Research and Public Health, 19*(17), 11143. https://doi.org/10.3390/ijerph191711143

Ikeda, H., Kubo, T., Izawa, S., Takahashi, M., Tsuchiya, M., Hayashi, N., & Kitagawa, Y. (2017). Impact of daily rest period on resting blood pressure and fatigue: A one-month observational study of daytime employees. *Journal of Occupational Environmental Medicine, 59*(4), 397–401.

Ikeda, H., Kubo, T., Sasaki, T., Liu, X., Matsuo, T., So, R., Matsumoto, S., Yamauchi, T., & Takahashi, M. (2018). Cross-sectional Internet-based survey of Japanese permanent daytime workers' sleep and daily rest periods. *Journal of Occupational Health, 60*(3), 229–235.

Ikeda, H., Kubo, T., Sasaki, T., Nishimura, Y., Liu, X., Matsuo, T., So, R., Matsumoto, S., & Takahashi, M. (2022). Prospective changes in sleep problems in response to the daily rest period among Japanese daytime workers: A longitudinal web survey. *Journal of Sleep Research, 31*(1), e13449. https://doi.org/10.1111/jsr.13449

International Air Transport Association. (2011). Fatigue risk management system (FRMS) implementation guide for operators. Retrieved April 18, 2023 from https://www.icao.int/safety/fatiguemanagement/frms%20tools/frms%20implementation%20guide%20for%20operators%20july%202011.pdf

Kallus, K. W., & Gaisbachgrabner, K. (2018). Stress and recovery in applied settings: Long working hours, recovery, and breaks. In M. Kellmann & J. Beckmann (Eds.), *Sport, recovery, and performance: Interdisciplinary insights* (pp. 233–246). Routledge.

Kellmann, M., Bertollo, M., Bosquet, L., Brink, M., Coutts, A. J., Duffield, R., Erlacher, D., Halson, S. L., Hecksteden, A., Heidari, J., Kallus, K. W., Meeusen, R., Mujika, I., Robazza, C., Skorski, S., Venter, R., & Beckmann, J. (2018). Recovery and performance in sport: Consensus statement. *International Journal of Sports Physiology and Performance, 13*(2), 240–245.

Kim, I., Koo, M. J., Lee, H. E., Won, Y. L., & Song, J. (2019). Overwork-related disorders and recent improvement of national policy in South Korea. *Journal of Occupational Health, 61*(4), 288–296.

Kivimäki, M., Jokela, M., Nyberg, S. T., Singh-Manoux, A., Fransson, E. I., Alfredsson, L., Bjorner, J. B., Borritz, M., Burr, H., Casini, A., Clays, E., De Bacquer, D., Dragano, N., Erbel, R., Geuskens, G. A., Hamer, M., Hooftman, W. E., Houtman, I. L., Jöckel, K. H., … IPD-Work Consortium. (2015). Long working hours and risk of coronary heart disease and stroke: A systematic review and meta-analysis of published and unpublished data for 603,838 individuals. *Lancet, 386*(10005), 1739–1746.

Kivimäki, M., Pentti, J., Ferrie, J. E., Batty, G. D., Nyberg, S. T., Jokela, M., Virtanen, M., Alfredsson, L., Dragano, N., Fransson, E. I., Goldberg, M., Knutsson, A., Koskenvuo, M., Koskinen, A., Kouvonen, A., Luukkonen, R., Oksanen, T., Rugulies, R., Siegrist, J., … IPD-Work Consortium. (2018). Work stress and risk of death in men and women with and without cardiometabolic disease: A multicohort study. *Lancet Diabetes Endocrinology, 6*(9), 705–713.

Kodama, S., Saito, K., Tanaka, S., Maki, M., Yachi, Y., Asumi, M., Sugawara, A., Totsuka, K., Shimano, H., Ohashi, Y., Yamada, N., & Sone, H. (2009). Cardiorespiratory fitness as a quantitative predictor of all-cause mortality and cardiovascular events in healthy men and women: A meta-analysis. *Journal of the American Medical Association, 301*(19), 2024–2035.

Kubo, T., Izawa, S., Ikeda, H., Tsuchiya, M., Miki, K., & Takahashi, M. (2021). Work e-mail after hours and off-job duration and their association with psychological detachment, actigraphic sleep, and saliva cortisol: A 1-month observational study for information technology employees. *Journal of Occupational Health, 63*(1), e12300. https://doi.org/10.1002/1348-9585.12300

Kubo, T., Izawa, S., Tsuchiya, M., Ikeda, H., Miki, K., & Takahashi, M. (2018). Day-to-day variations in daily rest periods between working days and recovery from fatigue among information technology workers: One-month observational study using a fatigue app. *Journal of Occupational Health, 60*(5), 394–403.

Kubo, T., Matsumoto, S., Sasaki, T., Ikeda, H., Izawa, S., Takahashi, M., Koda, S., Sasaki, T., & Sakai, K. (2021). Shorter sleep duration is associated with potential risks for overwork-related death among Japanese truck drivers: Use of the Karoshi prodromes from worker's compensation cases. *International Archives of Occupational Environmental Health, 94*(5), 991–1001.

Lin, R.-T., Lin, C.-K., Christiani, D. C., Kawachi, I., Cheng, Y., Verguet, S., & Jong, S. (2017). The impact of the introduction of new recognition criteria for overwork-related cardiovascular and cerebrovascular diseases: A cross-country comparison. *Scientific Reports, 7*(1), 167. https://doi.org/10.1038/s41598-017-00198-5

Liu, X., Ikeda, H., Oyama, F., & Takahashi, M. (2019). Haemodynamic responses to simulated long working hours in different age groups. *Occupational and Environmental Medicine, 76*(10), 754–757.

Matsuo, T., So, R., & Takahashi, M. (2020). Workers' physical activity data contribute to estimating maximal oxygen consumption: A questionnaire study to concurrently assess workers' sedentary behavior and cardiorespiratory fitness. *BMC Public Health, 20*(1), 22. https://doi.org/10.1186/s12889-019-8067-4

Ministry of Health Labour and Welfare Japan. (2001). *Revision of certification criteria for cerebro- or cardiovascular disease.* Retrieved March 25, 2023 from https://www.mhlw.go.jp/houdou/0112/h1212-1.html

Ministry of Health Labour and Welfare Japan. (2019). What is work-interval system? Retrieved March 25, 2023 from https://work-holiday.mhlw.go.jp/interval/

Ministry of Health Labour and Welfare Japan. (2021). *Overview of revisions to the occupational accident certification criteria for cerebro- or cardiovascular disease.* Retrieved March 25, 2023 from https://www.mhlw.go.jp/content/11201000/000832041.pdf

Ministry of Health Labour and Welfare Japan. (2022). *Work accident compensation situation such as death from overwork in 2021.* Retrieved January 1, 2023 from https://www.mhlw.go.jp/content/11402000/000955416.pdf

Ministry of Justice Japan. (2014). *Act promoting measures to prevent death and injury from overwork* [Japanese law translation]. Retrieved January 1, 2023 from https://www.japaneselawtranslation.go.jp/ja/laws/view/3258

North, S., & Morioka, R. (2016). Hope found in lives lost: Karoshi and the pursuit of worker rights in Japan. *Contemporary Japan, 28,* 59–80.

Occupational Safety and Health Administration, Ministry of Labor, Taiwan. (2021). *Reference guidelines for identifying occupational cardiovascular diseases.* Retrieved March 25, 2023 from https://www.osha.gov.tw/48110/48363/133456/48395/48405/52149/

Park, J., Kim, Y., Cheng, Y., & Horie, S. (2012). A comparison of the recognition of overwork-related cardiovascular disease in Japan, Korea, and Taiwan. *Industrial Health, 50*(1), 17–23.

Pega, F., Nafradi, B., Momen, N. C., Ujita, Y., Streicher, K. N., Pruss-Ustun, A. M., Technical Advisory, G., Descatha, A., Driscoll, T., Fischer, F. M., Godderis, L., Kiiver, H. M., Li, J., Magnusson Hanson, L. L., Rugulies, R., Sorensen, K., & Woodruff, T. J. (2021). Global, regional, and national burdens of ischemic heart disease and stroke attributable to exposure to long working hours for 194 countries, 2000–2016: A systematic analysis from the WHO/ILO Joint Estimates of the work-related burden of disease and injury. *Environment International, 154,* 106595. https://doi.org/10.1016/j.envint.2021.106595

Perez, M. V., Mahaffey, K. W., Hedlin, H., Rumsfeld, J. S., Garcia, A., Ferris, T., Balasubramanian, V., Russo, A. M., Rajmane, A., Cheung, L., Hung, G., Lee, J., Kowey, P., Talati, N., Nag, D., Gummidipundi, S. E., Beatty, A., Hills, M. T., Desai, S., … Turakhia, M. P. (2019). Large-scale assessment of a smartwatch to identify atrial fibrillation. *New England Journal of Medicine, 381*(20), 1909–1917.

Petrou, P., & Bakker, A. B. (2016). Crafting one's leisure time in response to high job strain. *Human Relations, 69*(2), 507–529.

Republic of Korea. (2021). *Enforcement decree of the industrial accident compensation insurance act.* Retrieved April 18, 2023 from https://law.go.kr/engLsSc.do?menuId=1&subMenuId=21&tabMenuId=117&query=%EC%82%B0%EC%97%85%EC%9E%AC%ED%95%B4%EB%B3%B4%EC%83%81%EB%B3%B4%ED%97%98%EB%B2%95#

Sakai, T., & Sasaki, T. (2018). 過労死等の実態解明と防止対策に関する総合的な労働安全衛生研究 [An analytical study for preventing and predicting Karoshi cases in transport and postal activities]. *Report of the industrial disease clinical research grants from the Ministry of Health, Labour and Welfare, Government of Japan* (pp. 102–132). https://www.jniosh.johas.go.jp/publication/houkoku/houkoku_overwork_2018.pdf

So, R., & Matsuo, T. (2020). Effects of using high-intensity interval training and calorie restriction in different orders on metabolic syndrome: A randomized controlled trial. *Nutrition, 75–76,* 110666. https://doi.org/10.1016/j.nut.2019.110666

Sonnentag, S., Arbeus, H., Mahn, C., & Fritz, C. (2014). Exhaustion and lack of psychological detachment from work during off-job time: Moderator effects of time pressure and leisure experiences. *Journal of Occupational Health Psychology, 19*(2), 206–216.

Sprajcer, M., Thomas, M. J. W., Sargent, C., Crowther, M. E., Boivin, D. B., Wong, I. S., Smiley, A., & Dawson, D. (2022). How effective are Fatigue Risk Management Systems (FRMS)? A review. *Accident Analysis & Prevention, 165*, 106398. https://doi.org/10.1016/j.aap.2021.106398

Takahashi, M. (2019). Sociomedical problems of overwork-related deaths and disorders in Japan. *Journal of Occupational Health, 61*(4), 269–277.

Tsuchiya, M., Takahashi, M., Miki, K., Kubo, T., & Izawa, S. (2017). Cross-sectional associations between daily rest periods during weekdays and psychological distress, non-restorative sleep, fatigue, and work performance among information technology workers. *Industrial Health, 55*(2), 173–179.

Uehata, T. (1991). Karoshi due to occupational stress-related cardiovascular injuries among middle-aged workers in Japan. *Journal of Science of Labour, 67*(1 Pt II), 20–28.

Vieten, L., Wöhrmann, A. M., & Michel, A. (2022). Boundaryless working hours and recovery in Germany. *International Archives of Occupational and Environmental Health, 95*(1), 275–292.

Winwood, P. C., Bakker, A. B., & Winefield, A. H. (2007). An investigation of the role of non-work-time behavior in buffering the effects of work strain. *Journal of Occupational and Environmental Medicine, 49*(8), 862–871.

Yamauchi, T., Sasaki, T., Yoshikawa, T., Matsumoto, S., Takahashi, M., Suka, M., & Yanagisawa, H. (2018). Differences in work-related adverse events by sex and industry in cases involving compensation for mental disorders and suicide in Japan from 2010 to 2014. *Journal of Occupational and Environmental Medicine, 60*(4), e178–e182.

14 Fostering recovery and well-being in a healthy lifestyle

A concluding summary

Jürgen Beckmann and Michael Kellmann

In today's fast-paced and demanding society, maintaining a healthy lifestyle has become a significant challenge. Work-related stress and the lack of balance between professional demands and family as well as other areas have detrimental effects on individuals' health and well-being. Stress has frequently been described as the central cause of impairment of health and well-being (Schneiderman et al., 2005). However, looking at stress alone is insufficient. A systemic view, in which stress is considered in connection with recovery is required. If individuals do not manage to recover from stress while stress accumulates a state of continued disbalance will eventually lead to a breakdown of sources of resistance entailing disease and/or performance impairment.

A systemic view was, however, almost not adopted in earlier research on stress. For health and well-being, it is crucial to take into consideration that the stress level can be compensated for by adequate recovery. The importance of this factor in prevention has only recently been addressed (Kellmann et al., 2023). Based on this perspective more comprehensive prevention programmes can be developed. Over the last decades, research in the sport context has provided numerous studies that show how to address recovery to find a balance between stress and recovery (Kellmann & Beckmann, 2022). Additionally, a preventive perspective has been developed in which recovery not only serves the function of resolving a disbalance but as well to prevent negative stress effects before they occur. Recovery is not restricted to regeneration processes but can also generate buffers against stress. A healthy lifestyle involves recovery processes that promote building resilience.

Adopting a holistic or systemic perspective is crucial for effectively managing stress and promoting recovery. Stress and recovery are integral components of well-being, and their interplay shapes individual health outcomes. Recognising the systemic nature of stress and recovery is vital for designing effective interventions and policies. By fostering a balance between stress and recovery across

Beckmann, J., & Kellmann, M. (2024). Fostering recovery and well-being in a healthy lifestyle: A concluding summary. In M. Kellmann & J. Beckmann (Eds.), *Fostering Recovery and Well-being in a Healthy Lifestyle: Psychological, Somatic, and Organizational Prevention Approaches* (pp. 218–222). Routledge.

DOI: 10.4324/9781003250654-18

physiological, psychological, and social dimensions, individuals and societies can cultivate resilience, promote optimal well-being, and mitigate the negative effects of chronic stress. This book addresses psychological, somatic, and organisational prevention strategies to foster recovery and a healthy lifestyle in society. It focuses on both research and applied counseling aspects to discuss recovery as an underestimated factor in various areas, particularly the work context.

The stress-recovery approach may remind of 'Work-Life-Balance' (WLB) which became a popular term since the 1970s. WLB contrasts a person's level of involvement in work to their participation in family or leisure activities, treating them as distinct and potentially conflicting aspects of life. The basic postulate is that a good balance or fit would increase life satisfaction or well-being and quality of life (APA Dictionary of Psychology, 2023). The WLB approach falls short because it does not take a differentiated look at the complex interaction of stress and recovery. WLB is based on assumptions that are too undifferentiated to derive generally applicable intervention measures. A fundamentally false claim is to consider work as a separate, dynamic aspect of life that does not require absolute commitment (Thijssen et al., 2008; Wey Smola & Sutton, 2002). Furthermore, demanding more balance between on- and off-job time implies the presupposition that work is primarily a negative domain that results in unhappiness, stress, and other negative states (de Jonge & Taris, this volume, Chapter 2; Eikhof et al., 2007) and that gaining more off-job time would reduce the negative effects of work by the positive benefits of personal life. This position ignores that work can be fulfilling and satisfying (Eikhof et al., 2007). However, it cannot be neglected that an almost exclusive focus on work can have negative effects on health and well-being. Kubo et al. (this volume, Chapter 13) address the *Karoshi* syndrome, death at work due to long working hours. *Karoshi* cannot be solely blamed on the long working hours, but rather the lack of adequate recovery and recuperation to compensate for them. Epidemiological and experimental evidence regarding the mechanisms of *Karoshi* cases is presented along with suggestions for organisational and individual strategic prevention measures. In a similar vein, Kuntz (this volume, Chapter 12) suggests building recovery into organisations to foster resilience. She describes the reciprocal influence of resilience and recovery in occupational contexts and elucidates how organisations could promote resilience and recovery through their practices and systems.

Another incorrect assumption in the 'Work-Life-Balance' approach is that more time outside the job would lead to a balance between the different roles in the work environment and family implying that leisure activities would more or less automatically result in the prevention of stress-related diseases, as well as increased well-being and quality of life. Reiter (2007) argues that 'balance' is subjective; instead of striving towards an absolute value of work-life-balance, it is better to strive towards optimal functioning within different life domains with as little conflict as possible between them. In line with this de Jonge and Taris (this volume, Chapter 2) address off-job and on-job recovery as predictors of health.

Recovery research has provided a far more differentiated model of what provides the chances for finding an equilibrium promoting prevention of diseases and the prospectives of well-being and good quality of life than the 'Work-Life-Balance' approach. Generally, instead of an artificial juxtaposition of 'work' and 'life', different systems in which individuals act are addressed. These different systems make different use of individual resources, e.g., in different physical activities versus mental activities. The activity in one system can help replenish resources in other systems. However, factors that determine people's capability of achieving recovery include:

- being aware of their specific needs and preferences
- their ability to self-regulate
- a self-determined initiation of recovery activities
- a perception of meaningfulness in what they do for recovery

The chapters in this book address how these preconditions can be met in different domains such as professional sports (Hogg, this volume, Chapter 5), organisations (Kubo et al., this volume, Chapter 13; Kuntz, this volume, Chapter 12), the military (Matthews et al., this volume, Chapter 11), and even social media use (Heidari & Kellmann, this volume, Chapter 7).

Balance of stress and recovery fluctuates over time. Sometimes the balance will shift to one system/context (e.g., the workplace); sometimes it will shift to another system/context (e.g., family). It is important to be aware of feelings about these different systems and contexts and to engage in behaviours that will prevent the negative effects of stress and imbalance when involvement shifts too much towards one particular system or context. When having to primarily focus on one system or context for a prolonged period it is important to perceive self-determined commitment (Ryan & Deci, 2017) and adopt a mindset that involves seeing chances for growth (Beckmann et al., this volume, Chapter 1; Dweck, 2006).

It must also be emphasised that balance is a crucial concept in this systemic approach. Most chapters in this book address an imbalance due to recovery that does not adequately offset the stress burden. We are dealing with underrecovery here. However, Kellmann and Kallus (2001) have already pointed out that there can also be too little stress. Of course, this does not mean burdensome distress, but too little eustress in the sense of Selye (1978). Boredom and emptiness can arise from a lack of eustress. This also is a case of imbalance which decreases well-being and quality of life. Many people face this situation after retirement when self-reported depression symptoms go up by 40% during the first few retirement years. Studies suggest, reliable financial resources, social networks, and marriage can mitigate negative health repercussions of retirement (Deeg & Bath, 2003). Particularly, people who worked on jobs with high demands and challenges may suffer from the 'empty-desk-syndrome' after retirement characterised by enduring psychological problems (Quadbeck & Roth, 2008).

According to Berlyne's (1960) theory, individuals seek to achieve or maintain an optimal level of stimulation (arousal potential) to feel good (hedonic value). If the arousal potential of the environment is too high, they will attempt to reduce it. If it is too low resulting in boredom, they will attempt to increase it.

For Berlyne the imbalance is accompanied by a high level of unpleasant internal activation. Assembly line work is mostly perceived as boring and not involving personal meaning. Interestingly, Csikszentmihalyi (1990) describes that even on a boring assembly line job the worker may find a way to experience a microflow which involves perception of meaning and helps to cope with the stress of boredom. As several chapters in this book address, there is plenty of room in organisational settings for the improvement of working conditions.

As described by Beckmann et al. (this volume, Chapter 1), higher stress levels with shorter periods of underrecovery are tolerable. The question is to what degree they negatively affect satisfaction with life and perceived quality of life. Different factors affect whether quality of life is possible despite unfavourable conditions or stressful periods in life. The mindset, i.e., a habitual or characteristic mental attitude that determines how a person defines and respond to situations is a crucial factor. Beckmann et al. (this volume, Chapter 1) address that even though stressors seem overwhelming and cannot be fully mastered as in chronic diseases, a good quality of life can still be achieved.

Nevertheless, it is important to be aware of recovery needs. Monitoring of the recovery-stress balance has previously mainly been addressed in the sport context. Individual monitoring is essential in an applied context because of large individual differences in stress reactivity and person-adequate recovery (Kallus, 2023). Various chapters in this book advocate the use of recovery and stress monitoring in the general population. Brüßler et al. (this volume, Chapter 3) point out that due to technological advancement, it is catching on lately with smartphone and smartwatches tracking.

Several factors in finding recovery are discussed in the book. A basic prerequisite appears to be detachment from a past activity, for example, stressful demands in high-performance areas such as sports as described by Balk (this volume, Chapter 4). Physical recovery and mental detachment from sport-related activities were found to prevent injury and enhance mental energy. For sport, but also the general population, debriefing (Hogg, this volume, Chapter 5), psychological relaxation techniques (Kellmann et al., this volume, Chapter 8), yoga (di Fronso et al., this volume, Chapter 9), and sleep (Kullik & Kiel, this volume, Chapter 10) play a major role as psychological and physical recovery strategies. Sleep is certainly one of the most important recovery means. Interestingly, Balk (this volume, Chapter 4) describes that sleep deprivation only partially mediated the relation between mental detachment and mental energy. Utilising detachment or relaxation techniques as recovery measures can be helpful in facilitating better sleep and improving sleep quality. Furthermore, creativity has not received attention in previous recovery research. Richard et al. (this volume, Chapter 6) point out that engaging in creative activities is a recovery approach that can promote health.

In conclusion, obtaining a recovery-stress balance is an essential component of a healthy lifestyle that supports well-being and health. By acknowledging the negative consequences of particularly underrecovery on physical and mental health, individuals need to become aware of recovery needs and adequate recovery activities.

References

APA Dictionary of Psychology. (2023). *Work-life-balance.* Retrieved July 14, 2023 from https://dictionary.apa.org/work-life-balance

Berlyne, D. E. (1960). *Conflict, arousal, and curiosity.* McGraw-Hill.

Csikszentmihalyi, M. (1990). *Flow: The psychology of optimal experience.* Harper & Row.

Deeg, D. J., & Bath, P. A. (2003). Self-rated health, gender, and mortality in older persons: Introduction to a special section. *The Gerontologist, 43*(3), 369–371.

Dweck, C. S. (2006). *Mindset: The new psychology of success.* Random House.

Eikhof, D. R., Warhurst, C., & Haunschild, A. (2007). Introduction: What work? What life? What balance? Critical reflections on the work-life balance debate. *Employee Relations, 29*(4), 325–333.

Kallus, K. W. (2023). Recovery and stress reactivity. In M. Kellmann, S. Jakowski, & J. Beckmann (Eds.), *The importance of recovery for physical and mental health: Negotiating the effects of underrecovery* (pp. 33–50). Routledge.

Kellmann, M., & Beckmann, J. (Eds.). (2022). *Recovery and well-being in sport and exercise.* Routledge.

Kellmann, M., Jakowski, S., & Beckmann, J. (Eds.). (2023). *The importance of recovery for physical and mental health: Negotiating the effects of underrecovery.* Routledge.

Kellmann, M., & Kallus, K. W. (2001). *The Recovery-Stress Questionnaire for Athletes. User manual.* Human Kinetics.

Quadbeck, O., & Roth, W. L. (2008). *Das "Empty-Desk"-Syndrom. Die Leere nach der Pensionierung: Wie Führungskräfte nach Beendigung der Erwerbsarbeit ihre psychischen Probleme bewältigen* [The "Empty Desk" syndrome. The post-retirement emptiness: How executives manage their mental health problems after ending gainful employment]. Pabst.

Reiter, N. (2007). Work life balance: What DO you mean? The ethical ideology underpinning appropriate application. *The Journal of Applied Behavioral Science, 43*(2), 273–294.

Ryan, R. M., & Deci, E. L. (2017). *Self-determination theory: Basic psychological needs in motivation, development and wellness.* Guilford Press.

Schneiderman, N., Ironson, G., & Siegel, S. D. (2005). Stress and health: Psychological, behavioral, and biological determinants. *Annual Review of Clinical Psychology, 1,* 607–628.

Selye, H. (1978). *The stress of life.* McGraw-Hill.

Thijssen, J. G., Van der Heijden, B. I., & Rocco, T. S. (2008). Toward the employability—link model: Current employment transition to future employment perspectives. *Human Resource Development Review, 7*(2), 165–183.

Wey Smola, K., & Sutton, C. D. (2002). Generational differences: Revisiting generational work values for the new millennium. *Journal of Organizational Behavior, 23*(4), 363–382.

Index

Pages in **bold** refer to tables and pages in *italics* refer to figures.

absenteeism 24
accelerometry 45
acceptance 6, 11–14, 17, 132–133, 137
Acceptance and Commitment Therapy (ACT) 13
activation 26–27, 45, 60, 76, 117–118, 120, 127, 136, 166, 184, 188, 191, 221
Acute Recovery and Stress Scale (ARSS) 42
adrenergic activity 123
Ambulatory Assessment (AA) 38, 40–46, 49–50
anger 41, 60, 79
anxiety 7–8, 45, 65, 67, 77, 93, 107, 117, 123, 132–134, 137–138, 147, 150, 152, 171, 173
arousal 118
Attributional Theory 75
autogenic training 120–122, 127
autonomy 9, 15, 25, 63, 76–78, 108, 185, 190–193

breaks 25, 27–28, 32–33, 39, 98, 119, 174, 183–184, 190, 193–194, 203, 210
breathing techniques 132–134, 136, 138
burnout 15, 24, 39, 59, 62, 68, 106, 166–167, 172, 176

caffeine 152–153, 155, 172
cardiorespiratory fitness 206, 210–211, 213
choking under pressure 121
chronic: disease 3–5, 8, 12, 16, 221; illness 3–5, 7, 9–17
chronotype 144, 146–148
circadian rhythm 144, 146–150, 173–174

Cognitive: Activation Theory of Stress 60; Fitness Framework (CF2) 169, 171; Fitness Model 169; gym 169; readiness 169, 171
competence 9, 15, 76, 127, 185
competition 38, 42, 48, 59, 62, 66–68, 74–75, 79–80, *82–84*, 87–88, 117–121, 123, 127, 136–138, 143, 152
comprehensibility 14, 109
concentration 26, 30–34, 48, *84*, 117, 120–122, 124–**125**, 127, 134–135, 138
congenital heart defect (CHD) 3, 6–8, 13
Conservation of Resources Theory (COR) 184–185
cortisol 95, 186, 188, *209*
COVID-19 27, 154, 199, 208, 210–211
creative: behaviour 92–93, 97; expression 93–96, 98–99; Potential System model 92, 95
creativity 63, 92–95, 221

dance 62, 64–66, 94
data: encryption 50; security 49
debriefing 67, 73–89, 121, **126**, 221
depression 7–8, 24, 93, 105, 131, 147–148, 150, 152, 220
Desert: Shield 168; Storm 168–169
detachment 25–34, 39, 59, 61–68, 96, 107–108, 110, 133–134, 136, 183–185, 192, 194, *209*, 211, 213, 221; antecedents of 65; cognitive 28, 30–33, 62, 66; emotional 28, 30–33, 62–64, 66, 133, 136; physical 25, 28–34, 61–62
diabetes 3–4, 147–148, 150, 205–206
digital: media 103–110; stress 107–108

digitisation 24, 48
disconnect from work 206, 208, 212
Dissonance Theory 6
Dual-Continuum Model 6–7, 16

Ecological Momentary Assessment
    (EMA) 40
Effort-Recovery Model (E-R) 25–26, 32,
    39, 184–185
Ego-Depletion Theory (EDT) 185
electronic media 152–153, 155
embeddedness 94, 98
emotional exhaustion 28, 30–34, 65
employees 24–30, 32–34, 59, 62–65, 68,
    96–97, 154, 193, 201, 203, 205,
    207–*209*, 211
empty-desk-syndrome 220
engulfment 11–13, 17
enrichment 11–13, 15, 17
external factors 76, 146, 151, 167, 171
extrinsically motivated 76

fatigue 9, 26, 28, 40, 61–63, 65–66, 68,
    94–95, 106, 117, 120, 133, 135,
    137–138, 150, 152, 165–169,
    171–176, 184, 187, 203, 206–210,
    212–213; physical 9, 61–62, 66, 68;
    Risk Management System (FRMS)
    210, 212
fear 77, 79, 85, 107, 109, **125**, 132, 171,
    200; of Missing Out 107, 109
feedback 73, 75, 77–78, 80–83, 85–88,
    105, 124, 191
fight-or-flight 166
flourishing 6, 11, 14, 92–94
frustration 79, 171

geolocation 41–42, 45, 49

health, predictors of 30, 219
Health-related Quality of Live (HRQOL)
    4, 17
heart rate 41, 46–49, 61, 123, 172, 194
hormone 146
Human Performance Optimisation
    (HPO) 175–176
hypnosis 119, 121–123

illness identity 9–11, 13, 17
immune function 146–147
individual sports 73–75, 86–87
Individual Zones of Optimal Functioning
    model (IZOF) 118

injury 39, 64, 132–133, 143, 189,
    199, 221
inner balance 119
insomnia 135, 147, 150, 153, 155, 166
Instagram 104, 106
interindividual 8, 118
internal factors 76
International Civil Aviation Organization
    210
International Labour Organization (ILO)
    199, 203
internet 103
intraindividual 39–40, 47, 106, 110
intrapersonal 41, 104, 182
intrinsically motivated 34, 76

jet lag 146, 148
job demands 32, 39, 59, 65, 183, 185,
    188–190

Karoshi 199–203, 205, 208–210,
    212–213, 219

languishing 6
leadership 74–75, 80, *82*, 86, 88, 171,
    189, 193
lifestyle 38, 106, 150–151, 153–154, 171,
    218–219, 221

mad-genius hypothesis 93
mastery 39, 76, 96, 107–108, 110,
    183–184, 189–190, 192, 194
meaning in life 4–5, 14–16
meaningfulness 5, 14–16, 220
melatonin 146–147, 150, 152
mental: cool-down 67–68; energy 61, 64,
    221; health 6–12, 15, 17, 38, 45, 93,
    106, 131, 133–134, 146–147,
    150–152, 154, 175, 203, 208, 221
microbreaks 83, 190, 193
military: environment 165–167, 172,
    175–176; operation 165, 168
mindfulness 12, 17, 67, 79, 110,
    131–134, 175–176; -Based-Stress-
    Reduction (MBSR) Model 175–176
moderator 12, 47, 99, 166
motivation 13, 15, 26, 61, 63–64, 76–77,
    80, 85, 184–186, 189–190
Motivation for Twitter Use Measure 104
motivational interviewing (MI) 13, 17
Motivations for Social Media Use
    Scale 104
motives 104, 110

Motives for Using Social Networking Sites 104
music 67, 93, 96–98, 103, 122–123

napping 155, 172, 174
National Sleep Foundation 144–146
non-REM (NREM) 144, 146, 148
nutrition 47, 106, 152, 154

organisation 25, 32, 34, 39, 49–50, 62–63, 68, 74, 95, 98–99, 103, 165, 175, 182–194, 205, 207, 210–212, 219–221
overload 33, 107, 167, 199–200

performance 24, 26, 34, 38–40, 48, 59–60, 62–67, 73–89, 95–99, 105–106, 117–123, 132–138, 143, 149, 151, 154, 165–169, 171–176, 182–185, 189, 192–193, 218; augmentation 171; cognitive 167, 171, 175
posture 132, 136
pranayama 132, 136–138
progressive muscle relaxation (PMR) 67, 119–**125**, 127, 137

Quality of Life (QOL) 3–4, 6, 8–10, 14, 16–17, 135, 219–221

Rapid eye movement (REM) 144, 168
reactivity 26, 44, 46, 186, 221
recovery: active 9, 106, 166; activities 24, 26, 28, 33–34, 39, 106, 182–194, 221; at-work 193; cognitive 171; enhancement 108, 134; experiences 34, 39, 42, 96, 108, 182–188, 190–192, 194; framework 184; holistic 106; media-induced 107–110; off-job 25, 27, 29–30, 32–34; off-work 192; on-job 24–25, 27–34, 219; optimal 39, 50, 132; outcome 61–62, 64, 183, 192, 211; passive 9, 120; pro-active 9, 106, 166; process 4, 9, 11–12, 25–28, 32, 34, 40, 44–45, 47, 60–62, 67, 78, 96, 106, 119–120, 122, 138, 183–187, 189, 218; resource 8–10, 13; tool 118–119; work 24–25, 31, 34, 39, 182–183, 208, 211
recovery-stress: balance 15, 40, 132, 134–135, 137–138, 221; continuum 47

Recovery-Stress Questionnaire (RESTQ) 40, 42
reflectiveness 94, 98
regeneration accelerator 119–120, 127
rejection 11–13, 17
relaxation 39, 41, 62, 67, 74, 96, 106–108, 110, 117–127, 133–138, 154, 183–184, 190, 192–194, 221
remote 183, 191, 210
resilience 3, 5, 9–10, 12–15, 17, 45, 74, 85, 131, 153, 172, 182, 184–193, 218–219; -recovery dynamic 188, 190
Resilient Mind Program (RMP) 171–172
rest-activity cycles 173–174
restoration 25, 32, 61, 106, 136, 171, 182, 190, 193
Royal Australian Navy Fleet 172
rumination 65–66, 120, 153, 183, *209*

salutogenic approach 14
Scissors-Model 38
self-: determination 3, 9–10, 16, 76; efficacy 12, 39, 76–77, 79, 154, 190; reflection 77–79, 89; regulation 4–5, 9–11, 16, 39, 117–121, 137, 184–185
Self-: Determination Theory (SDT) 15, 75–76, 185; Efficacy Theory 75–76
sense of coherence (SOC) 4–5, 13–14
Short Recovery and Stress Scale (SRSS) 42
sickness 24, 59
sleep: deprivation 149–151, 168, 221; disturbance 148, 151–152, 155, 200; duration 47, 105, 144–145, 148–149, 151–152, 154, 208; efficiency (SE) 145, 168; hygiene 154–155, 171; latency 135, 151; onset 145, 147, 150, 153–154; Onset Latency (SOL) 145, 147, 152; problems 28–34, 151, 153, 155; quality 28–29, 63, 65, 105, 120, 132–136, 145, 148, 151–155, 182, 208, 221; -wake cycle 146–147, 149
smartphone 34, 41, 44–45, 47, 49–50, 103, 108, 147, 152–153, 155, 221
social support 65, 151–152, 171, 186, 188, 191–192, 194
socialisation 94, 98, 183–184, 191, 193
stress-buffer hypothesis 46
Stressor-Detachment (S-D) Model 25–26, 61
supercompensation 138
systematic breathing 119–122, 124, 127

tablet 103, 106, 147
team sport 74–75, 80, *82*, 86–87
Three-Dimensional Model of physical
    health, mental illness, and well-being 8
time zones 148
tracking 42, 45, 49, 99, 109, 221
Transtheoretical Model of Behaviour
    Change 13

underrecovery trap 66
unwinding 25, 32, 182

vigour 25, 28, 63, 66
vulnerability 77, 88, 205

wake after sleep onset (WASO) 145, 152
wearables 47–48, 144

worker 28, 96, 135, 151, 166, 172, 174,
    183–194, 200, 202, 205
Work-Life-Balance (WLB) 219–220
workload 59, 96, 165, 167–168, 174,
    199–200, 203
work-related stress 24, 39, 151,
    154, 218
World Health Organization (WHO) 3–4,
    9, 16, 93, 199, 203
worry 65–67, *84*

yoga 96, 106, 131–138; Bali 133–134,
    137–138; Hatha 96, 132–133,
    137–138; Mindful 133–134, 137;
    Nidra 132–135, 137–138

zeitgeber 146–147